T0309613

New Insights into Rheumatoid Arthritis

Guest Editor

DAVID A. FOX, MD

RHEUMATIC DISEASE CLINICS OF NORTH AMERICA

www.rheumatic.theclinics.com

May 2010 • Volume 36 • Number 2

SAUNDERS an imprint of ELSEVIER, Inc.

W.B. SAUNDERS COMPANY

A Division of Elsevier Inc.

1600 John F. Kennedy Blvd., Suite 1800 • Philadelphia, PA 19103-2899

http://www.theclinics.com

RHEUMATIC DISEASE CLINICS OF NORTH AMERICA Volume 36, Number 2

May 2010 ISSN 0889-857X, ISBN 13: 978-1-4377-1870-6

Editor: Rachel Glover
Developmental Editor: Theresa Collier

Rheumatic Disease Clinics of North America (ISSN 0889-857X) is published quarterly by Elsevier Inc., 360 Park Avenue South, New York, NY 10010-1710. Months of issue are February, May, August, and November. Business and editorial offices: 1600 John F. Kennedy Boulevard, Suite 1800, Philadelphia, PA 19103-2899. Periodicals postage paid at New York, NY and additional mailing offices. Subscription prices are USD 264.00 per year for US individuals, USD 455.00 per year for US institutions, USD 132.00 per year for US students and residents, USD 311.00 per year for Canadian individuals, USD 563.00 per year for Canadian institutions, USD 369.00 per year for international individuals, USD 563.00 per year for international institutions, and USD 185.00 per year for Canadian and foreign students/residents. To receive student/resident rate, orders must be accompanied by name of affiliated institution, date of term, and the *signature* of program/residency coordinator on institution letterhead. Orders will be billed at individual rate until proof of status received. Foreign air speed delivery is included in all *Clinics* subscription prices. All prices are subject to change without notice. **POSTMASTER:** Send address changes to *Rheumatic Disease Clinics of North America*, Elsevier Health Sciences Division, Subscription Customer Service, 3251 Riverport Lane, Maryland Heights, MO 63043. **Customer Service: 1-800-654-2452 (US and Canada). From outside of the US and Canada: 314-453-7041. Fax: 314-453-5170. For print support, e-mail: JournalsCustomerService-usa@elsevier.com. For online support, e-mail: JournalsOnline Support-usa@elsevier.com.**

Reprints. For copies of 100 or more of articles in this publication, please contact the Commercial Reprints Department, Elsevier Inc., 360 Park Avenue South, New York, New York, 10010-1710; Tel.: (+1) 212-633-3813, Fax: (+1) 212-462-1935, and E-mail: reprints@elsevier.com.

Rheumatic Disease Clinics of North America is covered in *MEDLINE/PubMed (Index Medicus), Current Contents/Clinical Medicine, Science Citation Index, ISI/BIOMED,* and *EMBASE/Excerpta Medica.*

Printed in the United States of America

Transferred to Digital Printing, 2011

Contributors

GUEST EDITOR

DAVID A. FOX, MD
Professor and Chief, Division of Rheumatology and Rheumatic Diseases Research
Core Center; Department of Medicine, The University of Michigan Medical Center,
Ann Arbor, Michigan

AUTHORS

ISMAEL CALERO, MD
Resident in Internal Medicine, Internal Medicine Department, Hospital Virgen de la Luz,
Cuenca, Spain

KEVIN D. DEANE, MD
Division of Rheumatology, University of Colorado School of Medicine, Aurora, Colorado

DAVID A. FOX, MD
Professor and Chief, Division of Rheumatology and Rheumatic Diseases Research
Core Center; Department of Medicine, The University of Michigan Medical Center,
Ann Arbor, Michigan

ANGELICA GIERUT, MD
Rheumatology Fellow, Division of Rheumatology, Department of Medicine, Feinberg
School of Medicine, Northwestern University, Chicago, Illinois

ALISON GIZINSKI, MD
Lecturer, Division of Rheumatology and Rheumatic Diseases Research Core Center,
The University of Michigan, Ann Arbor, Michigan

JORG J. GORONZY, MD
Division of Immunology and Rheumatology, Department of Medicine, Stanford University,
Stanford, California

ELLEN M. GRAVALLESE, MD
Professor of Medicine, Chief, Division of Rheumatology, Department of Medicine,
University of Massachusetts Medical School, Worcester, Massachusetts

V. MICHAEL HOLERS, MD
Division of Rheumatology, University of Colorado School of Medicine, Aurora, Colorado

MARIANA J. KAPLAN, MD
Associate Professor of Internal Medicine, Division of Rheumatology, Department
of Internal Medicine, University of Michigan Medical School, Ann Arbor, Michigan

SOUGATA KARMAKAR, PhD
Postdoctoral Fellow, Division of Rheumatology, Department of Medicine, University of
Massachusetts Medical School, Worcester, Massachusetts

JONATHAN KAY, MD
Professor of Medicine, Division of Rheumatology, Department of Medicine, University of Massachusetts Medical School, Worcester, Massachusetts

TAMSIN M. LINDSTROM, PhD
Stanford Visiting Scholar, Geriatric Research Education and Clinical Center (GRECC), VA Palo Alto Health Care System, Palo Alto; Division of Immunology and Rheumatology, Stanford University School of Medicine, Stanford, California

STEVEN K. LUNDY, PhD
Assistant Professor, Division of Rheumatology and Rheumatic Diseases Research Core Center, The University of Michigan, Ann Arbor, Michigan

RACHEL MORGAN, BSc
Division of Rheumatology and Rheumatic Diseases Research Core Center, University of Michigan, Ann Arbor, Michigan

JOSE ANTONIO NIETO, MD
Section Chief, Internal Medicine Department, Hospital Virgen de la Luz, Cuenca, Spain

JILL M. NORRIS, MPH, PhD
Department of Epidemiology, Colorado School of Public Health, University of Colorado, Aurora, Colorado

HARRIS PERLMAN, PhD
Associate Professor, Division of Rheumatology, Department of Medicine, Feinberg School of Medicine, Northwestern University, Chicago, Illinois

ROBERT M. PLENGE, MD, PhD
Division of Rheumatology, Immunology and Allergy, Brigham and Women's Hospital, Harvard Medical School, Boston, Massachusetts

RICHARD M. POPE, MD
Mabel Greene Myers Professor of Medicine, Chief, Division of Rheumatology, Department of Medicine, Feinberg School of Medicine, Northwestern University, Chicago, Illinois

SOUMYA RAYCHAUDHURI, MD, PhD
Division of Rheumatology, Immunology and Allergy, Brigham and Women's Hospital, Harvard Medical School, Boston, Massachusetts

WILLIAM H. ROBINSON, MD, PhD
Staff Physician, Geriatric Research Education and Clinical Center (GRECC), VA Palo Alto Health Care System, Palo Alto; Assistant Professor of Medicine, Division of Immunology and Rheumatology, Stanford University School of Medicine, Stanford, California

IÑAKI SANZ, MD
Professor of Medicine, Department of Microbiology and Immunology, University of Rochester Medical Center; Chief, Division of Allergy, Immunology and Rheumatology, University of Rochester Medical Center, Rochester, New York

SUJATA SARKAR, MD
Section of Rheumatology, Department of Medicine, The University of Arizona, Tucson, Arizona

LAN SHAO, PhD
Division of Immunology and Rheumatology, Department of Medicine, Stanford University, Stanford, California

TUULIKKI SOKKA, MD, PhD
Arkisto/Tutkijat, Jyväskylä Central Hospital, Jyväskylä, Finland

CORNELIA M. WEYAND, MD
Division of Immunology and Rheumatology, Department of Medicine, Stanford University, Stanford, California

Contents

Rheumatoid arthritis (RA) likely develops in several phases, beginning with genetic risk, followed by asymptomatic autoimmunity, then finally, clinically apparent disease. Investigating the phases of disease that exist prior to the onset of symptoms (ie, the preclinical period of RA) will lead to understanding of the important relationships between genetic and environmental factors that may lead to disease, as well as allow for the development of predictive models for disease, and ultimately preventive strategies for RA.

Quantitative clinical monitoring of musculoskeletal conditions and inflammatory joint diseases is challenging. Traditional measures to assess rheumatoid arthritis (RA), such as joint assessment, laboratory, imaging, and patient self-report measures, have limitations and provide only a reflection of the underlying inflammatory process. A gold standard to define disease activity in RA does not exist and various indices of disease activity must be used. Standard quantitative monitoring with a treatment goal has been shown to be beneficial to patient outcomes in randomized clinical trials. Quantitative monitoring has also contributed to improved long-term outcomes for RA in clinical care. Challenges of the measures need to be recognized and hurdles identified that prevent quantitative monitoring in every-day clinical care concerning disease activity and beyond. These aspects are discussed in this article.

The purpose of this article is to place these genetic discoveries in the context of current and future therapeutic strategies for patients with RA. More specifically, this article focuses on (1) a brief overview of genetic studies, (2) human genetics as an approach to identify the Achilles heel of disease pathways, (3) humans as the model organism for functional studies of human mutations, (4) pharmacogenetic studies to gain insight into the mechanism of action of drugs, and (5) next-generation patient registries to enable large-scale genotype-phenotype studies.

Innate immunity, with macrophages playing a central role, is critically important in the pathogenesis of RA. Although environmental insults such as smoking have been implicated in the initiation of rheumatoid arthritis (RA) in patients who express the shared epitope, the understanding of the role of innate immunity in the pathogenesis of this disease is also expanding. As the understanding continues to expand, enticing targets for new therapeutic interventions continue to be identified. This article focuses on cells of myelomonocytic origin, their receptors, and factors that interact with them.

Immunologic models of rheumatoid arthritis (RA) have to take into account that the disease occurs at an age when immunocompetence is declining and in a host whose immune system shows evidence of accelerated immune aging. By several immune aging biomarkers, the immune system in patients with RA is prematurely aged by more than 20 years. One major pathogenetic mechanism is a defect in telomere maintenance and DNA repair that causes accelerated cell death. These findings in RA are reminiscent of murine autoimmunity models, in which lymphopenia was identified as a major risk factor for autoimmunity. Progress in the understanding of how accelerated immune aging is pathogenetically involved in RA may allow development of new therapeutic approaches that go beyond the use of anti-inflammatory agents and eventually could open new avenues for preventive intervention.

Understanding the pathogenesis of joint inflammation and destruction in rheumatoid arthritis involves dissection of the cellular and molecular interactions that occur in synovial tissue. Development of effective targeted therapies has been based on progress in achieving such insights. Safer and more specific approaches to treatment could flow from discovery of cell-cell interaction pathways that are specific to inflammation of the joint and less important in the defense against systemic infection. This article highlights selected cell-cell interactions in rheumatoid arthritis synovium that may be worthy of evaluation as future therapeutic targets.

Initially suggested by the presence of rheumatoid factor autoantibodies, multiple pathogenic roles for B cells (both antibody-mediated and antibody-independent) in rheumatoid arthritis (RA) now are supported by a growing body of experimental observations and human studies. The pathogenic significance of B cells in this disease also has been established conclusively by the proven benefit of Rituximab-induced B cell depletion in RA patients refractory to tumor necrosis factor (TNF) blockade. This article reviews the rationale for the use of B cell-targeting therapies in RA and discusses the caveats and limitations of indiscriminate B cell depletion as currently applied, ncluding incomplete depletion of pathogenic B cells and elimination of protective B cells. Finally, it presents alternative therapeutic strategies that exploit current knowledge of B cell activation, survival, and differentiation to provide more selective B cell and plasma cell targeting.

Identification of interleukin-17 (IL-17) as a powerful proinflammatory cytokine and the recent recognition of a T-helper cell subset that secretes it have focused attention on the role of IL-17 and Th17 cells in rheumatoid arthritis (RA) and other immune-mediated diseases. While understanding of its role in RA is still evolving, evidence from both animal models and human systems provides a compelling rationale for therapeutic targeting of IL-17 in RA. Both direct and indirect approaches to accomplish this are feasible. Mechanistic studies in the context of clinical trials will be required to understand why some strategies may be preferable from the perspectives of efficacy and safety.

Small-molecule kinase inhibitors are increasingly taking center stage in the quest for new drugs for the treatment of rheumatoid arthritis (RA). By targeting kinases, small-molecule inhibitors can exert potent anti-inflammatory and immunomodulatory effects; the success of small-molecule kinase inhibitors in the treatment of cancer has spurred efforts to identify kinases that could be targeted for the treatment of chronic inflammatory disorders, such as RA. Although many kinase inhibitors have proved efficacious in the treatment of inflammatory arthritis in animals few have been tested in RA clinical trials. This article discusses the challenges and progress in the pursuit of small-molecule kinase inhibitors for RA, including lessons learned from the failure of erstwhile frontrunner inhibitors and the promise of inhibitors making their debut on the RA stage.

In rheumatoid arthritis (RA), cells within the inflamed synovium and pannus elaborate a variety of cytokines, including tumor necrosis factor (TNF) α, interleukin (IL)-1, IL-6, and IL-17, that contribute to inflammation, and may directly affect bone. The receptor activator of NF-κB (RANK) ligand/

RANK/osteoprotegerin pathway plays a critical role in regulating osteoclastogenesis in articular bone erosions in RA. Proinflammatory cytokines
can modulate this pathway, and may also affect the ability of the osteoblast to repair bone at sites of articular erosion. In this review, the authors
discuss the current understanding of pathogenic mechanisms of bone erosion in RA and examine current therapeutic approaches to prevent this
damage.

Morbidity and mortality rates are higher in individuals with rheumatoid arthritis (RA) than in the general population. Ischemic heart disease and heart
failure now represent one of the most common causes of death in RA. Indeed, RA appears to represent an independent risk factor for ischemic
heart disease, similar to diabetes mellitus. However, no clear guidelines
with regard to cardiovascular disease diagnosis and prevention in RA
have been developed. This review highlights recent investigations on the
assessment, prevention, and treatment of cardiovascular disease in RA.

THE CLINICS ARE NOW AVAILABLE ONLINE!

Access your subscription at:
www.theclinics.com

Preface:
Rheumatoid
Arthritis—Halfway There

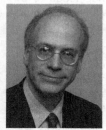

David A. Fox, MD
Guest Editor

Progress in the understanding and treatment of rheumatoid arthritis (RA) over the past three decades has been spectacular. Immunologic and molecular insights have directly led to a transformation of the treatment of RA, and the impact of these advances has resonated well beyond the field of rheumatology.

Despite these accomplishments, most of which are relevant specifically to the articular manifestations of RA, many challenges remain. We still do not know the cause of RA and lack a cure or well-validated prevention strategies. Thus, the three critical goals for any disease—cause, cure, and prevention—remain unattained. Even more unsettling, it seems that the undeniably impressive leaps forward in the treatment of RA may not yet be mitigating the survival disadvantage that this complex disease confers on its victims.

It is with these considerations in mind—remarkable progress as well as daunting challenges—that this issue of *Rheumatic Disease Clinics of North America* has been constructed. The authors of each article have been asked not only to consider the current state of the art but also to assess how the latest advances might affect treatment in the future. It is our hope that these links will prove interesting and compelling for clinical rheumatologists.

The article topics cover a wide range of subjects that reflect the spectrum of important issues in understanding, assessing, and managing RA. An article on preclinical RA integrates epidemiology, biomarkers, and aspects of pathogenesis to provide a conceptual basis for prevention strategies. An article on measurement of disease activity addresses issues that are critical to clinical research and patient care. The article on RA genetics updates and clarifies recent and rapid progress in this field. Articles that tie the pathophysiology of RA to current and future approaches to treatment focus on innate immunity, cellular senescence, Th17 cells, bone biology, and synovial cell interactions. Additional targets for therapeutics are considered in the articles on B cells and on kinases. The increasingly important topic of cardiovascular complications

Rheum Dis Clin N Am 36 (2010) xiii–xiv
doi:10.1016/j.rdc.2010.03.005
0889-857X/10/$ – see front matter © 2010 Elsevier Inc. All rights reserved.

rheumatic.theclinics.com

of RA is addressed in a separate article. Important topics have been omitted due to space constraints, but most of these are well reviewed in other recent publications.

No attempt has been made to reconcile or homogenize the diverse perspectives that individual authors have brought to their assigned topics. Instead, contrasting and well-supported points of view are presented that reflect the knowledge and judgment of the experts who have generously agreed to contribute to this issue. At a point in time when we are arguably approximately halfway towards what needs to be accomplished for patients with RA, it is my hope that this volume will help clarify an agenda of questions that need to be asked and answered in the years ahead.

David A. Fox, MD
Division of Rheumatology
University of Michigan Medical Center
1500 East Medical Center Drive
Ann Arbor, MI 48109, USA

E-mail address:
dfox@umich.edu

Preclinical Rheumatoid Arthritis: Identification, Evaluation, and Future Directions for Investigation

Kevin D. Deane, MD[a],*, Jill M. Norris, MPH, PhD[b],
V. Michael Holers, MD[a]

KEYWORDS
- Rheumatoid arthritis • Preclinical period
- Anticyclic citrullinated peptide antibodies

"When the rheumatic poison is in the system, any disturbing circumstance, even of temporary duration, such as over fatigue, anxiety, grief or anger, by rendering the system more susceptible of its influence, may prove the accidental or exciting cause of the disease"
  Henry William Fuller in "On Rheumatism, Rheumatic Gout, and Sciatica"
              Publishers: Samuel S & William Wood, New York, 1854.

The discovery of genetic and environmental factors associated with rheumatoid arthritis (RA), and elevations in autoantibodies and inflammatory markers prior to the onset of symptomatic disease, coupled with similar findings in other autoimmune diseases including type 1 diabetes mellitus (T1DM), has led to the creation of a shared model of autoimmune disease development. In this model, the development of RA follows a natural history divided into phases wherein genetic and environmental interactions initially lead to a period of asymptomatic autoimmunity, evidenced by the presence of RA-related autoantibodies, that later evolves into clinically apparent disease. It is the initial phases of risk and asymptomatic autoimmunity that encompass "preclinical" RA.

To understand the genetic and environmental influences that are important to the evolution of RA, as well as develop predictive models and preventive strategies for

[a] Division of Rheumatology, University of Colorado School of Medicine, 1775 Aurora Court, Mail Stop B-115, Aurora, CO 80045, USA
[b] Department of Epidemiology, Colorado School of Public Health, University of Colorado, 13001 East 17th Place, Aurora, CO 80045, USA
* Corresponding author.
E-mail address: Kevin.Deane@UCDenver.edu

Rheum Dis Clin N Am 36 (2010) 213–241
doi:10.1016/j.rdc.2010.02.001
0889-857X/10/$ – see front matter © 2010 Elsevier Inc. All rights reserved.

future symptomatic disease, this preclinical period must be investigated. Herein are discussed the following issues related to preclinical RA: (1) what is known about the preclinical development of autoimmunity and inflammation in RA as well as other autoimmune diseases that may follow a similar model of development as RA, (2) how RA development can be modeled based on studies in preclinical RA and other autoimmune diseases, (3) practical issues related to the challenge of defining for research studies "preclinical" RA, as compared with clinically apparent disease, and (4) what aspects of RA evolution including genetic and environmental influences, and predictive and preventive models, could be addressed in studies of the preclinical period. Finally, potential methodologies and areas of focus going forward for research into preclinical RA are discussed.

PART 1. AUTOANTIBODIES AND INFLAMMATION IN PRECLINICAL RHEUMATOID ARTHRITIS AS WELL AS OTHER AUTOIMMUNE DISEASES
Studies of Preclinical Rheumatoid Arthritis

Multiple studies have shown that RA-related autoantibodies are present years before the diagnosis of RA (**Table 1**).[1–11] del Puente and colleagues,[1] who investigated RA in the Pima Indians in the Southwestern United States, showed that rheumatoid factor was present before the onset of clinically apparent RA. Aho and colleagues,[2,12–14] who investigated preclinical RA in Finland using a biobank of stored prediagnosis samples, and Jonsson and colleagues,[15] who used Icelandic biobank samples, also demonstrated that rheumatoid factor (RF) (by various methodologies) was present prior to the onset of clinically apparent RA. Also, in a prospective study of initially healthy family members of patients with RA, Silman and colleagues[11] showed that the presence of RF preceded the onset of clinically apparent RA.

Later studies also showed preclinical RA positivity for RF, as well as positivity for the highly RA-specific antibodies to citrullinated protein antigens (ACPAs). Again using a Finnish biobank, Aho and colleagues[3,4] demonstrated preclinical RA positivity of antikeratin (AKA) and antiperinuclear factor (APF) antibodies, and antifillagrin antibodies (AFA)[6] — autoantibody targets that, based on later findings, represented citrullinated antigens.[16] Using stored blood samples available through the Medical Biobank of Northern Sweden, Rantapaa-Dahlqvist and colleagues[7] evaluated for elevations of RF isotypes (immunoglobulins [Ig] M, G and A) and the anticyclic citrullinated peptide (anti-CCP) antibody in 98 preclinical samples from 83 RA patients, collected a median of 2.5 years prior to symptomatic disease onset. In this study, approximately 34% of patients were positive for anti-CCP within 1.5 years prior to diagnosis of RA, and the prevalence of RF isotype positivity ranged from about 17% to 34% during this same period. In addition, in comparison to controls, a combination of both anti-CCP and any RF isotype was highly specific (99%) for the future development of classifiable RA. This report was followed by a similarly designed retrospective cohort study by Nielen and colleagues[8] that evaluated preclinical RA RF and anti-CCP positivity using pre-RA diagnosis samples stored in a Dutch blood donor biobank. In this study, 79 RA patients with stored prediagnosis samples were identified, with a median of 13 preclinical samples per case. Of these 79 cases, approximately 28% and 41% had pre-RA diagnosis elevation of RF (IgM isotype) or anti-CCP, respectively. RF was positive a median of 2.0 years prior to RA diagnosis (range 0.3–10.3 years), and anti-CCP was positive a median of 4.5 years prior to RA diagnosis (range 0.1–13.8 years).

Additional studies using stored biobank samples have also demonstrated preclinical RA positivity for autoantibodies. Using stored pre-RA samples from 83 United States military subjects with RA, Majka and colleagues[9] demonstrated pre-RA diagnosis positivity for RF and anti-CCP. In addition, they demonstrated that individuals that were older at the time of diagnosis of RA had longer duration of preclinical positivity of autoantibodies, a finding that was supported by work by Bos and colleagues.[17] Chibnik and colleagues[18] utilized the Nurses' Health Study (NHS) biobank to demonstrate anti-CCP positivity prior to RA diagnosis, and showed that a lower cut-off value for anti-CCP than the kit suggested was also highly specific for future RA.

Multiple studies have also evaluated elevations of inflammatory markers prior to diagnosis of RA, with varying results (see **Table 1**).[19–24] In their Finnish biobank study, Aho and colleagues[25] found no significant elevation of C-reactive protein (CRP) in pre-RA diagnosis samples, although the time of sample collection prediagnosis was not reported. Using the same Medical Biobank of Northern Sweden as in the study of pre-RA RF and anti-CCP positivity, Rantapaa-Dahlqvist and colleagues[21] showed a significant elevation of monocyte chemoattractant protein-1 (MCP-1) in 92 pre-RA cases versus controls, but not secretory phospholipase A2 (sPLA2), high-sensitivity CRP (hsCRP) or interleukin (IL)-6. Nielen and colleagues[19] demonstrated, in the Dutch pre-RA sample cohort described above, that CRP was elevated in the pre-RA period, most commonly about 2 years before diagnosis, regardless of prediagnosis autoantibody positivity, although these investigators were unable in this study to demonstrate the chronologic sequence of appearance of CRP versus autoantibodies. Nielen and colleagues[20] later additionally demonstrated pre-RA elevation of sPLA2 in this cohort, but were unable to determine whether CRP or sPLA2 preceded autoantibodies in the preclinical period, and they concluded that the temporal development of autoantibodies and these 2 markers were probably similar. Jorgensen and colleagues[24] utilized samples from a Norwegian biobank to examine in 49 cases with RA prediagnosis elevations of autoantibodies (RF and anti-CCP) and multiple cytokines. These investigators found that RF and anti-CCP were elevated in RA cases prediagnosis; however, they could not demonstrate any cytokine elevations prior to 5 years before disease onset, and only tumor necrosis factor α (TNFα) was statistically significantly elevated in cases (vs controls) during the 5-year period just before diagnosis of RA.[24] Using a single pre-RA diagnosis blood sample from 90 incident RA cases (case status confirmed by chart review) identified in the Women's Health Study (WHS), Shadick and colleagues[23] were unable to demonstrate significant elevations in CRP levels in cases versus controls (with case samples available a mean of 6.6 years prior to diagnosis), and they were unable to use a single CRP level to predict future RA. However, in a later study using 170 RA cases from a combination of the NHS and WHS cohorts, the same group[22] was able to demonstrate statistically significant elevations of soluble tumor necrosis factor receptor II (sTNFRII) prior to RA diagnosis, but not IL-6 or hsCRP. Most recently, Rantaapa-Dahlqvist and colleagues used an expanded sample set from their Swedish Biobank, to demonstrate elevations of multiple cytokines and chemokines prior to the diagnosis of RA, with these elevations likely indicating pre-clinical RA activity of Th1, Th2, and T regulatory processes.[26]

There are caveats when interpreting the data regarding pre-clinical elevations of biomarkers. Certainly the prospective studies by del Puente and colleagues[1] and Silman and colleagues[11] suggest that autoantibodies are truly elevated before the onset of clinically apparent disease. However, in the studies of preclinical autoantibody and inflammatory marker elevations using stored samples from biobanks, there were not detailed joint-directed questionnaires or examinations performed at baseline or over time to ensure that no clinically apparent arthritis was present at the time of presumed preclinical RA blood collections. As such, it may be that the duration of pre-RA diagnosis autoantibody positivity is overestimated in the studies utilizing stored biobank

Table 1
Summary of selected studies of preclinical rheumatoid arthritis (RA)

Study	Study Design	Biomarkers Assessed	Findings	Implications for Prediction of Future RA
del Puente et al, 1988[1]	Prospective; Native Americans, Southwest United States	RF	RF precedes diagnosis of RA	Increased incidence of RA in RF+ individuals. Rates 2.4–48.3 per 1000 person-years, with highest rates in those with highest RF titers at baseline
Silman et al, 1992[11]	Prospective; British; FDRs from families with ≥2 RA cases	RF	RF precedes diagnosis of RA	Average incidence of RA 8 per 1000 person-years in FDRs; highest rate in FDRs with RF+: 34.8 per 1000 person-years
Jonsson et al, 1992[15]	Retrospective; Icelandic; biobank	RF (isotypes)	RF isotype elevations precede diagnosis of RA	Not analyzed
Aho et al, 1985–1991[2,13,14]	Retrospective; Finnish; biobank	RF (isotypes)	RF precedes diagnosis of RA	Not analyzed
Aho et al, 1993, 2000[4,6]	Retrospective; Finnish; biobank	AKA, AFA, APF (later studies showed target antigens likely citrullinated)	AKA, AFA, APF precede diagnosis of RA	RA-related antibodies may be present in subjects who did not develop RA in follow-up period
Rantapaa-Dahlqvist et al, 2003[7]	Retrospective; Swedish; biobank; N = 83 RA cases	RF, anti-CCP	RF, anti-CCP precede diagnosis of RA; 34% anti-CCP+ ≤1.5 years prior to RA diagnosis; RF-isotypes+ in ~17%–34% of cases pre-RA diagnosis	PPV 22%for future RA if RF-IgA and anti-CCP positive (estimated population prevalence of RA of 1%)
Nielen et al, 2004[8]	Retrospective; Dutch; biobank; N = 79 RA cases	RF-IgM, anti-CCP	RF-IgM, anti-CCP precede RA diagnosis; 49% positive for RF-IgM and/or anti-CCP pre-RA. RF-IgM+ or anti-CCP+ median of 2.0 or 4.8 years prior to diagnosis of RA, respectively	PPV up to 100% for RA diagnosis within 5 years based on 5-year incidence rates of 0.001 (general population) or 3.9% (estimated from high-risk multicase RA families)

Reference	Population	Biomarkers	Findings	Genetic/Other findings
Majka et al, 2008[9]	Retrospective; United States Military; biobank; N = 83 RA cases	RF, anti-CCP	Pre-RA diagnosis: RF+ 57% of cases, median 6.0 years; anti-CCP+ 61% of cases, median 5.4 years	Increased age-at-diagnosis of RA associated with longer duration of preclinical autoantibody positivity (replicated by Bos et al[7])
Rantapaa-Dahlqvist et al, 2007[21]	Retrospective; Swedish; biobank	MCP-1, IL-6, CRP, sPLA2	After adjustment, only MCP-1 elevated prior to RA diagnosis	Not analyzed
Nielen et al, 2004, 2006[19,20]	Retrospective; Dutch; biobank	RF, anti-CCP, CRP, sPLA2	CRP and sPLA2 elevations precede RA diagnosis; CRP ~2 years prior; timing similar to RF/anti-CCP	Not analyzed
Jorgensen et al, 2008[24]	Retrospective; Norwegian; biobank; N = 49 RA cases	RF-IgM, anti-CCP, multiple cytokines	RF-IgM and/or anti-CCP precede RA diagnosis by as much as 20 years; anti-TNF elevated <5 years prior to diagnosis of RA. EBV and Parvovirus serologies not different between cases and controls	Suggests that cytokine elevation may indicate symptomatic disease within 5 years
Berglin et al, 2004[115]	Retrospective; Swedish; biobank; N = 59 RA cases	RF, anti-CCP, HLA-DRB1 alleles *0404, *0401		Anti-CCP + DRB1*0404 or 0401 high-risk for future RA (OR ~67)
Johansson et al, 2006[116]	Retrospective; Swedish; biobank; N = 92 RA cases	RF, anti-CCP; PTPN22 (1858T)		Anti-CCP + PTPN22: 100% specific for future RA, and high-risk (OR >132)

Abbreviations: AFA, antifilaggrin antibodies; AKA, antikeratin antibodies; anti-CCP, anticyclic citrullinated peptide antibodies; APF, antiperinuclear factor antibodies; CRP, C-reactive protein; FDR, first-degree relative of proband with RA; HLA, human leukocyte antigen; IL-6, interleukin-6; MCP-1, monocyte chemoattractant protein-1; OR, odds ratio; PPV, positive predictive value; PTPN22, protein phosphatase 22; RF, rheumatoid factor; sPLA2, secretory phospholipase A2.

samples, as subjects may have had mild or fluctuating inflammatory symptoms long before a confirmed diagnosis of RA. Also of importance, these pre-RA studies show that not all RA patients have detectable pre-RA diagnosis autoantibody positivity. Methodologic issues may in part explain these findings. For example, patients may not have a stored blood sample available for analysis from the correct time period to demonstrate their prediagnosis autoantibody positivity. Also, current assays for autoantibodies may not detect the earliest preclinical autoantibody specificities; perhaps an as-of-yet unknown citrullinated antigen is the earliest autoantibody target in preclinical RA? In addition, not all patients with RA may develop detectable circulating autoantibodies in the preclinical period. For example, some patients may develop circulating autoantibodies after clinically apparent disease develops. Of note, in the Nielen study, while only about 28% of patients with RA were RF-positive prediagnosis, about 67% of these same patients were positive for RF by 6 years post diagnosis, suggesting that circulating RF develops in some cases after symptomatic onset of RA.[8] All of these issues will need to be considered in studies of preclinical RA going forward.

The Contribution of Genetic and Environmental Factors Associated with Rheumatoid Arthritis to Understanding Preclinical Development

Although the exact etiology of RA is unknown, there are multiple genetic and environmental factors that have been associated with disease. Estimates of the genetic contribution to RA have ranged between 30% and 60%.[27,28] Of the known genetic factors associated with RA, a DRB1 allele containing the "shared epitope" is the most important genetic factor associated with RA.[29,30] Of the HLA alleles, *HLA-DRB1*0401* and *HLA-DRB1*0404* (within the *HLA-DR4* group) are the most strongly associated with RA, with an approximate relative risk for RA of almost 4 in Caucasians.[31] In addition, several genes outside the *HLA-DRB1* gene have recently been associated with RA. These genes include *PTPN22*, *TRAF1/C5*, *CTLA4*, and *STAT4*, and the list is rapidly growing.[32,33]

Several potential environmental factors that could play important roles in modifying either susceptibility to RA or disease severity have been identified. High levels of coffee consumption,[34] in particular decaffeinated coffee,[35] as well as a positive smoking history,[31,36] exposure to air pollution,[37] and environmental exposure to silica-containing dust[38,39] are also associated with increased risk for RA. In addition, infections have been associated with RA including pathogens such as the Epstein-Barr virus (EBV), *Mycoplasma* or *Proteus* species.[27,40–43] Finally, several factors have been identified as possibly protective against development of RA including a history of successful pregnancy,[44,45] oral contraceptive pill use,[46–48] and higher vitamin D intake.[49]

Several studies have examined the association of environmental factors with asymptomatic RA-related autoantibody positivity. These studies suggest that lack of oral contraceptive use and a history of heavy smoking are associated with an increased prevalence of RF,[50–52] whereas 25,hydroxyvitamin D levels are not associated with RF positivity in individuals without RA.[53] Active pulmonary infection with tuberculosis has also been associated with RF and anti-CCP positivity in individuals without clinically apparent synovitis.[54,55] These studies suggest that environmental factors affect RA-related autoimmunity, although prospective evaluation of future risk for RA in these types of autoantibody positive subjects is lacking.

Of recent interest regarding the pathogenesis of RA are interactions between genetic and environmental factors that may lead to RA-related autoimmunity and disease. For example, several studies have reported that smoking in individuals with specific HLA alleles is associated with ACPA-positive RA, suggesting that a gene-environment interaction leads to RA-related autoimmunity.[56–59]

However, while genetic and environmental factors have been associated with RA, the exact role that these factors play in the development of RA-related autoimmunity is not yet clear. Also, it is unclear whether these factors may lead to initial RA-related immune dysregulation or transition from asymptomatic autoimmunity to clinically apparent RA. It is important that, as discussed later, prospective study of the early phases of RA development should help to clarify these issues.

Preclinical Studies in Other Autoimmune Diseases

In addition to the information about preclinical RA available from RA-specific studies, much about the evolution of autoimmunity can be learned by examining the preclinical natural history of other autoimmune diseases including T1DM and systemic lupus erythematosus (SLE). In particular, prospective studies of T1DM have led to the development of a model of disease evolution that may be of importance to RA.

T1DM results from autoimmune-mediated destruction of the pancreatic β cells, and it affects approximately 1 in 300 children. Numerous studies of T1DM have established that there are specific high-risk HLA genotypes that predispose to disease.[60,61] Moreover, the autoimmune attack on the pancreatic β cells can be detected years before clinical onset of T1DM via the presence of any of the T1DM-related autoantibodies in the blood including antibodies to the following antigens: islet cell (ICA), insulin (IAA), protein tyrosine phosphatase (IA2), and glutamic acid decarboxylase (GAD65).[62,63]

Prospective studies of T1DM have established that T1DM exhibits several phases during its development.[63] The first phase is defined as the presence of genetic risk factors that, either alone or in combination, may predispose to the loss of self tolerance. The second phase is reached when transformation from the risk state to a state of immunologic autoreactivity occurs; this second phase of "asymptomatic autoimmunity" is measurable by testing for T1DM-related biomarkers, but this phase is not yet associated with the presence of clinically apparent hyperglycemia. This transition from genetic risk to asymptomatic autoimmunity occurs either because of the introduction of an environmental factor, or perhaps because of the stochastic nature of the immune response. In T1DM, this preclinical autoimmune phase is marked by initial immune reactivity to only a small number of autoantigens. The third phase of T1DM is the development of clinically apparent hyperglycemia; this final phase is characterized immunologically by autoreactivity to numerous antigens and extensive immune-mediated tissue destruction of islet cells caused by many proinflammatory pathways.

The presence of these 3 phases of diseases in T1DM is well established, as is the value of prospectively studying children with highly predictive autoantibodies in the preclinical phases of disease for epidemiologic and genetic associations.[60,64–70] Of importance, due to the strong association of T1DM with β-cell (or islet) autoimmunity (IA), defined as the presence of autoantibodies specific to β-cell autoantigens, IA has become an alternative end point to clinically apparent hyperglycemia in T1DM research. Advantages of this approach include the opportunity to study the pathologic process underlying T1DM in a preclinical state, and to verify that a candidate risk factor is not only related to diabetes but also to the alteration of immune function preceding clinical onset of disease. Studies using as end points both autoimmunity and clinically apparent diabetes have allowed for differentiation of the risk factors that initiate humoral autoimmunity from those that promote progression from subclinical autoimmunity to diabetes.[60,70] Of note, prospective studies using asymptomatic IA as an outcome measure have identified important findings regarding dietary and other factors in T1DM, including the lack of association of islet-cell autoimmunity with childhood vaccines,[68] and the important relationship of timing of cereal exposure during the first year of life to the later development of IA.[66] This latter finding has been of importance in terms of potentially reducing risk for T1DM based on dietary considerations.

The presence of autoantibodies can be also used in the prediction of future T1DM. In first-degree relatives (FDRs) of diabetic individuals, the presence of a single autoantibody on one occasion has been found to have a sensitivity and specificity of 95% and 99%, respectively, and a positive predictive value (PPV) of 46% for type 1 diabetes with 5 years of follow-up.[71] Of note, the number of unique T1DM-related autoantibodies that are positive also predicts risk for future T1DM. For example, a person who tests positive for multiple autoantibodies is at a much higher risk of developing T1DM than a person with a single detectable autoantibody.[72] However, T1DM-related autoantibodies may be transiently positive, and there are not yet enough longitudinal data to determine if all people that develop autoantibodies will eventually develop T1DM.[63,72,73] Although not 100% predictive of future T1DM development, IA still serves as a very useful intermediate end point when studying the autoimmune disease process and potential risk factors for T1DM. In terms of RA, given the high specificity of certain autoantibodies (notably ACPAs) for disease, using autoantibody positivity as a surrogate end point for autoimmunity in preclinical RA is likely to be of similar great value.

SLE is a multisystem autoimmune disease of unknown etiology. More than 98% of SLE patients are positive for antinuclear antibodies (ANA) and many SLE patients have additional reactivity to specific nuclear antigens including double-stranded DNA (dsDNA), Smith, ribonuclear proteins, and Ro and La.[74–77] Some of these autoantibodies are associated with specific clinical manifestations of disease. For example, autoantibodies to dsDNA are associated with nephritis, and levels of anti-dsDNA antibodies may fluctuate in conjunction with disease activity.[78,79] In addition, anti-Ro antibodies have also been shown to be associated with specific manifestations of SLE including skin disease and neutropenia.[75–77] Although these autoantibody systems have been extensively studied for more than 50 years, the initiating events for the development of these autoantibodies and the actual roles these antibody specificities play in clinical SLE are not known. However, these SLE-related autoantibodies are present in the serum of lupus patients many years prior to the first clinical evidence of disease.[80,81] Furthermore, the spectrum/number of autoantibody specificities increases up to the time of diagnosis.[82] The discovery of preclinical autoantibody positivity and evolution of antibody specificity has led to important investigations into potential etiologic agents such as EBV infection in SLE, investigations that could not be performed without preclinical studies.[83]

Animal Models and Preclinical Rheumatoid Arthritis

While animal models of arthritis are not an exact match to human disease, they have provided important insights into the preclinical period of arthritis development. In particular, investigations into the relationships between the major histocompatibility complex (MHC) class II dependence of disease, a requirement in some instances for the specific exposure to citrullinated autoantigen, and the timing between the evolution of ACPA and clinically apparent arthritis have been helpful in understanding important factors in preclinical arthritis. An early example was provided by evidence that citrullinated proteins are found in the synovium after immunization with bovine collagen type II in DBA/1j mice, a strain that is commonly used to study the type II collagen-induced arthritis (CIA) model of RA.[84] However, in this study no ACPAs were detected. In a second study of the same model, ACPAs were found to develop before clinically detectable joint inflammation.[85] In this latter study, 2 methods were used to show that the ACPAs are pathogenic: first, treatment of mice with a "tolerogenic" form of a citrullinated peptide decreased the arthritis disease severity by approximately 60% and decreased the levels of ACPAs and epitope spreading to other citrullinated peptides; and second, a mouse monoclonal antibody that recognized citrullinated peptides, and could be used as a representative example of an ACPA, was found to greatly amplify joint inflammation. This process occurred only following the administration of low doses of antibodies specific for type II collagen, which induced the generation of citrullinated target antigens, presumably through the actions of macrophages and neutrophils containing peptidyl arginine deiminase (PAD) enzymes that participated in the inflammatory response. This second experiment suggested that, in the absence of citrullinated target antigens, there is no target injury; however, when these antigens are present, such as during treatment with monoclonal antibodies specific for type II collagen, ACPAs can greatly amplify inflammation and damage. Recently, additional monoclonal antibodies reactive with citrullinated type II collagen, with or without cross-reactivity to other epitopes, were also found to amplify the development of arthritis in mice in vivo.[86] In addition, another study in rats has shown an increased incidence and severity of arthritis when collagen type II is citrullinated before immunization.[87]

Other animal studies have focused on the relationship between cellular and humoral autoimmunity to citrullinated antigens and the shared epitope and class II molecules. For example, immunization with citrullinated vimentin peptide leads to CD4[+] T-cell activation and proliferation in transgenic mice expressing human HLA-DRB1*0401.[88] In addition, immunization of human HLA-DRB1*0401-transgenic C57BL/6 mice with citrullinated human fibrinogen, but not native human fibrinogen or either form of mouse fibrinogen, resulted in the development of arthritis in a substantial proportion of animals.[89] In this setting, a relatively low level of inflammation was present, but this was accompanied by specific antibody responses to citrullinated human fibrinogen peptide, as well as T-cell responses to citrullinated protein. ACPA-positive arthritis was also found to develop in mice that are immunized with low doses of collagen type II and that have dysregulated MHC expression in the joints owing to transgenic expression of class II transactivator.[90] Finally, a particularly intriguing study has recently shown that immunization of a subset of strains of mice with human fibrinogen alone resulted in destructive arthritis as well as T- and B-cell reactivity to fibrinogen.[91] In this study, epitope spreading to citrullinated fibrinogen as well as many synovial citrullinated and noncitrullinated autoantigens developed. Remarkably, arthritis could be transferred to naïve mice with either serum or fibrinogen-reactive T cells from immunized mice.

PART 2. THE PHASES OF RHEUMATOID ARTHRITIS DEVELOPMENT: FROM GENETIC RISK TO CLINICALLY APPARENT DISEASE

Based on the above discussion, including the presence of preclinical RA-related autoantibodies and inflammatory markers, the genetic and environmental factors associated with RA, the models of autoimmune disease development established in prospective studies of T1DM, and the animal models of disease, it is likely that RA develops 3 phases, outlined as follows and in **Fig. 1A**. The initial phase (**Phase 1**) is characterized by genetic risk for RA, during which no biomarkers of active autoimmunity and inflammation or symptoms are present. This **Phase 1** is followed by environmental and additional genetic influences that lead to a **Phase 2** of disease development—asymptomatic autoimmunity—characterized by the presence of

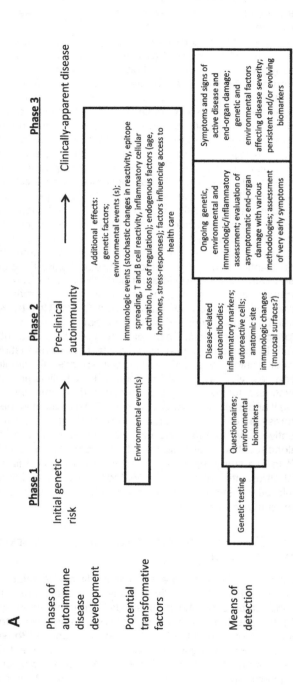

Fig. 1. A model of rheumatoid arthritis (RA) development. (A) Based on RA studies as well as prospective studies in other autoimmune disease (type 1 diabetes mellitus), RA may evolve through 3 phases of disease: Phase 1 = genetic risk, Phase 2 = asymptomatic autoimmunity (identified by presence of autoantibodies) and Phase 3 = clinically apparent disease. Transition between phases may be caused by interactions between genetic and environmental factors, and/or changes in immune reactivity. (B) RA-related factors that can be measured during the preclinical phases of disease development. (Adapted from Kolfenbach J, Deane KD, Derber LA, et al. A prospective approach to investigating the natural history of preclinical rheumatoid arthritis (RA) using first-degree relatives of probands with RA. Arthritis Rheum 2009;61(12):1735–4; with permission.)

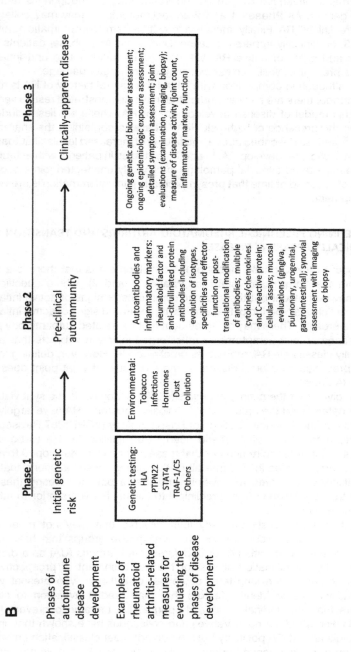

B

	Phase 1		**Phase 2**	**Phase 3**

Phases of autoimmune disease development

Initial genetic risk → Pre-clinical autoimmunity → Clinically-apparent disease

Examples of rheumatoid arthritis-related measures for evaluating the phases of disease development

Genetic testing: HLA PTPN22 STAT4 TRAF-1/C5 Others

Environmental: Tobacco Infections Hormones Dust Pollution

Autoantibodies and inflammatory markers: rheumatoid factor and anti-citrullinated protein antibodies including evolution of isotypes, specificities and effector function or post-translational modification of antibodies; multiple cytokines/chemokines and C-reactive protein; cellular assays; mucosal evaluations (gingiva, pulmonary, urogenital, gastrointestinal); synovial assessment with imaging or biopsy

Ongoing genetic and biomarker assessment; ongoing epidemiologic exposure assessment; detailed symptom assessment; joint evaluations (examination, imaging, biopsy); measure of disease activity (joint count, inflammatory markers, function)

Fig. 1. (continued)

RA-related autoantibodies and other immunologic factors such as T- and B-cell autoreactivity, and perhaps elevated inflammatory markers. **Phase 2** may be of variable length, perhaps influenced by genetic, environmental, or endogenous factors such as age or gender. As **Phases 1** and **2** are asymptomatic, they may collectively be termed "preclinical" RA. Finally, there is a transition from asymptomatic autoimmunity to **Phase 3**, or clinically apparent disease. During this final phase, patients will have symptoms and signs of active RA, with numerous autoimmune and inflammatory biomarkers present as well as clear evidence of end-organ damage.

Of note, although in comparison with T1DM the natural history of RA is much less well understood, there are several studies that have demonstrated results very consistent with this model of disease development for RA. These studies include several associating the presence of high-risk HLA-DR alleles containing the shared epitope with RA[29,30] and, as described above, the finding of increased levels of autoantibodies in individuals who later develop RA. In addition, studies in patients with established RA demonstrating altered synovial pathology in clinically unaffected joints suggest that there may be a period of time that presymptomatic joint inflammation is present during RA development.[92]

PART 3. DEFINING PRECLINICAL RHEUMATOID ARTHRITIS AND TRANSITION INTO CLINICALLY APPARENT DISEASE

A key aspect of this 3-phase model of RA development is that there is a transition period from the "preclinical" state (or **Phases 1** and **2**), where specific disease markers may be present but there are no symptoms or signs of active inflammatory disease, to a "clinical" period of RA, when symptoms and signs of active inflammatory disease are present. There may be agreement that RA-related autoantibody positivity, in the absence of joint symptoms or other organ injury, in subjects that eventually develop fully classifiable RA, represents preclinical RA. However, defining this transition from preclinical to clinical disease is more difficult: at what point does clinically apparent RA begin?

To date, given that the main anatomic site affected by RA is the synovial joint, the criteria for determining the presence of "clinically apparent" RA have largely focused on the joints. In the American College of Rheumatology (ACR) 1987 Revised Classification Criteria for RA, 4 of 7 criteria need to be fulfilled for RA to be defined.[93] However, it is important to remember that these criteria were developed to help standardize research studies in RA, that all of the disease manifestations that result in criteria fulfillment take time to develop, and that a patient meeting these criteria may have truly transitioned from preclinical to clinical RA years prior to fulfilling the ACR criteria for RA.[94,95]

In an attempt to investigate early joint disease that may not meet the 1987 Revised ACR Criteria, there are several investigative groups that have sought to classify inflammatory arthritis (IA) or undifferentiated arthritis (UA) as a distinct clinical entity. Such classification allows for the establishment of prospective clinical studies to determine the long-term outcomes of patients who present with such findings, as well as to identify factors that may predict evolution to classifiable and factors that may indicate that early aggressive therapy to prevent long-term disability is warranted. Of note, Verweij and colleagues have shown that, in patients with arthralgia and ACPA positivity but who do not meet classification criteria for RA, upregulation of certain genes in peripherally-circulating blood cells predicts risk for future development of fully-classificiable RA (by ACR criteria) within a defined time period.[96]

The most commonly utilized criteria for IA/UA are the Norfolk criteria and the Leiden criteria.[97–101] The Norfolk criteria define IA as 2 or more swollen joints of duration greater than 4 weeks.[97] In the Leiden criteria, IA/UA is defined as 1 or more joint with inflammatory findings confirmed by a rheumatologist, with the joint findings not otherwise classifiable (ie, gout or pseudogout).[98] In addition, together the ACR and the European League Against Rheumatism (EuLAR) are currently developing revised RA criteria, in part to address the need to link IA to the same long-term prognostic considerations and need for treatment, as are typical for RA as defined by the earlier ACR criteria.[102]

The Norfolk and Leiden criteria for UA/IA, and the new ACR/EuLAR criteria for RA, may be more useful than the current ACR RA criteria in identifying patients earlier in the transition from preclinical to clinical RA, and it will be important for studies in preclinical RA going forward to have clearly defined criteria for transition from preclinical disease in order to understand the evolution of RA, define when in the spectrum of clinical presentations therapeutic intervention may be necessary, and define a clinical outcome that is a suitable end point for prevention trials.

PART 4. WHAT CAN WE LEARN BY INVESTIGATING PRECLINICAL RHEUMATOID ARTHRITIS?
Genetic and Environmental Interactions in Preclinical Rheumatoid Arthritis

As discussed earlier, the genetic and environmental influences that lead to the preclinical phase of disease development are likely key features in the development of RA-related autoimmunity. However, given the observed length of time between the appearance of autoimmunity and diagnosis of RA, standard case-control study approaches using subjects with established RA may not optimally allow for the identification of environmental risk factors for RA or at what point the risk factors influence the development of autoimmunity and disease. For example, as mentioned earlier, there is now considerable data that supports that gene-environmental interactions between smoking and specific HLA alleles are associated with ACPA positivity in established RA.[36,56–59,103,104] However, investigating the relationship between these factors in the preclinical period would help determine whether HLA alleles, smoking, and ACPA positivity are associated in the absence of synovitis—a finding that would support a role for smoking as an initial and perhaps causative step in RA-related autoimmunity.

Inherent in the '**Phases**' model of RA development discussed above is that there is a physical location where genetic and environmental factors interact to lead to the initial RA-related immune dysregulation and break in tolerance. For example, given the strong association of smoking with RA, and in particular ACPA-positive RA, there is a theory that initial RA-related immune dysregulation occurs at the mucosal surfaces of the mouth (periodontal surfaces) or lung, with later spread of RA-related autoimmunity and inflammation to the joints resulting in clinically-apparent synovial disease.[37,39,57,58,105] Real-time prospective study of subjects with RA-related autoimmunity, evidenced by autoantibodies (either prevalent or incident) but no synovitis, would allow for detailed exploration of mucosal surface immune function. Supporting this approach, in preliminary work the authors have identified evidence of inflammatory lung injury, including airway and alveolar disease, using high-resolution computed tomography of the lungs of individuals with RA-related autoantibody positivity but without joint symptoms or findings, suggesting that RA-related inflammation may indeed occur initially in the lung.[106]

Evaluation of Autoantibody and Inflammatory Marker Evolution in the Preclinical Period of Rheumatoid Arthritis Development

There is a growing body of work suggesting that factors involving RA-related auto-antibodies including isotype switching, antigen specificity, posttranslational modification and effector function (such as autoantibody glycosylation) may be related to disease severity and perhaps evolution from UA to RA.[107–112] For example, Verpoort and colleagues[111] reported that patients who evolved from UA to RA had a broader spectrum of ACPA isotypes compared with those with persistent UA at follow-up. In addition, a study by Ioan-Facsinay and colleagues[113] comparing autoantibodies in North American natives with RA and their healthy FDRs showed ACPA reactivity in both groups (19% in healthy FDRs vs about 91% in RA cases); however, the fine specificities of ACPAs differed between RA cases and healthy controls, with reactivity to citrullinated fibrinogen and vimentin only seen in RA cases. Also in this study, ACPA isotypes were more limited in healthy FDRs compared with RA cases. As a whole, these findings suggest that ACPA isotype evolution and specificity may be important for disease development. As such, investigating the evolution of the isotype changes and specificity during the preclinical period when the possible transformations from nonpathogenic to pathogenic states may occur, may lead to key insights into RA development, and perhaps identification of the "original sin" in RA; that is, the initial autoantigen that leads to RA-related autoimmunity. In regard to this latter point, based on the work of several groups, ACPA reactivity to citrullinated α-enolase CEP-1 epitope may indicate that this citrullinated antigen most strongly links exposure to cigarette smoke and HLA risk alleles in RA.[59] If autoimmunity to this citrullinated antigen could be demonstrated in the preclinical period prior to other autoimmune responses to citrullinated antigens, the argument that this antigen is the initial one in RA would be compelling. In addition, prospective evaluation of cytokine/chemokine type (ie, IL-17, TNFα, or paradigm-specific small molecule profiles) may allow for identification of key inflammatory processes in RA development that may help to identify the inciting factors for this disease as well as allow us to specifically target aspects of the immune system for prevention.

Predictive Models for Future Rheumatoid Arthritis

Several prospective and retrospective studies suggest that autoantibodies or combinations of genetic factors and autoantibodies indicate high risk for future RA. In prospective evaluation (including joint examinations and radiographs of hands and feet approximately every 2 years) of approximately 2700 Pima and/or Papago Native Americans in Arizona, USA (a population with an overall prevalence rate of RA of approximately 5%), followed up to 19 years, del Puente and colleagues[1] demonstrated increased risk for incident RA in RF-positive (by sheep cell agglutination) individuals, with the highest risk of 48.3 cases per 1000 person-years seen in those with a titer of greater than 1:256 at baseline testing. Also in prospective evaluation of 370 FDRs from multicase RA families followed with periodic joint symptom assessment for a mean of 5 years, Silman and colleagues[11] found the overall rate for incident RA to be approximately 8 per 1000 person-years, with a rate of incident RA in subjects that were positive for RF at baseline of 34.8 cases per 1000 person-years (calculated from 4 incident cases of RA out of 24 individuals).

Retrospective biobank studies have also estimated risk for future RA, although these results are more limited due to lack of prospectively collected data. In their Swedish biobank study, Rantapaa-Dahlqvist and colleagues[7] estimated PPVs for future RA of 4% if RF-IgM positive alone, 16% if anti-CCP positive alone, and 22%

if anti-CCP and RF-IgA positive (these PPV calculations assumed a prevalence of RA in the general population of 1%). Nielen and colleagues[8] estimated a PPV for onset of classifiable RA within 5 years of 5.9% for subjects that were anti-CCP positive alone, assuming an incidence rate of RA over 5 years in the general population of 0.001%. However, this PPV increased to 69.4% if the incidence rate of RA in the population over 5 years used for calculation was 3.9%. Of note, this higher rate of incident RA (3.9% vs 0.001%) used by Nielen and colleagues in their PPV calculations was estimated from Silman and colleagues[11] 1992 study of incident RA in individuals from multicase RA families, in which a strong family history of RA (≥ 2 members with RA) may serve as a possible surrogate for additional genetic and/or environmental risk for RA. Also, in the Nielen study,[8] if both RF and anti-CCP were positive, the PPV for RA diagnosis within 5 years was 100%, regardless of which background incidence of RA was used for comparison.

Studies that have evaluated risk for future RA have shown that certain genetic factors, notably HLA alleles containing the "shared epitope," may increase risk for future RA.[114] However, the ability of genetic factors alone to predict future RA may be limited, in part due to the high prevalence of these factors in the population—in North American controls, at least one HLA allele containing the "shared epitope" is present in about 40% of the population, and PTPN22 risk alleles are present in about 16% of the population.[57] As such, prediction of risk for future RA will likely best be done using combinations of genetic, environmental, and autoantibody factors.

Several studies have already examined the relationship between genetic factors and autoantibodies in prediction of future RA. Berglin and colleagues,[115] using the Northern Sweden Health and Disease biobank, performed a nested case-control study to show a strong association between pre-RA diagnosis anti-CCP positivity and HLA-DRB1*0404 or *0401 alleles and risk for future RA (odds ratio 66.8, 95% confidence interval [CI] 8.3–539.4). In addition, using data from the same Swedish biobank and similar study design, Johansson and colleagues[116] showed a strong association of anti-CCP positivity and 2 copies of the 1858T variant allele of PTPN22 with future RA (odds ratio 132.0, 95% CI ~18–2721). Studies are also underway to use gene and environment interactions for prediction of RA, as well as prediction of preclinical RA-related autoantibody positivity as a surrogate outcome for evolving RA (Elizabeth Karlson, personal communication, 2009).

There may be other factors that act separately or in concert with genetic and environmental factors to influence transition from asymptomatic to symptomatic RA-related autoimmunity. Majka and colleagues[9] and Bos and colleagues[17] reported in their retrospective cohort analyses that subjects with older age at time of diagnosis of RA had longer duration of preclinical RA-related autoantibody positivity. These findings may be explained by differences in genetic or environmental exposures that vary by age, or by age-related immune senescence. In addition, these findings suggest that age or other endogenous factors such as gender may have relevance in predicting future onset of RA in at-risk populations.

Also, prospective studies of cohorts of patients initially with early symptomatic IA/UA have allowed for investigation of the effects of genetic and other factors in the persistence and evolution of symptomatic arthritis. Several Dutch studies have shown that factors such as age, sex, number of swollen joints, and autoantibody and CRP status may predict persistent IA at 1 year.[98,100,117] In addition, in separate studies, Feitsma and colleagues[118] and van der Helm-van Mil and colleagues[119] showed that the presence of PTPN22 or HLA risk alleles may not significantly increase risk of transition from UA to RA, but that these genetic risk factors do influence autoantibody presence (HLA) or level (PTPN22). Finally, several preclinical studies including those using the Swedish, Dutch, and NHS biobanks noted an increase in autoantibody titer and/or inflammatory marker levels in the time period immediately preceding diagnosis.[7,8,18,19,21,22] Regarding this latter point, prospective study of biomarker changes may also be of key interest in understanding the kinetics of preclinical RA and in predictive models for symptomatic disease.

Although these studies are supportive of the ability of predictive models to determine risk for future RA, it should be noted that estimates of risk for future RA using stored samples from biobanks are limited because such studies were not truly prospective. Of importance is that participants were not subjected to detailed baseline or follow-up joint examinations, and pre-RA diagnosis samples were assessed retrospectively in comparison with selected controls after RA had been diagnosed. For these reasons, the relationship between symptom onset and biomarker positivity is inexact.

Preclinical Prevention of Rheumatoid Arthritis

Several clinical trials have demonstrated that treatment with aggressive therapy in early RA (that meets 1987 ACR RA criteria) leads to improved clinical outcomes, and perhaps increased rates of drug-free remission.[120,121] As such, currently a major goal for RA treatment is early identification and treatment of disease.[122] In addition, several investigative groups have evaluated the efficacy of disease-modifying therapy in individuals who have UA/IA not yet meeting established ACR criteria for RA. For example, in the Probable Rheumatoid Arthritis Methotrexate versus Placebo Treatment (PROMPT) trial, in patients with UA of duration 2 years or less, use of methotrexate delayed progression to RA as defined by the 1987 ACR criteria, with the most benefit seen in anti-CCP positive subjects.[99] Another small study investigating abatacept in UA showed a trend toward decreased progression to classifiable RA.[123] Also, several studies utilizing immunomodulation to prevent progression of T1DM have been performed, and although T1DM has not yet been prevented, studies have shown that intervention may lead to decreased insulin usage, and decreased risk for death from ketoacidosis early in disease.[124] Finally, in SLE, a retrospective study of military patients with SLE by James and colleagues[125] found that treatment with hydroxychloroquine in early disease led to decreased progression of SLE-specific autoantibodies as well as clinical findings. Overall, the results from these studies suggest that intervention in an even earlier period of RA-related autoimmunity (ie, in the preclinical period) may lead to prevention of disease.

Unfortunately, as of yet there are no published results of preclinical RA prevention trials. However, interesting data obtained from database studies suggests that certain agents such as HMG-CoA reductase inhibitors (statins) that may have some benefit in treatment of active RA may modify future RA risk.[126–128] Jick and colleagues[129] have shown, using a national database in the United Kingdom (N = 313 RA cases and 1252 controls), a decreased risk for incident RA in patients using statins for hyperlipidemia (odds ratio 0.59, 95% CI 037–0.96).

Ultimately, these findings and further research may lead to preclinical pharmacologic immunomodulation to prevent disease. Alternatively, perhaps nonpharmacologic tolerization (based on murine models of disease) or risk factor modification in the preclinical period may be used to abrogate clinically apparent disease; for example, if a person at high-risk for future RA stopped smoking, this may decrease the risk for developing clinically apparent arthritis. However, while prevention of RA is of key importance, implementation of prevention trials will only be possible after researchers have first developed models in prospective studies to identify accurately those at high risk for future RA in a definable and relatively short time period necessary to conduct such studies.

PART 5. FUTURE RESEARCH IN PRECLINICAL RHEUMATOID ARTHRITIS

There are multiple approaches to investigate preclinical RA, and these are outlined in **Table 2**. The investigation of preclinical RA would ideally take an approach similar to the Framingham study, which followed a large population over time to investigate causes of cardiovascular disease using serial measures of biomarkers and clinical outcomes.[130] However, due to the low prevalence of RA, large-scale population studies at single centers may be impractical due to the cost of screening and relatively few outcomes of disease. As such, preclinical RA may best be investigated by using research models similar to those used in studies in T1DM, that is, using a multicenter approach and prospectively following subjects who are likely to be at higher risk for RA-related autoimmunity as well as development of clinically apparent disease. One example of a population at higher risk for RA is FDRs of RA probands, as these FDRs may have 5- to 7-fold increased risk for incident RA.[11] In a multicenter study in the United States, the authors are currently following prospectively a large cohort of FDRs of probands with RA (goal N = 2100).[131] To date, a substantial proportion (~14%, N~1200) of these FDRs exhibit RA-related autoantibody positivity.[131] In addition, in Canada, El-Gabalawy and colleagues[113,132,133] are currently prospectively following a cohort of North American Natives who are FDRs of probands with RA, and have demonstrated intriguing findings regarding differences in ACPA isotypes and specificities between RA cases and asymptomatic FDRs. These cohorts will be valuable in investigating the effects of genetic and environmental factors on RA-related autoimmunity, as well as in investigating the evolution of RA-related autoimmunity and inflammation over time. While identification of asymptomatic individuals with RA-related autoantibody positivity is of interest, these prospective cohort analyses will also allow for the identification of factors that impact the transition from **Phase 1** (genetic risk) to **Phase 2** (asymptomatic autoimmunity)—a transition during which the key early interactions leading to RA-related autoimmunity occur. Examples of RA-related measures that may be assessed prospectively in preclinical study are provided in **Fig. 1B**.

Also, based on the prior success of biobank studies of preclinical RA, additional samples from yet untapped existing biobanks may be evaluated for RA-related biomarkers. However, as these retrospective cohorts may lack detailed joint evaluations, the ability to investigate the relationship between immune parameters and symptomatic disease may be limited.

As an alternative to the prospective or biobank studies discussed earlier, a large general population could be screened for RA-related genetic traits or RA-related autoantibody positivity to identify those at high risk for disease. From this initial screening, a smaller group of individuals with high-risk genetic and/or autoantibody markers may be followed over time to evaluate the evolution of RA-related autoimmunity. For example, in a health-fair screen of approximately 5000 individuals, the authors have identified approximately 40 anti-CCP positive subjects without synovitis on examination, and these subjects are now being evaluated prospectively for evolution of RA-related autoimmunity.[134] Such population screening is complicated by cost issues and the potential for subjects participating in such screening to have existing symptomatic joint disease, thereby missing the "preclinical" window of disease. However, with appropriate methodologies, population screening may be a reasonable approach to identify individuals with asymptomatic RA-related autoimmunity.

Of note, given the growing availability of array technologies, it may be possible to screen large populations at risk of developing a wide variety of autoimmune diseases. By testing for multiple autoimmune diseases, this approach might also allow for

Table 2
Potential methodologies for investigating preclinical rheumatoid arthritis

Study Design	Examples	Strengths	Weaknesses
Retrospective case-control studies using stored prediagnosis samples (biobanks):	Finnish, Swedish, and Dutch biobank studies[6–8] United States Military/Department of Defense Serum Repository[9] Nurses' Health Study[18,22] Women's Health Study[22]	Biobanks already established and preclinical samples may be obtained from cases with known RA	Decreased ability to determine future risk for disease; unable to ascertain exact relationship between timing of appearance of RA-related biomarkers and symptoms; limited samples available
Prospective studies: Populations at high risk for RA (such as first-degree relatives of probands with RA, twin studies, or populations such as Native Americans with high prevalence of disease)	*Ongoing:* Holers et al[131]: Studies of the Etiologies of Rheumatoid Arthritis (SERA): prospective evaluation of first-degree relatives of probands with RA El-Gabalawy et al[113,132,133]: North American Native people in Central Canada (Cree and Ojibway) prospectively followed for evolution of RA-related autoimmunity. Background prevalence of RA in population ~2% *Prior:* Native American (Pima and Papago) studies[1]	Real-time evaluation of evolution of RA-related autoimmunity to determine timing of appearance of biomarkers in relationship to environmental exposures and development of symptomatic disease; possibility for detailed assessment of mucosal biology in preclinical RA	Costly in terms of money and time; relatively low prevalence of incident RA and prevalence of RA-related autoantibodies limits statistical power

Other prospective studies: Large-scale population screening to identify individuals with high-risk features for RA including genetic factors and RA-related autoantibody positivity	Health-fair screening in Colorado identifying anti-CCP positive asymptomatic individuals who are recruited for follow-up[134]	Potentially identifies subjects at risk for "sporadic RA"(as are most cases in population); may help to establish prevalence of RA-related autoantibodies in general populations	Expensive, and relatively low prevalence of RA-related autoantibodies requires large-scale screening to identify at-risk individuals
Coupling of prospective RA studies with other research projects (such as cardiovascular disease studies)	Multiple studies are likely available	Allows for coupling of research projects perhaps resulting in decreased costs	Costly in terms of money and effort to establish screening
Other approaches: Animal models of disease	Multiple	Allows for detailed evaluation of antigen interactions; may provide for testing of methodologies for tolerization	Animal models of arthritis have substantial differences from human disease
Population screening for multiple autoimmune diseases	Multiple	Multiple autoimmune diseases may be studied; array technology for multiple autoantibody testing	Expensive; optimal diagnostic accuracy and reproducibility of testing would need to be established

a more cost-effective way to identify individuals at risk for RA-related autoimmunity as well as those at risk for other autoimmune diseases that also exhibit preclinical disease-related autoantibodies, including T1DM and SLE already mentioned, as well as autoimmune thyroid disease (Graves disease and Hashimoto thyroiditis), primary biliary cirrhosis, and celiac disease.[135,136] With regard to such a strategy, it is important to understand that in aggregate these diseases affect up to 7% of the population.[135,136] Also, there are data to support the possibility that risk for cardiovascular disease (CVD), the leading cause of death in RA patients, may be increased even in the preclinical period of RA.[137] As such, preclinical evaluation of RA may not only identify RA-specific factors but also lead to a better understanding of CVD risk in RA, and perhaps CVD prevention.

In addition to the design and implementation of prospective studies to investigate the preclinical period of RA development, several other issues regarding research methodologies in preclinical RA need to be addressed. First, what constitutes positivity for RA-related autoantibodies? At present there are multiple methodologies for testing RFs and ACPAs, with each kit having different cut-offs for positivity resulting in a variety of sensitivities and specificities. As such, standardized methodologies for testing RFs and ACPAs as well as for determining what result is considered positive will need to be established in order to homogenize testing results and development of predictive models for future RA. International studies in T1DM have already adopted standardized autoantibody testing, and these tests are performed in a limited number of research laboratories to ensure accuracy and reproducibility of testing. Second, as discussed earlier, we will need to define what constitutes "preclinical" RA as well as what constitutes transition from asymptomatic RA-related autoimmunity to clinically apparent disease. Likely this will need standardized symptom and joint count assessments, as well as potentially standardized techniques for imaging of the synovium using magnetic resonance imaging and/or ultrasound, and standardized synovial biopsy techniques and tissue processing. Also, it may be useful in preclinical studies to establish biomarker end points that could be employed in prevention trials. Such profiles, which may include autoantibodies and inflammatory markers, may be used as surrogate outcomes for increased risk for future RA. For example, if an asymptomatic individual in a prevention trial has RA-related autoantibodies suggesting high risk for future RA as well as an elevated CRP suggesting active inflammation, a decrease of CRP in this individual due to a pharmacologic intervention (in absence of joint symptoms) may be considered a clinically appropriate success in prevention of disease. This approach is aimed at allowing for a more timely assessment of intervention success, as joint symptoms may take years to develop. Of note, in terms of symptoms or examination findings, swollen joints may not be the first indication of transition from preclinical RA to clinical RA, and perhaps patient-reported measures such as stiffness or pain in absence of detectable swelling are the first indications of symptomatic RA. Detailed studies of the preclinical period, closely examining joint symptoms, and perhaps investigating asymptomatic organ injury using synovial biopsy to discover asymptomatic synovitis, or joint or lung imaging to detect asymptomatic RA-related injury, may be necessary to understand truly the evolution from preclinical to clinical RA. Third, what phenotype of RA will be best to investigate? Will it be best to focus on seropositive disease, as it will be easier to identify preclinical seropositive RA due to the presence of specific autoantibodies? Given that seronegative RA may be distinct from seropositive RA in terms of genetic and environmental risk factors, it may be worthwhile to focus efforts going forward on seropositive disease.[138] Fourth, to understand the predictive power of RA-related biomarkers for future disease, relevant control populations for prospective studies of preclinical RA need to be established. This factor is of particular importance when considering that several preclinical studies in RA have already shown that not all subjects with RA-related auto-antibody positivity, including ACPAs, may develop symptomatic RA.[4,15] Finally, standardized approaches for assessing epidemiologic exposures that might impact RA development will need to be established.

In addition to studies in humans, animal models of autoimmune disease may yield important insights into preclinical autoimmunity. In particular, animal models may be utilized to understand initial citrullinated protein-specific autoimmunity, or the role of mucosal surfaces in the generation of autoimmunity. Also, animal models may help to identify methods to tolerize individuals to citrullinated or other antigens important to RA in the preclinical period of RA development, a time period in which nonpharmaceutical, immunomodulatory strategies may be more effective prior to the extensive epitope spreading that has occurred in RA by the time clinical symptoms and signs of disease appear. Animal studies may also allow the determination of whether novel treatments focused on the citrullination process itself may be beneficial.

SUMMARY

Based on multiple studies in RA as well as other autoimmune diseases, RA likely develops in phases exhibited by genetic risk, asymptomatic autoimmunity and, finally, clinically apparent disease, with transformations between these phases occurring due to combinations of genetic, environmental, and immunologic factors. Investigating the preclinical phases of RA development will provide key insights into the factors that lead to disease, as well as allow for development of predictive models for disease, and ultimately prevention strategies for RA. Going forward, studies of preclinical RA may use bio-repositories, but the most effective approach will likely be the use of prospective cohort studies, with subjects chosen from populations at greater risk for RA such as FDRs or twin studies, or those identified with high-risk markers for RA, either genetic or autoantibody, through community screening. In addition to design and implementation of such prospective studies, the rheumatology community will need to define with greater clarity what constitutes the transition from preclinical to clinical RA, as well as standardize autoantibody and inflammatory marker testing. Although these latter tasks are daunting, investigation of preclinical RA likely gives us the greatest hope for curing or preventing this disease.

REFERENCES

1. del Puente A, Knowler WC, Pettitt DJ, et al. The incidence of rheumatoid arthritis is predicted by rheumatoid factor titer in a longitudinal population study. Arthritis Rheum 1988;31(10):1239–44.
2. Aho K, Heliovaara M, Maatela J, et al. Rheumatoid factors antedating clinical rheumatoid arthritis. J Rheumatol 1991;18(9):1282–4.
3. Kurki P, Aho K, Palosuo T, et al. Immunopathology of rheumatoid arthritis. Anti-keratin antibodies precede the clinical disease. Arthritis Rheum 1992;35(8): 914–7.
4. Aho K, von Essen R, Kurki P, et al. Antikeratin antibody and antiperinuclear factor as markers for subclinical rheumatoid disease process. J Rheumatol 1993;20(8):1278–81.
5. Aho K, Heliovaara M, Knekt P, et al. Serum immunoglobulins and the risk of rheumatoid arthritis. Ann Rheum Dis 1997;56(6):351–6.

6. Aho K, Palosuo T, Heliovaara M, et al. Antifilaggrin antibodies within "normal" range predict rheumatoid arthritis in a linear fashion. J Rheumatol 2000; 27(12):2743–6.
7. Rantapaa-Dahlqvist S, de Jong BA, Berglin E, et al. Antibodies against cyclic citrullinated peptide and IgA rheumatoid factor predict the development of rheumatoid arthritis. Arthritis Rheum 2003;48(10):2741–9.
8. Nielen MM, van Schaardenburg D, Reesink HW, et al. Specific autoantibodies precede the symptoms of rheumatoid arthritis: a study of serial measurements in blood donors. Arthritis Rheum 2004;50(2):380–6.
9. Majka DS, Deane KD, Parrish LA, et al. Duration of preclinical rheumatoid arthritis-related autoantibody positivity increases in subjects with older age at time of disease diagnosis. Ann Rheum Dis 2008;67(6):801–7.
10. MacGregor AJ, Silman AJ. Rheumatoid factors as predictors of rheumatoid arthritis. J Rheumatol 1991;18(9):1280–1.
11. Silman AJ, Hennessy E, Ollier B. Incidence of rheumatoid arthritis in a genetically predisposed population. Br J Rheumatol 1992;31(6):365–8.
12. Aho K, Palosuo T, Heliovaara M. Predictive significance of rheumatoid factor. J Rheumatol 1995;22(11):2186–7.
13. Aho K, Palosuo T, Raunio V, et al. The timing of rheumatoid factor seroconversions. Arthritis Rheum 1987;30(6):719–20.
14. Aho K, Palosuo T, Raunio V, et al. When does rheumatoid disease start? Arthritis Rheum 1985;28(5):485–9.
15. Jonsson T, Thorsteinsson J, Kolbeinsson A, et al. Population study of the importance of rheumatoid factor isotypes in adults. Ann Rheum Dis 1992;51(7): 863–8.
16. van Venrooij WJ, Pruijn GJ. Citrullination: a small change for a protein with great consequences for rheumatoid arthritis. Arthritis Res 2000;2(4):249–51.
17. Bos WH, Nielen MM, Dijkmans BA, et al. Duration of pre-rheumatoid arthritis anti-cyclic citrullinated peptide positivity is positively associated with age at seroconversion. Ann Rheum Dis 2008;67(11):1642.
18. Chibnik LB, Mandl LA, Costenbader KH, et al. Comparison of threshold cut-points and continuous measures of anti-cyclic citrullinated peptide antibodies in predicting future rheumatoid arthritis. J Rheumatol 2009;36(4):706–11.
19. Nielen MM, van Schaardenburg D, Reesink HW, et al. Increased levels of C-reactive protein in serum from blood donors before the onset of rheumatoid arthritis. Arthritis Rheum 2004;50(8):2423–7.
20. Nielen MM, van Schaardenburg D, Reesink HW, et al. Simultaneous development of acute phase response and autoantibodies in preclinical rheumatoid arthritis. Ann Rheum Dis 2006;65(4):535–7.
21. Rantapaa-Dahlqvist S, Boman K, Tarkowski A, et al. Up regulation of monocyte chemoattractant protein-1 expression in anti-citrulline antibody and immunoglobulin M rheumatoid factor positive subjects precedes onset of inflammatory response and development of overt rheumatoid arthritis. Ann Rheum Dis 2007; 66(1):121–3.
22. Karlson EW, Chibnik LB, Tworoger SS, et al. Biomarkers of inflammation and development of rheumatoid arthritis in women from two prospective cohort studies. Arthritis Rheum 2009;60(3):641–52.
23. Shadick NA, Cook NR, Karlson EW, et al. C-reactive protein in the prediction of rheumatoid arthritis in women. Arch Intern Med 2006;166(22):2490–4.
24. Jorgensen KT, Wiik A, Pedersen M, et al. Cytokines, autoantibodies and viral antibodies in premorbid and postdiagnostic sera from patients with rheumatoid

arthritis: case-control study nested in a cohort of Norwegian blood donors. Ann Rheum Dis 2008;67(6):860–6.

25. Aho K, Palosuo T, Knekt P, et al. Serum C-reactive protein does not predict rheumatoid arthritis. J Rheumatol 2000;27(5):1136–8.

26. Kokkonen H, Soderstrom I, Rocklow J, et al. Up-regulation of cytokines and chemokines predates the onset of rheumatoid arthritis. Arthritis Rheum 2010;62(2): 383–91.

27. Silman AJ. Epidemiology of rheumatoid arthritis. APMIS 1994;102(10):721–8.

28. Alarcon GS. Epidemiology of rheumatoid arthritis. Rheum Dis Clin North Am 1995;21(3):589–604.

29. Reveille JD. The genetic contribution to the pathogenesis of rheumatoid arthritis. Curr Opin Rheumatol 1998;10(3):187–200.

30. Nepom GT, Nepom BS. Prediction of susceptibility to rheumatoid arthritis by human leukocyte antigen genotyping. Rheum Dis Clin North Am 1992;18(4): 785–92.

31. Karlson EW, Chang SC, Cui J, et al. Gene-environment interaction between HLA-DRB1 shared epitope and heavy cigarette smoking in predicting incident rheumatoid arthritis. Ann Rheum Dis 2010;69(1):54–60.

32. Plenge RM. Rheumatoid arthritis genetics: 2009 update. Curr Rheumatol Rep 2009;11(5):351–6.

33. Barton A, Worthington J. Genetic susceptibility to rheumatoid arthritis: an emerging picture. Arthritis Rheum 2009;61(10):1441–6.

34. Heliovaara M, Aho K, Knekt P, et al. Coffee consumption, rheumatoid factor, and the risk of rheumatoid arthritis. Ann Rheum Dis 2000;59(8):631–5.

35. Mikuls TR, Cerhan JR, Criswell LA, et al. Coffee, tea, and caffeine consumption and risk of rheumatoid arthritis: results from the Iowa Women's Health Study. Arthritis Rheum 2002;46(1):83–91.

36. Padyukov L, Silva C, Stolt P, et al. A gene-environment interaction between smoking and shared epitope genes in HLA-DR provides a high risk of seropositive rheumatoid arthritis. Arthritis Rheum 2004;50(10):3085–92.

37. Hart JE, Laden F, Puett RC, et al. Exposure to traffic pollution and increased risk of rheumatoid arthritis. Environ Health Perspect 2009;117(7):1065–9.

38. Parks CG, Conrad K, Cooper GS. Occupational exposure to crystalline silica and autoimmune disease. Environ Health Perspect 1999;107(Suppl 5): 793–802.

39. Koeger AC, Lang T, Alcaix D, et al. Silica-associated connective tissue disease. A study of 24 cases. Medicine (Baltimore) 1995;74(5):221–37.

40. Blaschke S, Schwarz G, Moneke D, et al. Epstein-Barr virus infection in peripheral blood mononuclear cells, synovial fluid cells, and synovial membranes of patients with rheumatoid arthritis. J Rheumatol 2000;27(4):866–73.

41. Oliver JE, Silman AJ. Risk factors for the development of rheumatoid arthritis. Scand J Rheumatol 2006;35(3):169–74.

42. Dixon B. Bacteria and arthritis. BMJ 1990;301(6759):1043.

43. Ebringer A. Rheumatoid arthritis and proteus. Clin Med 2005;5(4):420–1.

44. Silman AJ, Hochberg MC. Rheumatoid arthritis. In: Silman AJ, Hochberg MC, editors. Epidemiology of the rheumatic diseases. New York: Oxford University Press; 1993. p. 7–68.

45. Spector TD, Silman AJ. Is poor pregnancy outcome a risk factor in rheumatoid arthritis? Ann Rheum Dis 1990;49(1):12–4.

46. Pladevall-Vila M, Delclos GL, Varas C, et al. Controversy of oral contraceptives and risk of rheumatoid arthritis: meta-analysis of conflicting studies and review

of conflicting meta-analyses with special emphasis on analysis of heterogeneity. Am J Epidemiol 1996;144(1):1–14.

47. Spector TD, Hochberg MC. The protective effect of the oral contraceptive pill on rheumatoid arthritis: an overview of the analytic epidemiological studies using meta-analysis. J Clin Epidemiol 1990;43(11):1221–30.

48. Doran MF, Crowson CS, O'Fallon WM, et al. The effect of oral contraceptives and estrogen replacement therapy on the risk of rheumatoid arthritis: a population based study. J Rheumatol 2004;31(2):207–13.

49. Merlino LA, Curtis J, Mikuls TR, et al. Vitamin D intake is inversely associated with rheumatoid arthritis: results from the Iowa Women's Health Study. Arthritis Rheum 2004;50(1):72–7.

50. Bhatia SS, Majka DS, Kittelson JM, et al. Rheumatoid factor seropositivity is inversely associated with oral contraceptive use in women without rheumatoid arthritis. Ann Rheum Dis 2007;66(2):267–9.

51. Korpilahde T, Heliovaara M, Knekt P, et al. Smoking history and serum cotinine and thiocyanate concentrations as determinants of rheumatoid factor in non-rheumatoid subjects. Rheumatology (Oxford) 2004;43(11):1424–8.

52. Tuomi T, Heliovaara M, Palosuo T, et al. Smoking, lung function, and rheumatoid factors. Ann Rheum Dis 1990;49(10):753–6.

53. Feser M, Derber LA, Deane KD, et al. Plasma 25, OH vitamin D concentrations are not associated with rheumatoid arthritis (RA)-related autoantibodies in individuals at elevated risk for RA. J Rheumatol 2009;36(5):943–6.

54. Elkayam O, Caspi D, Lidgi M, et al. Auto-antibody profiles in patients with active pulmonary tuberculosis. Int J Tuberc Lung Dis 2007;11(3):306–10.

55. Elkayam O, Segal R, Lidgi M, et al. Positive anti-cyclic citrullinated proteins and rheumatoid factor during active lung tuberculosis. Ann Rheum Dis 2006;65(8): 1110–2.

56. Criswell LA, Saag KG, Mikuls TR, et al. Smoking interacts with genetic risk factors in the development of rheumatoid arthritis among older Caucasian women. Ann Rheum Dis 2006;65(9):1163–7.

57. Kallberg H, Padyukov L, Plenge RM, et al. Gene-gene and gene-environment interactions involving HLA-DRB1, PTPN22, and smoking in two subsets of rheumatoid arthritis. Am J Hum Genet 2007;80(5):867–75.

58. Klareskog L, Stolt P, Lundberg K, et al. A new model for an etiology of rheumatoid arthritis: smoking may trigger HLA-DR (shared epitope)-restricted immune reactions to autoantigens modified by citrullination. Arthritis Rheum 2006;54(1):38–46.

59. Mahdi H, Fisher BA, Kallberg H, et al. Specific interaction between genotype, smoking and autoimmunity to citrullinated alpha-enolase in the etiology of rheumatoid arthritis. Nat Genet 2009;41(12):1319–24.

60. Steck AK, Zhang W, Bugawan TL, et al. Do non-HLA genes influence development of persistent islet autoimmunity and type 1 diabetes in children with high-risk HLA-DR, DQ genotypes? Diabetes 2009;58(4):1028–33.

61. Sheehy MJ. HLA and insulin-dependent diabetes. A protective perspective. Diabetes 1992;41(2):123–9.

62. Taplin CE, Barker JM. Autoantibodies in type 1 diabetes. Autoimmunity 2008; 41(1):11–8.

63. Achenbach P, Bonifacio E, Koczwara K, et al. Natural history of type 1 diabetes. Diabetes 2005;54(Suppl 2):S25–31.

64. Norris JM, Beaty B, Klingensmith G, et al. Lack of association between early exposure to cow's milk protein and beta-cell autoimmunity. Diabetes Autoimmunity Study in the Young (DAISY). JAMA 1996;276(8):609–14.

65. Ziegler AG, Schmid S, Huber D, et al. Early infant feeding and risk of developing type 1 diabetes-associated autoantibodies. JAMA 2003;290(13):1721–8.
66. Norris JM, Barriga K, Klingensmith G, et al. Timing of initial cereal exposure in infancy and risk of islet autoimmunity. JAMA 2003;290(13):1713–20.
67. Graves PM, Rotbart HA, Nix WA, et al. Prospective study of enteroviral infections and development of beta-cell autoimmunity. Diabetes autoimmunity study in the young (DAISY). Diabetes Res Clin Pract 2003;59(1):51–61.
68. Graves PM, Barriga KJ, Norris JM, et al. Lack of association between early childhood immunizations and beta-cell autoimmunity. Diabetes Care 1999;22(10):1694–7.
69. Norris JM, Yin X, Lamb MM, et al. Omega-3 polyunsaturated fatty acid intake and islet autoimmunity in children at increased risk for type 1 diabetes. JAMA 2007;298(12):1420–8.
70. Lamb MM, Yin X, Barriga K, et al. Dietary glycemic index, development of islet autoimmunity, and subsequent progression to type 1 diabetes in young children. J Clin Endocrinol Metab 2008;93(10):3936–42.
71. Verge CF, Gianani R, Kawasaki E, et al. Number of autoantibodies (against insulin, GAD or ICA512/IA2) rather than particular autoantibody specificities determines risk of type I diabetes. J Autoimmun 1996;9(3):379–83.
72. Taplin CE, Barker JM. Natural evolution, prediction, and prevention of type 1 diabetes in youth. Endocr Res 2008;33(1–2):17–33.
73. Kishiyama CM, Chase HP, Barker JM. Prevention strategies for type 1 diabetes. Rev Endocr Metab Disord 2006;7(3):215–24.
74. Maddison PJ, Reichlin M. Quantitation of precipitating antibodies to certain soluble nuclear antigens in SLE. Arthritis Rheum 1977;20(3):819–24.
75. Lee LA, Gaither KK, Coulter SN, et al. Pattern of cutaneous immunoglobulin G deposition in subacute cutaneous lupus erythematosus is reproduced by infusing purified anti-Ro (SSA) autoantibodies into human skin-grafted mice. J Clin Invest 1989;83(5):1556–62.
76. Miranda-Carus ME, Askanase AD, Clancy RM, et al. Anti-SSA/Ro and anti-SSB/La autoantibodies bind the surface of apoptotic fetal cardiocytes and promote secretion of TNF-alpha by macrophages. J Immunol 2000;165(9):5345–51.
77. Kurien BT, Newland J, Paczkowski C, et al. Association of neutropenia in systemic lupus erythematosus (SLE) with anti-Ro and binding of an immunologically cross-reactive neutrophil membrane antigen. Clin Exp Immunol 2000;120(1):209–17.
78. Hahn BH. Antibodies to DNA. N Engl J Med 1998;338(19):1359–68.
79. Davis P, Percy JS, Russell AS. Correlation between levels of DNA antibodies and clinical disease activity in SLE. Ann Rheum Dis 1977;36(2):157–9.
80. Arbuckle MR, McClain MT, Rubertone MV, et al. Development of autoantibodies before the clinical onset of systemic lupus erythematosus. N Engl J Med 2003;349(16):1526–33.
81. McClain MT, Arbuckle MR, Heinlen LD, et al. The prevalence, onset, and clinical significance of antiphospholipid antibodies prior to diagnosis of systemic lupus erythematosus. Arthritis Rheum 2004;50(4):1226–32.
82. Arbuckle MR, James JA, Dennis GJ, et al. Rapid clinical progression to diagnosis among African-American men with systemic lupus erythematosus. Lupus 2003;12(2):99–106.
83. Gross AJ, Hochberg D, Rand WM, et al. EBV and systemic lupus erythematosus: a new perspective. J Immunol 2005;174(11):6599–607.
84. Vossenaar ER, Nijenhuis S, Helsen MM, et al. Citrullination of synovial proteins in murine models of rheumatoid arthritis. Arthritis Rheum 2003;48(9):2489–500.

85. Kuhn KA, Kulik L, Tomooka B, et al. Antibodies against citrullinated proteins enhance tissue injury in experimental autoimmune arthritis. J Clin Invest 2006;116(4):961–73.
86. Uysal H, Bockermann R, Nandakumar KS, et al. Structure and pathogenicity of antibodies specific for citrullinated collagen type II in experimental arthritis. J Exp Med 2009;206(2):449–62.
87. Lundberg K, Nijenhuis S, Vossenaar ER, et al. Citrullinated proteins have increased immunogenicity and arthritogenicity and their presence in arthritic joints correlates with disease severity. Arthritis Res Ther 2005;7(3):R458–67.
88. Hill JA, Southwood S, Sette A, et al. Cutting edge: the conversion of arginine to citrulline allows for a high-affinity peptide interaction with the rheumatoid arthritis-associated HLA-DRB1*0401 MHC class II molecule. J Immunol 2003;171(2):538–41.
89. Hill JA, Bell DA, Brintnell W, et al. Arthritis induced by posttranslationally modified (citrullinated) fibrinogen in DR4-IE transgenic mice. J Exp Med 2008;205(4):967–79.
90. Kanazawa S, Ota S, Sekine C, et al. Aberrant MHC class II expression in mouse joints leads to arthritis with extraarticular manifestations similar to rheumatoid arthritis. Proc Natl Acad Sci U S A 2006;103(39):14465–70.
91. Ho PP, Lee LY, Zhao X, et al. Autoimmunity against fibrinogen mediates inflammatory arthritis in mice. J Immunol 2010;184(1):379–90.
92. Kraan MC, Versendaal H, Jonker M, et al. Asymptomatic synovitis precedes clinically manifest arthritis. Arthritis Rheum 1998;41(8):1481–8.
93. Arnett FC, Edworthy SM, Bloch DA, et al. The American Rheumatism Association 1987 revised criteria for the classification of rheumatoid arthritis. Arthritis Rheum 1988;31(3):315–24.
94. Aletaha D, Breedveld FC, Smolen JS. The need for new classification criteria for rheumatoid arthritis. Arthritis Rheum 2005;52(11):3333–6.
95. Silman AJ, Symmons DP. Selection of study population in the development of rheumatic disease criteria: comment on the article by the American College of Rheumatology Diagnostic and Therapeutic Criteria Committee. Arthritis Rheum 1995;38(5):722–3.
96. van Baarsen LG, Bos WH, Rustenburg F, et al. Gene expression profiling in auto-antibody-positive patients with arthralgia predicts development of arthritis. Arthritis Rheum 2010;62(3):694–704.
97. Symmons DP, Silman AJ. The Norfolk Arthritis Register (NOAR). Clin Exp Rheumatol 2003;21(5 Suppl 31):S94–9.
98. van der Helm-van Mil AH, le Cessie S, van Dongen H, et al. A prediction rule for disease outcome in patients with recent-onset undifferentiated arthritis: how to guide individual treatment decisions. Arthritis Rheum 2007;56(2):433–40.
99. van Dongen H, van Aken J, Lard LR, et al. Efficacy of methotrexate treatment in patients with probable rheumatoid arthritis: a double-blind, randomized, placebo-controlled trial. Arthritis Rheum 2007;56(5):1424–32.
100. Verpoort KN, van Dongen H, Allaart CF, et al. Undifferentiated arthritis–disease course assessed in several inception cohorts. Clin Exp Rheumatol 2004;22(5 Suppl 35):S12–7.
101. van Aken J, van Bilsen JH, Allaart CF, et al. The Leiden early arthritis clinic. Clin Exp Rheumatol 2003;21(5 Suppl 31):S100–5.
102. Panel ACoRAaELARE, editor. New rheumatoid arthritis criteria. American College of Rheumatology Annual Meeting. Philadelphia, PA, 2009.

103. Pedersen M, Jacobsen S, Garred P, et al. Strong combined gene-environment effects in anti-cyclic citrullinated peptide-positive rheumatoid arthritis: a nationwide case-control study in Denmark. Arthritis Rheum 2007;56(5):1446–53.
104. Verpoort KN, Papendrecht-van der Voort EA, van der Helm-van Mil AH, et al. Association of smoking with the constitution of the anti-cyclic citrullinated peptide response in the absence of HLA-DRB1 shared epitope alleles. Arthritis Rheum 2007;56(9):2913–8.
105. Smolik I, Robinson D, El-Gabalawy HS, et al. Periodontitis and rheumatoid arthritis: epidemiologic, clinical, and immunologic associations. Compend Contin Educ Dent 2009;30(4):188–90 [92, 94 passim; quiz: 98, 210].
106. Deane KD, Simonian PL, Lynch DA, et al. Rheumatoid arthritis (RA)-related autoantibodies are associated with pulmonary airway abnormalities in individuals without RA [abstract 340]. Arthritis Rheum 2008;58(9):S292.
107. Aho K, Tuomi T, Heliovaara M, et al. Rheumatoid factors and rheumatoid arthritis. Scand J Rheumatol Suppl 1988;74:41–4.
108. Dorner T, Egerer K, Feist E, et al. Rheumatoid factor revisited. Curr Opin Rheumatol 2004;16(3):246–53.
109. van der Helm-van Mil AH, Verpoort KN, Breedveld FC, et al. Antibodies to citrullinated proteins and differences in clinical progression of rheumatoid arthritis. Arthritis Res Ther 2005;7(5):R949–58.
110. Verpoort KN, Cheung K, Ioan-Facsinay A, et al. Fine specificity of the anti-citrullinated protein antibody response is influenced by the shared epitope alleles. Arthritis Rheum 2007;56(12):3949–52.
111. Verpoort KN, Jol-van der Zijde CM, Papendrecht-van der Voort EA, et al. Isotype distribution of anti-cyclic citrullinated peptide antibodies in undifferentiated arthritis and rheumatoid arthritis reflects an ongoing immune response. Arthritis Rheum 2006;54(12):3799–808.
112. Malhotra R, Wormald MR, Rudd PM, et al. Glycosylation changes of IgG associated with rheumatoid arthritis can activate complement via the mannose-binding protein. Nat Med 1995;1(3):237–43.
113. Ioan-Facsinay A, Willemze A, Robinson DB, et al. Marked differences in fine specificity and isotype usage of the anti-citrullinated protein antibody in health and disease. Arthritis Rheum 2008;58(10):3000–8.
114. Gregersen PK, Silver J, Winchester RJ. The shared epitope hypothesis. An approach to understanding the molecular genetics of susceptibility to rheumatoid arthritis. Arthritis Rheum 1987;30(11):1205–13.
115. Berglin E, Padyukov L, Sundin U, et al. A combination of autoantibodies to cyclic citrullinated peptide (CCP) and HLA-DRB1 locus antigens is strongly associated with future onset of rheumatoid arthritis. Arthritis Res Ther 2004;6(4):R303–8.
116. Johansson M, Arlestig L, Hallmans G, et al. PTPN22 polymorphism and anti-cyclic citrullinated peptide antibodies in combination strongly predicts future onset of rheumatoid arthritis and has a specificity of 100% for the disease. Arthritis Res Ther 2006;8(1):R19.
117. van der Helm-van Mil AH, Detert J, le Cessie S, et al. Validation of a prediction rule for disease outcome in patients with recent-onset undifferentiated arthritis: moving toward individualized treatment decision-making. Arthritis Rheum 2008; 58(8):2241–7.
118. Feitsma AL, Toes RE, Begovich AB, et al. Risk of progression from undifferentiated arthritis to rheumatoid arthritis: the effect of the PTPN22 1858T-allele in anti-citrullinated peptide antibody positive patients. Rheumatology (Oxford) 2007;46(7):1092–5.

119. van der Helm-van Mil AH, Verpoort KN, Breedveld FC, et al. The HLA-DRB1 shared epitope alleles are primarily a risk factor for anti-cyclic citrullinated peptide antibodies and are not an independent risk factor for development of rheumatoid arthritis. Arthritis Rheum 2006;54(4):1117–21.
120. Allaart CF, Breedveld FC, Dijkmans BA. Treatment of recent-onset rheumatoid arthritis: lessons from the BeSt study. J Rheumatol Suppl 2007;80: 25–33.
121. Goekoop-Ruiterman YP, de Vries-Bouwstra JK, Allaart CF, et al. Clinical and radiographic outcomes of four different treatment strategies in patients with early rheumatoid arthritis (the BeSt study): a randomized, controlled trial. Arthritis Rheum 2008;58(Suppl 2):S126–35.
122. Cush JJ. Early rheumatoid arthritis—is there a window of opportunity? J Rheumatol Suppl 2007;80:1–7.
123. Emery P, Durez P, Dougados M, et al. Impact of T-cell costimulation modulation in patients with undifferentiated inflammatory arthritis or very early rheumatoid arthritis: a clinical and imaging study of abatacept (the ADJUST trial). Ann Rheum Dis 2010;69(3):510–6.
124. Rewers M, Gottlieb P. Immunotherapy for the prevention and treatment of type 1 diabetes: human trials and a look into the future. Diabetes Care 2009;32(10): 1769–82.
125. James JA, Kim-Howard XR, Bruner BF, et al. Hydroxychloroquine sulfate treatment is associated with later onset of systemic lupus erythematosus. Lupus 2007;16(6):401–9.
126. Endres M. Statins: potential new indications in inflammatory conditions. Atheroscler Suppl 2006;7(1):31–5.
127. McInnes IB, McCarey DW, Sattar N. Do statins offer therapeutic potential in inflammatory arthritis? Ann Rheum Dis 2004;63(12):1535–7.
128. Klareskog L, Hamsten A. Statins in rheumatoid arthritis—two birds with one stone? Lancet 2004;363(9426):2011–2.
129. Jick SS, Choi H, Li L, et al. Hyperlipidaemia, statin use and the risk of developing rheumatoid arthritis. Ann Rheum Dis 2009;68(4):546–51.
130. Dawber TR, Meadors GF, Moore FE Jr. Epidemiological approaches to heart disease: the Framingham Study. Am J Public Health Nations Health 1951; 41(3):279–81.
131. Kolfenbach JR, Deane KD, Derber LA, et al. A prospective approach to investigating the natural history of preclinical rheumatoid arthritis (RA) using first-degree relatives of probands with RA. Arthritis Rheum 2009;61(12):1735–42.
132. Oen K, Robinson DB, Nickerson P, et al. Familial seropositive rheumatoid arthritis in North American Native families: effects of shared epitope and cytokine genotypes. J Rheumatol 2005;32(6):983–91.
133. El-Gabalawy HS, Robinson DB, Hart D, et al. Immunogenetic risks of anticyclical citrullinated peptide antibodies in a North American Native population with rheumatoid arthritis and their first-degree relatives. J Rheumatol 2009; 36(6):1130–5.
134. Deane KD, Striebich CC, Goldstein BL, et al. Identification of undiagnosed inflammatory arthritis in a community health fair screen. Arthritis Rheum 2009; 61(12):1642–9.
135. Bizzaro N. The predictive significance of autoantibodies in organ-specific autoimmune diseases. Clin Rev Allergy Immunol 2008;34(3):326–31.
136. Rose NR. Predictors of autoimmune disease: autoantibodies and beyond. Autoimmunity 2008;41(6):419–28.

137. Maradit-Kremers H, Crowson CS, Nicola PJ, et al. Increased unrecognized coronary heart disease and sudden deaths in rheumatoid arthritis: a population-based cohort study. Arthritis Rheum 2005;52(2):402–11.
138. Alarcon GS, Koopman WJ, Acton RT, et al. Seronegative rheumatoid arthritis. A distinct immunogenetic disease? Arthritis Rheum 1982;25(5):502–7.

How Should Rheumatoid Arthritis Disease Activity Be Measured Today and in the Future in Clinical Care?

Tuulikki Sokka, MD, PhD

KEYWORDS

• Rheumatoid arthritis • Disease activity
• Clinical evaluation • Outcomes

Quantitative clinical monitoring of musculoskeletal conditions and inflammatory joint diseases is challenging compared with quantitative monitoring of conditions such as hypertension or hyperlipidemia, for which single measures can be used as an indicator of disease status and change. Traditional measures to assess rheumatoid arthritis (RA), such as joint assessment, laboratory, imaging, and patient self-report measures, have limitations and provide only a reflection of the underlying inflammatory process. A gold standard to define disease activity in RA does not exist and various indices of disease activity must be used.

Quantitative monitoring of RA as part of daily clinical practice has certainly improved since Dr Wright's observation in 1983 that "clinicians may all too easily spend years writing 'doing well' in the notes of a patient who has become progressively crippled before their eyes...."[1] Standard quantitative monitoring with a treatment goal has been shown to be beneficial to patient outcomes in randomized clinical trials. Quantitative monitoring has also contributed to improved long-term outcomes for RA in clinical care.

One of the earliest proposals for an active monitoring and treatment strategy for RA was expressed by Luukkainen and colleagues[2] in 1978 "... In our opinion gold treatment ought to be started in the early stages of RA, before the development of erosions. We are treating not only the actual inflammation of the joints but also the quality of the patient's life for many decades in the future." Although benefits of quantitative monitoring of RA are obvious, challenges of the measures need to be recognized

Jyväskylä Central Hospital, 40620 Jyväskylä, Finland
E-mail address: tuulikki.sokka@ksshp.fi

Rheum Dis Clin N Am 36 (2010) 243–257
doi:10.1016/j.rdc.2010.02.007
0889-857X/10/$ – see front matter © 2010 Elsevier Inc. All rights reserved.

rheumatic.theclinics.com

and hurdles identified that prevent quantitative monitoring in every-day clinical care concerning disease activity and beyond. These aspects are discussed in this article.

MEASURING OF DISEASE ACTIVITY LEADS TO LESS DISEASE ACTIVITY

Most clinical trials are designed to analyze differences between active and control treatments rather than to attain a certain clinical status. A traditional clinical trial involves an extensive battery of measures of disease activity and other measures at study visits, which are simply used to document patient status but not to guide therapies. However, a few trials can be called strategy trials because they involve a treatment goal, and response/disease activity level at each study visit influences treatment doses.

The Finnish Combination Treatment Trial (FIN-RACo) was the first clinical trial with remission as the primary outcome measure.[3] During the 2-year study, treatments had to be adjusted if remission was not met. At the end of the study, disease activity score (DAS28) remission rates were 68% in the combination arm and 41% in the monotherapy arm, and American College of Rheumatology (ACR) remission rates were 42% versus 20% in the 2 groups, among the highest ever seen in clinical trials or clinical care.[4]

The TICORA (Tight Control of RA) study aimed at low disease activity of DAS <2.4 in the strategy arm, with frequent clinical visits and escalation of treatments.[5] At the end of the trial, 65% of patients were in DAS remission of DAS <1.6 in the strategy arm versus 16% in the routine care arm. The Behandelstrategieën voor Reumatoide Artritis (BeSt [Treatment Strategies for RA]) study had a treatment goal of DAS ≤2.4; 38% to 46% of patients in the 4 arms were in DAS remission at the end of the intervention.[6] In the 2-year CAMERA (an open-label strategy trial), 50% of patients were in DAS28 remission in an intensively computer-assisted monitoring group versus 37% in the conventional group.[7] Similarly, in the CIMESTRA (Cyclosporine, Methotrexate, Steroid in RA) trial, 2-year radiographic and clinical results were better in the strategy group versus the control group.[8] Fransen and colleagues[9] compared a strategy group designed with routine disease activity measurements and the aim of DAS28 ≤3.2 with a usual care group with no routine measuring. For 24 weeks, patients in the strategy group received more antirheumatic drugs and had better outcomes than patients in the usual care group.

These clinical trials indicate that the practice of quantitative monitoring of RA leads to better outcomes than routine care without quantitative monitoring. Furthermore, a treatment target and quantitative monitoring have obviously played a role in clinics that have reported favorable long-term outcomes of RA.[10–12] However, quantitative monitoring of RA involves challenges that may prevent implementation of these measures in routine clinical care (**Table 1**).

CHALLENGES OF CLINICAL MEASURES OF RA DISEASE ACTIVITY
No Single Gold Standard

A single gold standard for patient assessment, such as blood pressure or serum cholesterol level, which can be used to assess all individual patients in clinical trials, clinical research, and clinical care, is not available for any rheumatic disease. Therefore, different types of measures are used in assessment of patients with rheumatic diseases. Measures used in assessment of RA disease activity include formal joint counts by the physician, laboratory tests, and patient self-report questionnaire measures of physical function, pain, global status, fatigue, and others. Each of these measures seems effective to document changes of status with treatment in groups of patients, but no single measure can serve as a gold standard to document changes in each individual patient.

Table 1
Challenges of disease activity measures of rheumatoid arthritis

Method	Challenges
Physician measures: joint counts	Poorly reproducible
	More likely to improve with placebo treatment than the other disease activity measures
	Not as sensitive to detect inflammatory activity as ultrasound or magnetic resonance imaging
	Time-consuming and tedious
Laboratory measures: ESR and CRP	Normal in a considerable proportion of patients with clinical RA
	Not specific for RA
	Different methods to measure ESR and CRP challenge comparison of patient status across clinics
Patient self-report measures	Patient questionnaires are not specific to the degree of inflammatory activity
	Gender differences are obvious in patient-report measures
	Normative values of patient-reported measures are rarely reported
	Cultural differences in interpretation of questions and data
	Motivation of patients and health professionals
Indices of disease activity	Challenges of the components

Abbreviations: CRP, C-reactive protein; ESR, erythrocyte sedimentation rate; RA, rheumatoid arthritis.

CHALLENGES IN PHYSICIAN MEASURES: JOINT ASSESSMENT

A careful joint examination is required to establish a diagnosis of RA[13]; quantitative counts of swollen and tender joints are the most specific measures for patient assessment.[14–17] The number of swollen and tender joints is regarded as the most important measure for RA clinical trials to distinguish active and control treatments,[18] and the best measure of status in usual clinical care.[19] The joint count is included in a core data set[20–22] and in disease activity indices (discussed later). Nonetheless, several limitations of the joint count have been described, as summarized here and described in greater detail elsewhere.[23,24]

Joint Counts are Poorly Reproducible

Joint counts are poorly reproducible in formal studies.[25–37] Variation in joint count results can be reduced by training rheumatologists or other assessors to standardize scores.[31,35,36] Nonetheless, all protocols for clinical trials and other clinical research studies in RA require that a joint count must be performed by the same observer at each assessment. Most measures such as temperature, pulse, or even blood pressure are regarded as ascertainable by any trained health professional at any time.

The need for the same person to perform each joint count in a given patient presents a considerable limitation to the use of joint counts as rigorous indicators of the need for changes in therapy, responses to therapy, or to document quality of care. Possible collaborative care between rheumatologists and family practitioners or other health professionals to manage patients is limited by a requirement for the same observer, as joint counts by different observers cannot be compared reliably.

Joint count measures are at least as likely or more likely to improve with placebo treatment compared with other disease activity measures. In clinical trials, patients who receive placebo or control treatments almost always show improvement in swollen and tender joint counts as great as or greater than in other core data set measures.[38] For example, in a clinical trial of leflunomide or methotrexate versus placebo,[39] placebo treatment resulted in improvement in patient status of 21% for swollen joint count, 20% for tender joint count, 12% for physician global estimate of status, and 12% for patient global estimate of status; worsening of status of 20% was seen for pain, 9% for physical function, and 22% for erythrocyte sedimentation rate (ESR). These data are typical of analyses of other clinical trials that indicate that swollen and tender joint counts improve with placebo or control treatments as much as or more than other core data set measures.

Joint Counts are Not as Sensitive for Detecting Inflammatory Activity as Ultrasound or Magnetic Resonance Imaging

Several studies indicate that formal swollen and tender joint counts are not as sensitive as ultrasonography or magnetic resonance imaging for detecting synovitis. In a study of 80 patients with early untreated oligoarthritis,[40] 1470 joints were clinically examined. Of these joints, 185 had clinical synovitis. Ultrasound detected synovitis in 150 (33%) of 459 joints that were painful but not swollen, as well as 107 (13%) of 826 joints that were clinically normal. The findings indicate that patients have synovitis that is not detectable by clinical examination in a substantial number of affected joints. These studies indicate that tender and swollen joint count may be limited for optimal detection of synovitis or response to therapy, explained in part by poor reliability, as discussed earlier.

CHALLENGES IN THE USE OF LABORATORY TESTS

The discovery in the 1940s of rheumatoid factor[41,42] led to hopes that laboratory tests could serve as gold standard measures in rheumatic diseases. In many diseases, laboratory tests provide the most definitive information in diagnosis, management, prognosis, and documentation of course of the disease. According to a biomedical model, laboratory tests are often seen as the most important information from a rheumatology visit.

Most patients with RA have an increased ESR and C-reactive protein (CRP) level.[43] An abnormal ESR or CRP are often used as inclusion criteria for clinical trials.[44] An ESR less than 30 mm/h in a woman and less than 20 mm/h in a man is required to meet ACR remission criteria.[45] Reductions in ESR and CRP are seen in groups of patients in all successful clinical trials of RA therapies that indicate efficacy of an active treatment compared with a control treatment.

ESR and CRP are Normal in a Considerable Proportion of Patients with Clinical RA

ESR and CRP are normal in about 40% of patients with RA, reported initially in 1994 by Wolfe and Michaud[46] from Wichita, Kansas, USA, and confirmed recently at 2 sites, 1 in Nashville, TN, USA and the other in Jyväskylä, Finland.[47] Mean ESR levels have declined from 50 mm/h in RA cohorts at baseline in 1954–1980, to 41 mm/h in 1981–1984, to 35 mm/h after 1985.[48] Furthermore, although a decline in ESR or CRP is seen concomitantly with clinical improvement in many patients and in most groups of patients in clinical trials, ESR and CRP tend to remain at similar levels in many other patients, even with clinical improvement.[49]

ESR and CRP are Not Specific for RA

Comorbidities are common in patients with RA, including comorbidities with increased laboratory markers for inflammation.[50] Furthermore, higher ESR levels are considered normal in women than men, especially in older age groups.[51]

Different Methods to Measure ESR and CRP Challenge Comparison of Patient Status Across Clinics

ESR is traditionally measured according to the Westergren method, which has now been replaced in some laboratories with more modern methods. In some clinics, CRP has replaced ESR in the assessment of RA. Different methods to assess CRP involve different normal values and different presentation of results. This introduces challenges in the calculation of disease activity indices; for example, a normal CRP may be reported as <10; CRP values of 0 to 9.9 provide different values in disease activity scores from CRP = 10, especially on low disease activity levels approaching criteria for remission.[52]

Laboratory research is essential to provide new insights into pathogenesis and new treatments for rheumatic diseases. However, in usual clinical care, laboratory tests often have limited sensitivity and sensitivity, with high levels of false-positive and false-negative results. Physicians and patients may attribute disproportionate importance to laboratory tests in rheumatic diseases.

CHALLENGES OF PATIENT SELF-REPORTED MEASURES

Patient self-reporting has become prominent in rheumatology assessment, as the patient is the only source for information concerning functional capacity, pain, global health, fatigue, psychological distress, and so forth. The Health Assessment Questionnaire (HAQ)[53] is the most commonly used tool for physical function and includes 20 activities of daily living (ADL) in 8 categories to assess functional disability. Several modifications have been developed to provide simplified scoring in routine clinical care and allow the clinician to visualize an ADL score. The most widely used modifications are the modified HAQ (MHAQ) which includes only 1 question in each of 8 categories,[54] and the multidimensional HAQ (MDHAQ), which also includes 3 psychological items.[55–57] Pain, global health, and fatigue are generally assessed on a 10-cm visual analog scale.

Patient questionnaires concerning functional status provide the most significant prognostic clinical measure for all important long-term outcomes of RA, including functional status,[58,59] work disability[60–62] costs,[63] joint replacement surgery,[64] and premature death.[58,65–71] Questionnaire data concerning physical function predict RA mortality at levels comparable with blood pressure, cholesterol, and smoking, as risk factors for premature cardiovascular death.[67] Physical fitness and performance are universal predictors for survival in diseased and nondiseased populations[72] and can be measured using approaches ranging from simple patient self-report questionnaires to full scale performance tests, among which patient self-report is the most convenient in various settings.

In RA, inflammation of joints and other systems affects patient functional status, and causes pain, fatigue, and other symptoms, which resolve as inflammation responds to treatments. Therefore, patient-reported outcomes (PROs) perform well as measures of disease activity. However, several aspects need to be taken into account in the interpretation of PROs as RA disease activity measures.

Patient Questionnaires are Not Specific to the Degree of Inflammatory Activity

A patient's pain score might improve or decline considerably because of developments other than direct changes in inflammatory status; for example, a score might improve as a result of good news, but could be higher (more pain) as a result of severe back pain, an injury, and so forth. This phenomenon emphasizes that any measure, whether a questionnaire score, laboratory test, or radiographic score, must be interpreted by a clinician when formulating clinical decisions.

Gender Differences in Patient-report Measures

In general, women are known to report more symptoms and poor scores on most questionnaires,[73] including scores for pain,[74] depression, and other health-related items.[75,76] Furthermore, throughout the history of the HAQ, women have been found to report poorer scores than men.[77–82] This is understandable as women have lesser strength than men,[83,84] which has a major effect on functional status of patients with RA and in a healthy population.[85]

Normative Values of PROs?

Interpretation of the relative level of PROs might need normative age- and gender-adjusted values. For example, if a 35-year-old man or an 85-year-old woman with RA had a HAQ score of 1, would that mean that the level of the disability was the same for both? Both experience at least some difficulties in most ADL, but without reference values from the background population, it is not possible to determine whether the level of the disability in these example cases was different from that of people of the same age and sex in general.[81,85] In the Central Finland population the authors found that the HAQ scores of older patients with RA were similar to the HAQ scores of the age- and sex-adjusted population, while the effect of disability caused by RA appeared greater in younger and middle-aged people.[81]

Cultural Differences and PROs

Patient questionnaires can be subject to cultural and linguistic differences; for example, in one study, Hispanic patients had higher pain scores than Whites, whereas Asian patients had lower pain scores than Caucasians.[86] Furthermore, some patients may have difficulty completing questionnaires because of issues of literacy.

Motivation

Motivation of a patient and especially of health professionals is the greatest hurdle of PROs as RA disease activity measures. PROs are considered as subjective measures versus objective laboratory- or physician-assessed measures. Administration of a patient questionnaire at each visit as an infrastructure of daily clinical work seems routine in a minority of rheumatology clinics.

INDICES TO MEASURE RA DISEASE ACTIVITY

Indices of 3 to 7 measures are used in clinical assessment of RA disease activity, based on a core data set of 7 measures including 3 from a health professional (swollen joint count, tender joint count, global estimate of status), 1 from a laboratory (ESR or CRP), and 3 from the patient (physical function, pain, patient global estimate of status). The earliest use of an index was defined by the ACR as a 20%, 50%, or 70% improvement in swollen and tender joint count plus 3 of the other 5 measures, known as ACR20, ACR50, and ACR70 responses.[21,87] The ACR criteria measure change compared with baseline, rather than absolute status. Therefore, a 50% improvement can be achieved when tender and swollen joint counts decrease from 20 to 10, or when a joint counts decrease from 4 to 2 (provided that 3 of 5 other ACR core data set measures also improve 50%).

Inflammatory activity can be assessed according to absolute indices of efficacy or disease state, which may be defined as a measurable, cross-sectional level of disease activity. The most widely used index, the disease activity score (DAS/DAS28)[88–90] includes swollen joint count, tender joint count, ESR or CRP, and patient global estimate, calculated using a computer Web site or a DAS calculator. A simplified disease activity index (SDAI)[91] includes 5 measures: the 4 DAS28 measures plus a physician assessment of global status. The clinical disease activity index (CDAI)[92] deletes the CRP from the SDAI. Other RA indices have been developed: the mean overall index for rheumatoid arthritis (MOI-RA)[93] which includes all 7 core data set measures; and the LUNDEX,[94] an index designed to incorporate patients' adherence to therapy.

Indices have also been designed based entirely on PRO measures such as a routine assessment of patient index data 3 (RAPID3).[95,96] An index of physical function, pain, and patient global status distinguishes active and control treatment in clinical trials involving traditional[97,98] and biologic therapies.[99]

Challenges of indices reflect those of the components. An issue of the effect of gender on disease activity at levels close to remission has emerged recently, at a time when patient clinical status is improved compared with earlier decades, because of better treatment strategies and biologic agents.[100] Remissions are seen more frequently than in earlier decades, although this is influenced by the definition of remission that is used.[52,101] Some studies suggest that male gender is a major predictor of remission in early RA[102,103] and some others that men have better responses to treatments with biologic agents than women.[104–106]

All biologic clinical trials use DAS28 for the definition of remission.[101] The influence of gender on DAS28 remission was studied in the multinational Quantitative Standard Monitoring of Patients with Rheumatoid Arthritis (QUEST-RA) database in more than 6000 patients. Overall, 30% of men and 17% of women were in DAS28 remission.[52,82] Gender differences were most pronounced in patients who had no swollen joints: fewer women than men (42% vs 58%) met DAS28 remission. These observations indicate that lower remission rates in women are accounted for by components of the indices other than the number of swollen joints, such as number of tender joints, patient self-report scores, and higher normal ESR in women.[51] Higher DAS28 remission rates in men might reflect, at least in part, gender differences in indices rather than true gender differences in RA disease activity.

DISCONNECT OF INFLAMMATORY ACTIVITY, DAMAGE, AND OUTCOMES

Disease activity measures are sensitive to change in a period of weeks to months and are regarded as short-term surrogate markers for long-term joint damage (such as joint deformity and radiographic progression) and clinical outcomes (such as work disability, joint replacement surgery, and premature mortality[67]), which develop over years to decades.

However, it was recognized in the mid-1980s that short-term drug efficacy was not necessarily translated into long-term effectiveness.[58] Several studies have indicated progression of radiographic damage and decline of physical function over 5 to 10 years although measures of inflammatory activity were stable or improved (reviewed in Ref.[107]). One of the recent examples is the FIN-RACo trial, which documented suppression of inflammation at a level of 20% or 50% (ie, ACR20 or ACR50) does not provide optimal improvement in outcomes. Among patients whose inflammation was controlled to a status of remission at 6 months, no patient was receiving work disability payments 4.5 years later. By contrast, 22% of patients who had ACR20 or ACR50 responses, and 54% of patients who did not have ACR20 responses, were receiving work disability payments at 5 years after baseline.[108] Therefore, improvements greater than 50% in RA disease activity measures are needed to prevent adverse long-term outcomes.

QUANTITATIVE MEASURING BEYOND DISEASE ACTIVITY

As suggested earlier, disease activity is only one dimension of manifestations of RA and may not be sufficient to provide an overall picture of patient status over time. A standard format for efficient collection of data in patients with RA has been developed, called a standard protocol to evaluate rheumatoid arthritis (SPERA).[109,110] This format has proved useful to collect data in several studies on prognosis and monitoring of patients, including development of a 28-joint count[33]; observation of radiographic damage in most patients within the first 2 years of disease[111]; recognition that patient question-naires are correlated significantly with joint counts, radiographic scores, and laboratory tests[112] and provide more significant predictors of work disability[60] and mortality[67,69] than traditional measures; and observations that a relatively small proportion of patients was eligible for clinical trials in contemporary care of RA.[44,113] The SPERA format was used to establish that patients with RA in 2000 had considerably better status than all patients seen in 1985 in the same clinical setting.[56] SPERA has been used to collect comprehensive baseline clinical data in more than 8000 patients in 32 countries for the QUEST-RA program.[82,114–117]

SPERA includes data from the patient and clinician. The patient completes a standard self-report questionnaire: a HAQ,[53] MDHAQ,[95,96] or a variant for physical function and questions about pain, global status, fatigue, self-report joint count, duration of morning stiffness, years of education, height and weight for body mass index, lifestyle choices such as smoking and physical exercise, and work status.

The clinician completes a SPERA, which addresses

1. Review of clinical features, including classification criteria, extraarticular features, comorbidities, and relevant surgeries
2. All previous and present disease-modifying antirheumatic drugs, their adverse events, and reasons for discontinuation
3. A 42-joint count[118] that includes swollen and tender joints, as well as joints with limited motion or deformity.

The first 2 SPERA documents are designated as permanent documents that can be updated if needed. The SPERA protocol captures most of the important baseline infor-mation a clinician needs to know about a patient who might have RA, as well as baseline information for a clinical trial or observational research study. It incorporates the 5 core domains listed in a consensus for long-term observational studies from an Outcome Measures in Rheumatoid Arthritis Clinical Trials (OMERACT) conference in 1998: health status, disease process, damage, mortality, and toxicity/adverse reactions.[119]

SUMMARY

A database such as the SPERA could be used at baseline for all clinical trials and in standard care to facilitate analyses of long-term outcomes of rheumatic diseases beyond disease activity measures.

REFERENCES

1. Smith T. Questions on clinical trials [editorial]. Br Med J 1983;287:569.
2. Luukkainen R, Kajander A, Isomäki H. Treatment of rheumatoid arthritis [letter]. Br Med J 1978;2:1501.
3. Möttönen T, Hannonen P, Leirisalo-Repo M, et al. Comparison of combination therapy with single-drug therapy in early rheumatoid arthritis: a randomised trial. FIN-RACo trial group. Lancet 1999;353:1568–73.
4. Makinen H, Kautiainen H, Hannonen P, et al. Sustained remission and reduced radiographic progression with combination disease modifying antirheumatic drugs in early rheumatoid arthritis. J Rheumatol 2007;34(2):316–21.

5. Grigor C, Capell H, Stirling A, et al. Effect of a treatment strategy of tight control for rheumatoid arthritis (the TICORA study): a single-blind randomised controlled trial. Lancet 2004;364:263–9.
6. Goekoop-Ruiterman YP, de Vries-Bouwstra JK, Allaart CF, et al. Clinical and radiographic outcomes of four different treatment strategies in patients with early rheumatoid arthritis (the BeSt study): a randomized, controlled trial. Arthritis Rheum 2005;52:3381–90.
7. Verstappen SM, Jacobs JW, van der Veen MJ, et al. Intensive treatment with methotrexate in early rheumatoid arthritis: aiming for remission. Computer Assisted Management in Early Rheumatoid Arthritis (CAMERA, an open-label strategy trial). Ann Rheum Dis 2007;66(11):1443–9.
8. Hetland ML, Stengaard-Pedersen K, Junker P, et al. Aggressive combination therapy with intra-articular glucocorticoid injections and conventional disease-modifying anti-rheumatic drugs in early rheumatoid arthritis: second-year clinical and radiographic results from the CIMESTRA study. Ann Rheum Dis 2008;67:815–22.
9. Fransen J, Moens HB, Speyer I, et al. Effectiveness of systematic monitoring of rheumatoid arthritis disease activity in daily practice: a multicentre, cluster randomised contolled trial. Ann Rheum Dis 2005;64:1294–8.
10. Sokka T, Kautiainen H, Häkkinen K, et al. Radiographic progression is getting milder in patients with early rheumatoid arthritis. Results of 3 cohorts over 5 years. J Rheumatol 2004;31:1073–82.
11. Pincus T, Sokka T, Kautiainen H. Patients seen for standard rheumatoid arthritis care have significantly better articular, radiographic, laboratory, and functional status in 2000 than in 1985. Arthritis Rheum 2005;52:1009–19.
12. Uhlig T, Heiberg T, Mowinckel P, et al. Rheumatoid arthritis is milder in the new millennium: health status in patients with rheumatoid arthritis 1994–2004. Ann Rheum Dis 2008;67(12):1710–5.
13. Pincus T. The DAS is the most specific measure, but a patient questionnaire is the most informative measure to assess rheumatoid arthritis. J Rheumatol 2006; 33:834–7.
14. Cooperating Clinics Committee of the American Rheumatism Association. A seven-day variability study of 499 patients with peripheral rheumatoid arthritis. Arthritis Rheum 1965;8:302–35.
15. Ritchie DM, Boyle JA, McInnes JM, et al. Clinical studies with an articular index for the assessment of joint tenderness in patients with rheumatoid arthritis. New Series. Q J Med 1968;37:393–406.
16. American Rheumatism Association. Dictionary of the rheumatic diseases, vol. I: signs and symptoms. New York: Contact Associates International; 1982.
17. Decker JL. American Rheumatism Association nomenclature and classification of arthritis and rheumatism. Arthritis Rheum 1983;26:1029–32.
18. Bombardier C, Tugwell P, Sinclair A, et al. Preference for endpoint measures in clinical trials: results of structured workshops. J Rheumatol 1982;9: 798–801.
19. Wolfe F, Pincus T, Thompson AK, et al. The assessment of rheumatoid arthritis and the acceptability of self-report questionnaires in clinical practice. Arthritis Care Res 2003;49(1):59–63.
20. Boers M, Tugwell P, Felson DT, et al. World Health Organization and International League of Associations for Rheumatology core endpoints for symptom modifying antirheumatic drugs in rheumatoid arthritis clinical trials. J Rheumatol 1994;21(Suppl 41):86–9.

21. Felson DT, Anderson JJ, Boers M, et al. The American College of Rheumatology preliminary core set of disease activity measures for rheumatoid arthritis clinical trials. Arthritis Rheum 1993;36:729–40.

22. American College of Rheumatology Committee to Reevaluate Improvement Criteria. A proposed revision to the ACR20: the hybrid measure of American College of Rheumatology response. Arthritis Rheum 2007;57(2):193–202.

23. Pincus T. Limitations of a quantitative swollen and tender joint count to assess and monitor patients with rheumatoid arthritis. Bull NYU Hosp Jt Dis 2008; 66(3):216–23.

24. Sokka T, Pincus T. Joint counts to assess rheumatoid arthritis for clinical research and usual clinical care: advantages and limitations. Rheum Dis Clin North Am 2009;35(4):713, vi.

25. Lansbury J, Baier HN, McCracken S. Statistical study of variation in systemic and articular indexes. Arthritis Rheum 1962;5:445–56.

26. Eberl DR, Fasching V, Rahlfs V, et al. Repeatability and objectivity of various measurements in rheumatoid arthritis: a comparative study. Arthritis Rheum 1976;19:1278–86.

27. Hanson MT, Keiding S, Lauritzen SL, et al. Clinical assessment of disease activity in rheumatoid arthritis. Scand J Rheumatol 1979;8:101–5.

28. Hart LE, Tugwell P, Buchanan WW, et al. Grading of tenderness as a source of interrater error in the Ritchie articular index. J Rheumatol 1985;12:716–7.

29. Thompson PW, Kirwan JR. Observer variation and the Ritchie articular index. J Rheumatol 1986;13:836–7.

30. Lewis PA, O'Sullivan MM, Rumfeld WR, et al. Significant changes in Ritchie scores. Br J Rheumatol 1988;27:32–6.

31. Klinkhoff AV, Bellamy N, Bombardier C, et al. An experiment in reducing interobserver variability of the examination for joint tenderness. J Rheumatol 1988;15: 492–4.

32. Thompson PW, Kirwan JR, Currey HLF. A comparison of the ability of 28 articular indices to detect an induced flare of joint inflammation in rheumatoid arthritis. Br J Rheumatol 1988;27:375–80.

33. Fuchs HA, Brooks RH, Callahan LF, et al. A simplified twenty-eight joint quantitative articular index in rheumatoid arthritis. Arthritis Rheum 1989;32:531–7.

34. Thompson PW, Hart LE, Goldsmith CH, et al. Comparison of four articular indices for use in clinical trials in rheumatoid arthritis: patient, order and observer variation. J Rheumatol 1991;18:661–5.

35. Bellamy N, Anastassiades TP, Buchanan WW, et al. Rheumatoid arthritis antirheumatic drug trials. 1. Effects of standardization procedures on observer dependent outcome measures. J Rheumatol 1991;18:1893–900.

36. Scott DL, Choy EH, Greeves A, et al. Standardising joint assessment in rheumatoid arthritis. Clin Rheumatol 1996;15:579–82.

37. Lassere MN, van der Heijde D, Johnson KR, et al. Reliability of measures of disease activity and disease damage in rheumatoid arthritis: implications for smallest detectable difference, minimal clinically important difference, and analysis of treatment effects in randomized controlled trials. J Rheumatol 2001;28(4): 892–903.

38. Tugwell P, Wells G, Strand V, et al. Clinical improvement as reflected in measures of function and health-related quality of life following treatment with leflunomide compared with methotrexate in patients with rheumatoid arthritis: sensitivity and relative efficiency to detect a treatment effect in a twelve-month, placebo-controlled trial. Arthritis Rheum 2000;43(3):506–14.

39. Strand V, Cohen S, Crawford B, et al. Patient-reported outcomes better discriminate active treatment from placebo in randomized controlled trials in rheumatoid arthritis. Rheumatology 2004;43:640–7.

40. Wakefield RJ, Green MJ, Marzo-Ortega H, et al. Should oligoarthritis be reclassified? Ultrasound reveals a high prevalence of subclinical disease. Ann Rheum Dis 2004;63:382–5.

41. Waaler E. On the occurrence of a factor in human serum activating the specific agglutination of sheep blood corpuscles. Acta Pathol Microbiol Scand 1940;17:172–8.

42. Rose HM, Ragan C, Pearce E, et al. Differential agglutination of normal and sensitized sheep erythrocytes by sera of patients with rheumatoid arthritis. Proc Soc Exp Biol Med 1948;68:1–6.

43. Abelson B, Rupel A, Pincus T. Limitations of a biomedical model to explain socioeconomic disparities in mortality of rheumatic and cardiovascular diseases. Clin Exp Rheumatol 2008;26(5 Suppl 51):S25–34.

44. Sokka T, Pincus T. Most patients receiving routine care for rheumatoid arthritis in 2001 did not meet inclusion criteria for most recent clinical trials or American College of Rheumatology criteria for remission. J Rheumatol 2003;30(6):1138–46.

45. Pinals RS, Masi AT, Larsen RA, et al. Preliminary criteria for clinical remission in rheumatoid arthritis. Arthritis Rheum 1981;24:1308–15.

46. Wolfe F, Michaud K. The clinical and research significance of the erythrocyte sedimentation rate. J Rheumatol 1994;21:1227–37.

47. Sokka T, Pincus T. Erythrocyte sedimentation rate, C-reactive protein, or rheumatoid factor are normal at presentation in 35%–45% of patients with rheumatoid arthritis seen between 1980 and 2004: analyses from Finland and the United States. J Rheumatol 2009;36(7):1387–90.

48. Abelson B, Sokka T, Pincus T. Declines in erythrocyte sedimentation rates in patients with rheumatoid arthritis over the second half of the 20th century. J Rheumatol 2009;36(8):1596–9.

49. Wolfe F, Pincus T. The level of inflammation in rheumatoid arthritis is determined early and remains stable over the longterm course of the illness. J Rheumatol 2001;28(8):1817–24.

50. Isomäki HA, Hakulinen T, Joutsenlahti U. Excess risk of lymphomas, leukemia and myeloma in patients with rheumatoid arthritis. J Chronic Dis 1978;31:691–6.

51. Miller A, Green M, Robinson D. Short rule for calculating normal erythrocyte sedimentation rate. Br Med J 1983;286:266.

52. Sokka T, Hetland ML, Makinen H, et al. Remission and rheumatoid arthritis: data on patients receiving usual care in twenty-four countries. Arthritis Rheum 2008;58(9):2642–51.

53. Fries JF, Spitz P, Kraines RG, et al. Measurement of patient outcome in arthritis. Arthritis Rheum 1980;23:137–45.

54. Pincus T, Summey JA, Soraci SA Jr, et al. Assessment of patient satisfaction in activities of daily living using a modified Stanford health assessment questionnaire. Arthritis Rheum 1983;26:1346–53.

55. Pincus T, Swearingen C, Wolfe F. Toward a multidimensional health assessment questionnaire (MDHAQ): assessment of advanced activities of daily living and psychological status in the patient friendly health assessment questionnaire format. Arthritis Rheum 1999;42:2220–30.

56. Pincus T, Sokka T, Kautiainen H. Further development of a physical function scale on a multidimensional health assessment questionnaire for standard care of patients with rheumatic diseases. J Rheumatol 2005;32:1432–9.

57. Pincus T, Yazici Y, Bergman M. Development of a multi-dimensional health assessment questionnaire (MDHAQ) for the infrastructure of standard clinical care. Clin Exp Rheumatol 2005;23:S19–28.
58. Pincus T, Callahan LF, Sale WG, et al. Severe functional declines, work disability, and increased mortality in seventy-five rheumatoid arthritis patients studied over nine years. Arthritis Rheum 1984;27:864–72.
59. Wolfe F, Cathey MA. The assessment and prediction of functional disability in rheumatoid arthritis. J Rheumatol 1991;18:1298–306.
60. Callahan LF, Bloch DA, Pincus T. Identification of work disability in rheumatoid arthritis: physical, radiographic and laboratory variables do not add explanatory power to demographic and functional variables. J Clin Epidemiol 1992;45:127–38.
61. Wolfe F, Hawley DJ. The longterm outcomes of rheumatoid arthritis: work disability: a prospective 18 year study of 823 patients. J Rheumatol 1998;25:2108–17.
62. Sokka T, Kautiainen H, Möttönen T, et al. Work disability in rheumatoid arthritis 10 years after the diagnosis. J Rheumatol 1999;26:1681–5.
63. Lubeck DP, Spitz PW, Fries JF, et al. A multicenter study of annual health service utilization and costs in rheumatoid arthritis. Arthritis Rheum 1986;29:488–93.
64. Wolfe F, Zwillich SH. The long-term outcomes of rheumatoid arthritis: a 23-year prospective, longitudinal study of total joint replacement and its predictors in 1,600 patients with rheumatoid arthritis. Arthritis Rheum 1998;41:1072–82.
65. Wolfe F, Kleinheksel SM, Cathey MA, et al. The clinical value of the Stanford Health Assessment Questionnaire Functional Disability Index in patients with rheumatoid arthritis. J Rheumatol 1988;15:1480–8.
66. Leigh JP, Fries JF. Mortality predictors among 263 patients with rheumatoid arthritis. J Rheumatol 1991;18:1307–12.
67. Pincus T, Brooks RH, Callahan LF. Prediction of long-term mortality in patients with rheumatoid arthritis according to simple questionnaire and joint count measures. Ann Intern Med 1994;120:26–34.
68. Callahan LF, Cordray DS, Wells G, et al. Formal education and five-year mortality in rheumatoid arthritis: mediation by helplessness scale scores. Arthritis Care Res 1996;9:463–72.
69. Callahan LF, Pincus T, Huston JW III, et al. Measures of activity and damage in rheumatoid arthritis: depiction of changes and prediction of mortality over five years. Arthritis Care Res 1997;10:381–94.
70. Söderlin MK, Nieminen P, Hakala M. Functional status predicts mortality in a community based rheumatoid arthritis population. J Rheumatol 1998;25:1895–9.
71. Sokka T, Hakkinen A, Krishnan E, et al. Similar prediction of mortality by the health assessment questionnaire in patients with rheumatoid arthritis and the general population. Ann Rheum Dis 2004;63:494–7.
72. Sokka T, Hakkinen A. Poor physical fitness and performance as predictors of mortality in normal populations and patients with rheumatic and other diseases. Clin Exp Rheumatol 2008;26(5 Suppl 5):14–20.
73. Barsky AJ, Peekna HM, Borus JF. Somatic symptom reporting in women and men. J Gen Intern Med 2001;16(4):266–75.
74. Keogh E, Herdenfeldt M. Gender, coping and the perception of pain. Pain 2002;97(3):195–201.
75. Loge JH, Kaasa S. Short form 36 (SF-36) health survey: normative data from the general Norwegian population. Scand J Soc Med 1998;26(4):250–8.

76. Bowling A, Bond M, Jenkinson C, et al. Short Form 36 (SF-36) Health Survey questionnaire: which normative data should be used? Comparisons between the norms provided by the Omnibus Survey in Britain, the Health Survey for England and the Oxford Healthy Life Survey. J Public Health Med 1999;21(3):255–70.
77. Katz PP, Criswell LA. Differences in symptom reports between men and women with rheumatoid arthritis. Arthritis Care Res 1996;9(6):441–8.
78. Sherrer YS, Bloch DA, Mitchell DM, et al. Disability in rheumatoid arthritis: comparison of prognostic factors across three populations. J Rheumatol 1987;14:705–9.
79. Thompson PW, Pegley FS. A comparison of disability measured by the Stanford Health Assessment Questionnaire disability scales (HAQ) in male and female rheumatoid outpatients. Br J Rheumatol 1991;30(4):298–300.
80. McKenna F, Tracey A, Hayes J. Assessment of disability in male and female rheumatoid patients. Br J Rheumatol 1991;30(6):477.
81. Sokka T, Krishnan E, Häkkinen A, et al. Functional disability in rheumatoid arthritis patients compared with a community population in Finland. Arthritis Rheum 2003;48(1):59–63.
82. Sokka T, Toloza S, Cutolo M, et al. Women, men, and rheumatoid arthritis: analyses of disease activity, disease characteristics, and treatments in the QUEST-RA Study. Arthritis Res Ther 2009;11(1):R7.
83. Hakkinen A, Kautiainen H, Hannonen P, et al. Muscle strength, pain, and disease activity explain individual subdimensions of the health assessment questionnaire disability index, especially in women with rheumatoid arthritis. Ann Rheum Dis 2006;65(1):30–4.
84. Hallert E, Thyberg I, Hass U, et al. Comparison between women and men with recent onset rheumatoid arthritis of disease activity and functional disability over two years (the TIRA project). Ann Rheum Dis 2003;62:667–70.
85. Krishnan E, Sokka T, Hakkinen A, et al. Normative values for the Health Assessment Questionnaire disability index: benchmarking disability in the general population. Arthritis Rheum 2004;50:953–60.
86. Yazici Y, Kautiainen H, Sokka T. Differences in clinical status measures in different ethnic/racial groups with early rheumatoid arthritis: implications for interpretation of clinical trial data. J Rheumatol 2007;34(2):311–5.
87. Felson DT, Anderson JJ, Boers M, et al. American College of Rheumatology preliminary definition of improvement in rheumatoid arthritis. Arthritis Rheum 1995;38:727–35.
88. van der Heijde DM, van't Hof MA, van Riel PL, et al. Judging disease activity in clinical practice in rheumatoid arthritis: first step in the development of a disease activity score. Ann Rheum Dis 1990;49:916–20.
89. van der Heijde DM, van't Hof M, van Riel PL, et al. Development of a disease activity score based on judgment in clinical practice by rheumatologists. J Rheumatol 1993;20:579–81.
90. Prevoo ML, van't Hof MA, Kuper HH, et al. Modified disease activity scores that include twenty-eight-joint counts: development and validation in a prospective longitudinal study of patients with rheumatoid arthritis. Arthritis Rheum 1995; 38:44–8.
91. Smolen JS, Breedveld FC, Schiff MH, et al. A simplified disease activity index for rheumatoid arthritis for use in clinical practice. Rheumatology (Oxford) 2003;42: 244–57.
92. Aletaha D, Nell VP, Stamm T, et al. Acute phase reactants add little to composite disease activity indices for rheumatoid arthritis: validation of a clinical activity score. Arthritis Res Ther 2005;7:R796–806.

93. Makinen H, Kautiainen H, Hannonen P, et al. A new disease activity index for rheumatoid arthritis: Mean Overall Index for Rheumatoid Arthritis (MOI-RA). J Rheumatol 2008;35(8):1522–7.

94. Kristensen LE, Saxne T, Geborek P, et al. A new index of drug efficacy in clinical practice: results of a five-year observational study of treatment with infliximab and etanercept among rheumatoid arthritis patients in southern Sweden. Arthritis Rheum 2006;54(2):600–6.

95. Pincus T, Bergman MJ, Yazici Y, et al. An index of only patient-reported outcome measures, routine assessment of patient index data 3 (RAPID3), in two abatacept clinical trials: similar results to disease activity score (DAS28) and other RAPID indices that include physician-reported measures. Rheumatology (Oxford) 2008;47(3):345–9.

96. Pincus T, Swearingen CJ, Bergman M, et al. RAPID3 (routine assessment of patient index data 3), a rheumatoid arthritis index without formal joint counts for routine care: proposed severity categories compared to DAS and CDAI categories. J Rheumatol 2008;35:2136–47.

97. Pincus T, Strand V, Koch G, et al. An index of the three core data set patient questionnaire measures distinguishes efficacy of active treatment from placebo as effectively as the American College of Rheumatology 20% response criteria (ACR20) or the disease activity score (DAS) in a rheumatoid arthritis clinical trial. Arthritis Rheum 2003;48(3):625–30.

98. Pincus T, Amara I, Koch GG. Continuous indices of Core Data Set measures in rheumatoid arthritis clinical trials: lower responses to placebo than seen with categorical responses with the American College of Rheumatology 20% criteria. Arthritis Rheum 2005;52:1031–6.

99. Pincus T, Chung C, Segurado OG, et al. An index of patient self-reported outcomes (PRO Index) discriminates effectively between active and control treatment in 4 clinical trials of adalimumab in rheumatoid arthritis. J Rheumatol 2006;33:2146–52.

100. Sokka T. Long-term outcomes of rheumatoid arthritis. Curr Opin Rheumatol 2009;21(3):284–90.

101. Makinen H, Hannonen P, Sokka T. Definitions of remission for rheumatoid arthritis and review of selected clinical cohorts and randomized clinical trials for the rate of remission. Clin Exp Rheumatol 2006;24(S43):S22–8.

102. Forslind K, Hafstrom I, Ahlmen M, et al. Sex: a major predictor of remission in early rheumatoid arthritis? Ann Rheum Dis 2007;66(1):46–52.

103. Mancarella L, Bobbio-Pallavicini F, Ceccarelli F, et al. Good clinical response, remission, and predictors of remission in rheumatoid arthritis patients treated with tumor necrosis factor-alpha blockers: the GISEA study. J Rheumatol 2007;34(8):1670–3.

104. Hyrich KL, Watson KD, Silman AJ, et al. British Society for Rheumatology Biologics Register. Predictors of response to anti-TNF-{alpha} therapy among patients with rheumatoid arthritis: results from the British Society for Rheumatology Biologics Register. Rheumatology (Oxford) 2006;45(12):1558–65.

105. Yamanaka H, Tanaka Y, Sekiguchi N, et al. Retrospective clinical study on the notable efficacy and related factors of infliximab therapy in a rheumatoid arthritis management group in Japan (RECONFIRM). Mod Rheumatol 2007;17(1):28–32.

106. Kvien TK, Uhlig T, Odegard S, et al. Epidemiological aspects of rheumatoid arthritis: the sex ratio. Ann N Y Acad Sci 2006;1069:212–22.

107. Pincus T, Sokka T, Kavanaugh A. Relative versus absolute goals of therapies for RA: ACR 20 or ACR 50 responses versus target values for "near remission" of DAS or single measures. Clin Exp Rheumatol 2004;22(Suppl 35):S50–6.
108. Puolakka K, Kautiainen H, Möttönen T, et al. Early suppression of disease activity is essential for maintenance of work capacity in patients with recent-onset rheumatoid arthritis: five-year experience from the FIN-RACo trial. Arthritis Rheum 2005;52(1):36–41.
109. Pincus T, Brooks RH, Callahan LF. A proposed standard protocol to evaluate rheumatoid arthritis (SPERA) that includes measures of inflammatory activity, joint damage, and longterm outcomes. J Rheumatol 1999;26:473–80.
110. Pincus T, Sokka T. A three-page Standard Protocol to Evaluate Rheumatoid Arthritis (SPERA) for efficient capture of essential data from patients and health professionals in standard clinical care and clinical research. Best Pract Res Clin Rheumatol 2007;21(4):677–85.
111. Fuchs HA, Kaye JJ, Callahan LF, et al. Evidence of significant radiographic damage in rheumatoid arthritis within the first 2 years of disease. J Rheumatol 1989;16:585–91.
112. Pincus T, Callahan LF, Brooks RH, et al. Self-report questionnaire scores in rheumatoid arthritis compared with traditional physical, radiographic, and laboratory measures. Ann Intern Med 1989;110:259–66.
113. Sokka T, Pincus T. Eligibility of patients in routine care for major clinical trials of anti-tumor necrosis factor alpha agents in rheumatoid arthritis. Arthritis Rheum 2003;48(2):313–8.
114. Sokka T, Kautiainen H, Toloza S, et al. QUEST-RA: quantitative clinical assessment of patients with rheumatoid arthritis seen in standard rheumatology care in 15 countries. Ann Rheum Dis 2007;66:1491–6.
115. Sokka T, Kautiainen H, Pincus T, et al. Disparities in rheumatoid arthritis disease activity according to gross domestic product in 25 countries in the QUEST-RA database. Ann Rheum Dis 2009;68:1666–72.
116. Khan NA, Yazici Y, Calvo-Alen J, et al. Reevaluation of the role of duration of morning stiffness in the assessment of rheumatoid arthritis activity. J Rheumatol 2009;36:2435–42.
117. Naranjo A, Sokka T, Descalzo M, et al. Cardiovascular disease in patients with rheumatoid arthritis: results from the QUEST-RA study. Arthritis Res Ther 2008; 10:R30.
118. Sokka T, Pincus T. Quantitative joint assessment in rheumatoid arthritis. Clin Exp Rheumatol 2005;23:S58–62.
119. Wolfe F, Lassere M, van der Heijde D, et al. Preliminary core set of domains and reporting requirements for longitudinal observational studies in rheumatology. Omeract IV: outcome measures in rheumatology. Cancun, Mexico, April 16–20, 1998. J Rheumatol 1999;26:484–9.

Leveraging Human Genetics to Develop Future Therapeutic Strategies in Rheumatoid Arthritis

Robert M. Plenge, MD, PhD*, Soumya Raychaudhuri, MD, PhD

KEYWORDS

• Locus • Allele • Mutation • Human genetics

Despite decades of research, the biologic pathways that initiate rheumatoid arthritis (RA) are unknown.[1,2] Without knowing the specific pathways that lead to RA, it is very difficult to develop novel therapies. Because genetic mutations are inherited before disease onset, human genetics provides prima facie evidence that a pathway is important in pathogenesis. Moreover, because human genetic strategies can be applied genome wide, they offer an unbiased search of the human genome for an insight into RA pathogenesis.

Since the 1970s, more than 20 RA risk loci have been identified (**Table 1**). The first locus associated with RA risk was the major histocompatibility (MHC) locus, identified by mixed lymphocyte cultures between patients and controls with RA.[3,4] Subsequently, Gregersen and colleagues[5] advanced the hypothesis that the multiple RA risk alleles within the *HLA-DRB1* gene share a conserved amino acid sequence. This is now widely known as the "shared epitope" hypothesis, and the risk alleles are known as shared epitope alleles.[6] With the sequence of the human genome[7] and improved understanding of human genetic diversity[8] came many additional genetic discoveries.[9] Between 2003 and 2005, common alleles within the *PADI4*, *PTPN22*, and *CTLA4* genes were found to be reproducibly associated with risk of RA.[10–12] Genome-wide association studies (GWASs), which in the contemporary form test hundreds of thousands of single nucleotide polymorphisms (SNPs) across the genome, have been systematically performed in large case-control collections. These GWASs have identified more than 20 common alleles (where an allele is 1 of the 2 base pairs of an SNP) that confer a 10% to 20% increase in disease risk per

Division of Rheumatology, Immunology and Allergy, Brigham and Women's Hospital, Harvard Medical School, 77 Avenue Louis Pasteur, Suite 168, Boston, MA 02115, USA
* Corresponding author.
E-mail address: rplenge@partners.org

Rheum Dis Clin N Am 36 (2010) 259–270
doi:10.1016/j.rdc.2010.03.002
0889-857X/10/$ – see front matter © 2010 Elsevier Inc. All rights reserved.

rheumatic.theclinics.com

Table 1
Known RA SNP associations

SNP	Locus	Candidate Gene	OR	Allele Frequency	References
rs3890745	1p36.2	TNFSF14	0.920	0.320	Raychaudhuri et al,[15] 2008
rs2240340	1p36.13	PADI4	1.40	0.373	Suzuki et al,[10] 2003
rs2476601	1p13.2	PTPN22	1.750	0.100	Begovich et al,[11] 2004
rs11586238	1p13.1	CD2, IGSF2, CD58	1.120	0.227	Raychaudhuri et al,[16] 2009
rs7528684	1q23.1	FCLR3	1.2	0.35	Kochi et al,[69] 2005
rs12746613	1q23.2	FCGR2A	1.100	0.124	Raychaudhuri et al,[16] 2009
rs3766379	1q23.3	CD244	1.31	0.53	Suzuki et al,[73] 2008
rs10919563	1q31.3	PTPRC	0.900	0.132	Raychaudhuri et al,[16] 2009
rs13031237	2p16.1	REL	1.207	0.340	Gregersen et al,[23] 2009
rs934734	2p14	SPRED2	1.13	0.51	Stahl et al,[74] 2010
rs10865035	2q11.2	AFF3	1.140	0.460	Barton et al,[19] 2009
rs7574865	2q32.3	STAT4	1.320	0.180	Remmers et al,[17] 2007
rs1980422	2q33.2	CD28	1.100	0.238	Raychaudhuri et al,[16] 2009
rs3087243	2q33.2	CTLA4	1.136	0.560	Plenge et al,[12] 2005
rs13315591	3p14	PXK	1.13	0.08	Stahl et al,[74] 2010
rs874040	4p15	RBPJ	1.18	0.30	Stahl et al,[74] 2010
rs6822844	4q27	IL2/IL21	1.389	0.710	Zhernakova et al,[18] 2007
rs6859219	5q11	ANKRD55	0.85	0.22	Stahl et al,[74] 2010
rs26232	5q21	C5orf13	0.93	0.32	Stahl et al,[74] 2010
rs2395175 (and others)	6p21.32	MHC	1.000	0.021	Gregersen et al,[6] 1987
rs548234	6q21	PRDM1	1.100	0.322	Raychaudhuri et al,[16] 2009
rs10499194	6q23.3	TNFAIP3	1.220	0.220	Plenge et al,[13] 2007
rs6920220	6q23.3	TNFAIP3	1.333	0.610	Thomson et al,[22] 2007
rs5029937	6q23.3	TNFAIP3	1.34	0.04	Orozco et al,[70] 2009
rs394581	6q25.3	TAGAP	0.930	0.286	Raychaudhuri et al,[16] 2009
rs3093023	6q27	CCR6	1.11	0.43	Stahl et al,[74] 2010
rs10488631	7q32	IRF5	1.25	0.10	Stahl et al,[74] 2010
rs2736340	8p23.1	BLK	1.122	0.243	Gregersen et al,[23] 2009
rs2812378	9p13.3	CCL21	1.100	0.355	Raychaudhuri et al,[15] 2008
rs951005	9p13.3	CCL21	0.87	0.15	Stahl et al,[74] 2010
rs3761847	9q33.1	TRAF1	1.100	0.440	Plenge et al,[14] 2007; Kurreeman et al,[71] 2007
rs2104286	10p15.1	IL2RA	0.92	0.28	Thomson et al,[22] 2007; Kurreeman et al,[72] 2009
rs706778	10p15.1	IL2RA	1.11	0.40	Stahl et al,[74] 2010
rs4750316	10p15.1	PRKCQ	0.910	0.183	Raychaudhuri et al,[15] 2008; Barton et al,[21] 2008
rs540386	11p12	RAG1, TRAF6	0.920	0.144	Raychaudhuri et al,[16] 2009
rs1678542	12q13.3	KIF5A	0.890	0.351	Barton et al,[21] 2008; Raychaudhuri et al,[15] 2008
rs4810485	20q13.12	CD40	0.910	0.231	Raychaudhuri et al,[15] 2008
rs3218253	22q12.3	IL2RB	1.110	0.730	Barton et al,[21] 2008

copy of the risk allele.[13–23] Collectively, these risk alleles explain approximately 15% to 20% of the overall disease burden.[15,16]

The purpose of this article is to place these genetic discoveries in the context of current and future therapeutic strategies for patients with RA. More specifically, this article focuses on (1) a brief overview of genetic studies, (2) human genetics as an approach to identify the Achilles heel of disease pathways, (3) humans as the model organism for functional studies of human mutations, (4) pharmacogenetic studies to gain insight into the mechanism of action of drugs, and (5) next-generation patient registries to enable large-scale genotype-phenotype studies.

BRIEF OVERVIEW OF HUMAN GENETICS: FROM SNP TO CAUSAL ALLELE

There are approximately 10 million common SNPs in the human genome.[8] A fundamental challenge in human genetics is to systematically test each of these 10 million common SNPs for its role in disease. Advances in genomic technology have made this feasible.[24] Contemporary GWASs test several hundred thousand SNPs across the entire human genome, most of which are common (minor allele frequency >5%) in the general, healthy population. To test the remaining more than 9 million common SNPs, the GWAS approach relies on the correlation structure of nearby SNPs.[24] That is, 9 of 10 SNPs are highly correlated, and testing 1 SNP serves to tag the remaining 9 nearby SNPs. This concept is known as linkage disequilibrium (LD).

But the properties of LD that make it powerful for gene mapping also underscore the challenges that remain once an SNP is associated with disease risk; it is unknown if the SNP genotyped (and associated with risk in the genetic study) is the actual causal allele or whether the genotyped/associated SNP is simply in LD with the causal allele. Here causal allele is the single genetic mutation that is responsible for disrupting gene function and giving rise to the phenotype of interest. Given the sheer number of common alleles, the genotyped/associated SNP is most likely just a proxy for the actual causal allele. An example of the correlation structure of an RA risk locus is shown in **Fig. 1**.[14]

There is often more than 1 gene in the region of LD that harbors the genotyped/associated SNP, which makes it difficult to pinpoint definitively which gene is the causal gene. On the other hand, there may be no nearby gene in the region of LD. Here causal gene is the single gene that is altered by a mutation to give rise to the phenotype of interest (eg, risk of RA). For convenience, the best biologic gene, based on its known function, is often nominated as the "causal gene." **Fig. 1** illustrates that there are 3 genes in a region of LD at the locus on chromosome 9, 2 of which are very strong biologic candidate genes: *TRAF1* (encoding tumor necrosis factor (TNF) α receptor–associated factor 1) and *C5* (encoding complement component 5). Thus, this locus is referred to as the *TRAF1-C5* RA risk locus.

For most of the 20 RA risk alleles shown in **Table 1**, the causal mutation and the causal gene are yet to be identified. Outside of the MHC, the 1 exception is *PTPN22* in which the associated mutation alters protein structure and function.[25,26] Although it may be reasonable to nominate the most likely biologic candidate gene to be the causal gene, direct evidence is not yet available.

There are at least 2 reasons why it is important to identify (or "fine map") the causal mutation. First, knowing the causal mutation helps guide functional studies. For drug discovery, it is crucial to understand if the risk allele is a gain-of-function or loss-of-function allele. Second, knowing the causal allele provides more accurate estimates of risk that could facilitate disease prediction. If the associated SNP is highly but not perfectly correlated with the causal allele, then risk estimates will be deflated.

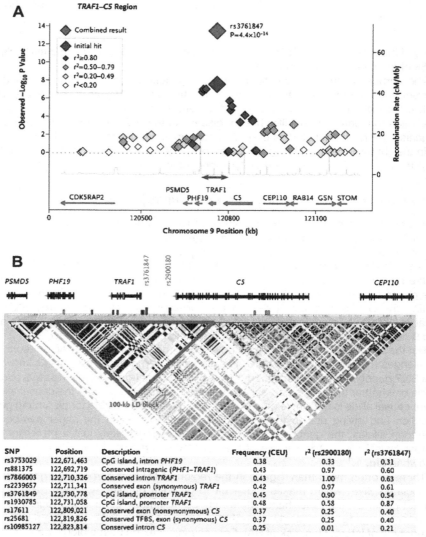

A

TRAF1–C5 Region

rs3761847
P=4.4×10⁻¹⁴

- Combined result
- Initial hit
- $r^2 \geq 0.80$
- $r^2 = 0.50-0.79$
- $r^2 = 0.20-0.49$
- $r^2 < 0.20$

SNP	Position	Description	Frequency (CEU)	r² (rs2900180)	r² (rs3761847)
rs3753029	122,671,463	CpG island, intron *PHF19*	0.38	0.33	0.31
rs881375	122,692,719	Conserved intragenic (*PHF1–TRAF1*)	0.43	0.97	0.60
rs7866003	122,710,326	Conserved intron *TRAF1*	0.43	1.00	0.63
rs2239657	122,711,341	Conserved exon (synonymous) *TRAF1*	0.42	0.97	0.61
rs3761849	122,730,778	CpG island, promoter *TRAF1*	0.45	0.90	0.54
rs1930785	122,731,058	CpG island, promoter *TRAF1*	0.48	0.58	0.87
rs17611	122,809,021	Conserved exon (nonsynonymous) *C5*	0.37	0.25	0.40
rs25681	122,819,826	Conserved TFBS, exon (synonymous) *C5*	0.37	0.25	0.40
rs10985127	122,823,814	Conserved intron *C5*	0.25	0.01	0.21

Fig. 1. Case-control association results and LD structure in the TRAF1-C5 locus. Panel A shows results for SNPs genotyped across 1 Mb as part of the original genome-wide association scan in samples from 1522 case subjects with anti–CCP-positive RA and 1850 control subjects. Each diamond indicates a genotyped SNP; the color of each diamond is based on the correlation coefficient (r²), with the CEPH (Centre d'Etude du Polymorphisme Humain) from Utah (CEU) HapMap with the most significant SNP in the study (rs3761847). The blue diamond indicates the *P* value for all samples in the study (the original scan plus replication samples) as determined by the Cochran-Mantel-Haenszel method in the samples of both the North American Rheumatoid Arthritis Consortium (NARAC) and the Epidemiological Investigation of Rheumatoid Arthritis (EIRA). The recombination rate (in cM/Mb) with the CEU HapMap is shown in light blue along the x axis; the red arrow indicates the block of LD shown in panel B. The blue arrows indicate gene location. Panel B shows the LD structure across 200 kb of the TRAF1-C5 locus, based on pairwise r² with the CEU HapMap. The intron-exon structure of each gene is at the top of the figure. Putative functional SNPs in LD with either rs3761847 or rs2900180 are indicated by hatched bars in which red indicates r²>0.80 and pink indicates r² = 0.20 to 0.80; the specific SNPs, frequency, pairwise r² with the CEU HapMap, and the putative annotated function are listed at the bottom of the figure. CpG denotes cytidine and guanosine joined by a phosphodiester bond. (*Modified from* Plenge RM, Seielstad M, Padyukov L, et al. TRAF1-C5 as a risk locus for rheumatoid arthritis—a genomewide study. N Engl J Med 2007;357(12):119–209; with permission.)

A limitation of contemporary GWASs is that they only test common SNPs. For every common allele (defined as having an allele frequency of >5% in the general population), there is at least 1, and likely many more, rare alleles (frequency <5%).[8] In addition, there are other forms of genetic variation besides SNPs, including copy number variants (in which a gene may be duplicated or deleted). Next-generation sequencing and genotyping technologies are required to identify and test rare variants and structural variants.

DRUG DISCOVERY: RISK ALLELES IDENTIFY THE ACHILLES HEEL OF BIOLOGIC PATHWAYS

There are several effective drugs used to treat patients with active RA. Nonetheless, there are needs that are unmet in the current pharmacologic armamentarium. First, no single drug is effective in all patients, and most drugs induce disease remission in only one-third of patients. As a consequence, identifying the right medication for each patient continues to be a painstaking exercise in trial and error. Because irreversible erosive damage occurs early in the disease course, it is important to start patients with RA on the right drug at disease onset to minimize long-term disability. Second, even among those drugs that are effective, many have unacceptable side effects (eg, increased susceptibility to potentially life-threatening infections). Third, many of the drugs are extremely expensive, which places a large burden on families and the health care system. And finally, there is no drug that prevents or cures RA. Such a drug would radically change clinical practice.

How might Human Genetics Help Fill These Unmet Needs?

An important concept is that human mutations that confer a modest increase in the risk of disease pinpoint critical components of disease pathways. To understand why, first consider 2 extreme examples of human mutations and their effect on biologic pathways. If a gene is absolutely essential to a pathway, then a human mutation that alters gene function will likely be highly deleterious to the person carrying the mutation. Consequently, such a mutation is subject to negative evolutionary selection. In contrast, if a gene is not important at all to a pathway, then a human mutation will not exert any meaningful phenotype. Now consider the desired target of a drug. If a drug targets a pathway that is essential to survival, then the drug will likely have untoward side effects. And if a drug targets a pathway that is inconsequential, it will have no biologic effect. Finally, consider common genetic variants that predispose to disease. These variants must affect the Achilles heel of a critical disease pathway because they predispose to disease, but at the same time, these mutations have survived negative selection and therefore have modest effects. These mutations are not so severe that they are highly deleterious to the individual who carries them, but they are also within a gene that is important to a disease-relevant biologic pathway.

Effectively, human evolution has done the natural experiment by introducing 10 million common mutations throughout the genome in an unbiased manner. It is up to geneticists to determine which of those 10 million common mutations are relevant to disease.

There is a precedent for the concept that common alleles with a modest effect on disease risk identify effective drug targets. In each example below, the drug was developed before the genetic association was established. Still, these examples suggest that other human genetic mutations might identify the Achilles heel of a biologic pathway and that in turn, these genetic mutations identify effective drug targets.

In RA, a common allele within the *CTLA4* gene is known to increase risk of RA by approximately 15% per copy of the risk allele (which corresponds to an odds ratio of approximately 1.15).[12,23] Abatacept, which is a fusion protein composed of the extracellular domain of *CTLA4* and an immunoglobulin domain, is very effective in treating RA patients with active disease.[27] After T-cell activation, *CTLA4* expression is upregulated. The protein product traffics to the T-cell membrane, where it binds and inhibits costimulatory molecules CD80 and CD86 (which are also known as B7 proteins) on the surface of antigen-presenting cells (APCs).[28] Abatacept is thought to exert its effect through a high-affinity binding site for B7 molecules on the surface of APCs, thereby inhibiting the costimulatory signal to T cells.[29] Alternative splicing produces 2 CTLA4 protein isoforms: a full-length protein and a shorter, soluble isoform that is secreted from activated T cells. Functional studies demonstrate that the *CTLA4* risk allele results in lower mRNA levels of the soluble isoform of CTLA4.[30] Common alleles in the costimulatory genes *CD28* and *CD40* have also been implicated in RA pathogenesis, indicating that these pathways are critical in RA pathogenesis.[16,31]

There are also examples in nonautoimmune diseases in which common alleles of modest effect on phenotype identify effective drug targets. A common allele in the 3-hydroxy-3-methylglutaryl coenzyme A reductase gene is associated with low-density lipoprotein cholesterol levels in the general population.[32] Statins are highly effective cholesterol-lowering drugs that inhibit this enzyme, which is the rate-limiting enzyme of the mevalonate pathway of cholesterol synthesis. A common allele of *PPARG* is associated with risk of type 2 diabetes (T2D).[33,34] Thiazolidinediones, a class of drugs used to treat T2D, act by binding to the *PPARG* gene product inside the cell nucleus. Sulfonylureas, another class of drugs to treat T2D, bind to an adenosine triphosphate–dependent potassium channel on the cell membrane of pancreatic beta cells. A common allele in the gene that codes for this receptor, *KCNJ11*, is associated with risk of T2D.[35] Common alleles in genes associated with bone mineral density (*RANKL* and *OPG*) identify drugs (eg, denosumab) that show promise in clinical trials.[36–38]

GENOTYPE TO FUNCTION: HUMANS AS THE MODEL ORGANISM FOR TRANSLATIONAL IMMUNOLOGY

To turn genetic studies into effective medications, a major challenge is to take the expanding list of RA risk alleles and understand their effect on gene function. For example, it is important to understand whether the risk allele increases or decreases gene function (ie, whether it is a gain-of-function or loss-of-function allele) and to understand the most relevant cell type. Armed with this insight, it should be possible to target novel therapies for clinically relevant biologic pathways.

To go from genotype to function, there is a growing awareness of the importance of conducting experiments in human tissues of immunologic relevance.[39,40] Essentially, a goal should be to use humans as the model organism for translational immunology. To do this, novel resources are becoming available.

Biorepositories have now been established to study the functional consequences of common genetic mutations in blood cells from healthy control subjects.[41] Human immune cells are easily accessible through a simple blood draw. These immune cells are of direct relevance to pathogenesis of RA and other autoimmune diseases.[1,42] Human immune cells derived from healthy control subjects have been used successfully to gain insight into function of common mutations at several autoimmune genes: the missense mutation at *PTPN22* has been shown to alter secretion of interleukin (IL) 2 from T cells stimulated via the T-cell receptor[25]; a common multiple sclerosis risk mutation at *CD58* can explain approximately 40% of the variance of CD58 cell-surface expression on peripheral blood mononuclear cells[43]; and a common type 1 diabetes mutation in *IL2RA* alters IL2RA cell-surface expression on CD4[+] memory T cells.[44]

Another novel approach is to generate induced pluripotent stem (iPS) cells from patients who carry specific genetic mutations. First described in 2006,[45] several studies have shown that iPS cells can be derived from patients with human mutations.[46] Protocols have been developed to differentiate human embryonic stem cells into B cells, T cells, natural killer cells, and other immune lineages.[47–54] Whether iPS cells derived from patients with RA will be useful for functional studies of human genetic mutations is a hypothesis that needs to be rigorously tested.

PHARMACOGENETICS: INSIGHT INTO MECHANISMS OF TREATMENT FAILURE

Although the general mechanism of action of many RA drugs is known (for example, drugs that target the inflammatory cytokine TNF-α), it is still not known why some patients respond and other patients do not. Given that most RA drugs induce remission in only one-third of patients, it would be very useful to identify genetic predictors of treatment response. Moreover, the exact mechanisms of action of other drugs, including the most commonly prescribed RA drug, methotrexate (MTX), are not entirely clear. Once these mechanisms are illuminated, it should be possible to develop more effective drugs.

Pharmacogenetics is at a much earlier state than the field of genetic predictors of disease risk.[55] In short, there is no reproducible genetic variant that is associated with response to any drugs used to treat RA. Several studies have identified alleles in the enzyme 5,10-methylenetetrahydrofolate reductase that reduce enzyme activities (C677T and A1298C) and that have suggestive associations with efficacy or toxicity of MTX. However, these studies have been small and have not achieved overwhelming evidence of statistical significance.[56–62] Several studies have identified alleles associated with response to anti-TNF therapy (reviewed in the article by Plenge and Criswell[55]). As with the MTX studies, these studies have identified only suggestive but no confirmed associations.

Although it might be possible to use human genetics to help target the right therapy to the right patient (so-called personalized medicine), the predictive value of common alleles of modest effect sizes are likely to have little discriminating value.[63] As an example, a composite genetic risk score (GRS) based on all known RA susceptibility alleles is able to risk-stratify patients across a 10-fold range. However, a GRS has little clinical application in patients without symptoms (as there are no preventative measures). Once alleles that influence treatment response are identified, it will be important to determine whether or not they add to predictive models of treatment response.

NEXT-GENERATION PATIENT REGISTRIES: ENABLING LARGE-SCALE GENOTYPE-PHENOTYPE STUDIES

Currently, the main bottleneck in pharmacogenetic and other genotype-phenotype studies is access to large sample collections that have both DNA and detailed clinical data. The largest pharmacogenetic studies to date, conducted by the Biologics in Rheumatoid Arthritis Genetics and Genomics Study Syndicate (BRAGGSS) based in the United Kingdom, have analyzed just more than 1000 patients with RA.[64–66] Most genetic studies of patient outcomes (eg, cardiovascular events, infections, malignancy) are conducted on fewer patients. In contrast, the largest genetic association studies of RA susceptibility have been conducted in more than 20,000 combined case-control samples.[16]

Traditional patient registries and clinical trials, the workhorse for sample collection during the past decades, are unlikely to achieve the size required to obtain thousands of patient samples with DNA and detailed clinical data. Novel approaches (next-generation registries) are required to break this bottleneck. In theory, it should be possible to collect data as part of routine patient care. Medical informatics tools are available to collect basic clinical information (eg, components of the disease activity score 28, medications, adverse events) every time a physician sees a patient.[67,68] Increased use of electronic medical records (EMRs)[69] and novel approaches to mine clinical data from EMRs[70] represent one exciting approach to expand sample collections.

SUMMARY

The greatest effect of human genetics will likely be insight into the Achilles heel of biologic pathways that lead to RA and a better understanding of mechanism of action of drugs to treat RA. For drug discovery, it will be important to understand the functional relevance of the risk alleles identified to date (and the many alleles that remain to be discovered). This requires using humans as a model organism for translational immunology. For pharmacogenetic studies, novel resources are required to build large patient registries with detailed clinical data linked with biospecimens for genomic studies.

REFERENCES

1. Firestein GS. Evolving concepts of rheumatoid arthritis. Nature 2003;423(6937): 356–61.
2. Klareskog L, Catrina AI, Paget S. Rheumatoid arthritis. Lancet 2009;373(9664): 659–72.
3. Stastny P. Mixed lymphocyte cultures in rheumatoid arthritis. J Clin Invest 1976; 57(5):1148–57.
4. Stastny P. Association of the B-cell alloantigen DRw4 with rheumatoid arthritis. N Engl J Med 1978;298(16):869–71.
5. Gregersen PK, Moriuchi T, Karr RW, et al. Polymorphism of HLA-DR beta chains in DR4, -7, and -9 haplotypes: implications for the mechanisms of allelic variation. Proc Natl Acad Sci U S A 1986;83(23):9149–53.
6. Gregersen PK, Silver J, Winchester RJ. The shared epitope hypothesis. An approach to understanding the molecular genetics of susceptibility to rheumatoid arthritis. Arthritis Rheum 1987;30(11):1205–13.
7. Lander ES, Linton LM, Birren B, et al. Initial sequencing and analysis of the human genome. Nature 2001;409(6822):860–921.
8. Consortium IH, Frazer KA, Ballinger DG, et al. A second generation human haplotype map of over 3.1 million SNPs. Nature 2007;449(7164):851–61.
9. Altshuler D, Daly MJ, Lander ES. Genetic mapping in human disease. Science 2008;322(5903):881–8.
10. Suzuki A, Yamada R, Chang X, et al. Functional haplotypes of PADI4, encoding citrullinating enzyme peptidylarginine deiminase 4, are associated with rheumatoid arthritis. Nat Genet 2003;34(4):395–402.
11. Begovich AB, Carlton VE, Honigberg LA, et al. A missense single-nucleotide polymorphism in a gene encoding a protein tyrosine phosphatase (PTPN22) is associated with rheumatoid arthritis. Am J Hum Genet 2004;75(2):330–7.
12. Plenge RM, Padyukov L, Remmers EF, et al. Replication of putative candidate-gene associations with rheumatoid arthritis in >4,000 samples from North

America and Sweden: association of susceptibility with PTPN22, CTLA4, and PADI4. Am J Hum Genet 2005;77(6):1044–60.

13. Plenge RM, Cotsapas C, Davies L, et al. Two independent alleles at 6q23 associated with risk of rheumatoid arthritis. Nat Genet 2007;39:1477–82.

14. Plenge RM, Seielstad M, Padyukov L, et al. TRAF1-C5 as a Risk Locus for Rheumatoid Arthritis – A Genomewide Study. N Engl J Med 2007;357(12):1199–209.

15. Raychaudhuri S, Remmers EF, Lee AT, et al. Common variants at CD40 and other loci confer risk of rheumatoid arthritis. Nat Genet 2008;40(10):1216–23.

16. Raychaudhuri S, Thomson BP, Remmers EF, et al. Genetic variants at CD28, PRDM1 and CD2/CD58 are associated with rheumatoid arthritis risk. Nat Genet 2009;41(12):1313–8.

17. Remmers EF, Plenge RM, Lee AT, et al. STAT4 and the risk of rheumatoid arthritis and systemic lupus erythematosus. N Engl J Med 2007;357(10):977–86.

18. Zhernakova A, Alizadeh BZ, Bevova M, et al. Novel association in chromosome 4q27 region with rheumatoid arthritis and confirmation of type 1 diabetes point to a general risk locus for autoimmune diseases. Am J Hum Genet 2007;81(6): 1284–8.

19. Barton A, Eyre S, Ke X, et al. Identification of AF4/FMR2 family, member 3 (AFF3) as a novel rheumatoid arthritis susceptibility locus and confirmation of two further pan-autoimmune susceptibility genes. Hum Mol Genet 2009; 18(13):2518–22.

20. Barton A, Thomson W, Ke X, et al. Re-evaluation of putative rheumatoid arthritis susceptibility genes in the post-genome wide association study era and hypothesis of a key pathway underlying susceptibility. Hum Mol Genet 2008;17:2274–9.

21. Barton A, Thomson W, Ke X, et al. Rheumatoid arthritis susceptibility loci at chromosomes 10p15, 12q13 and 22q13. Nat Genet 2008;40(10):1156–9.

22. Thomson W, Barton A, Ke X, et al. Rheumatoid arthritis association at 6q23. Nat Genet 2007;39:1431–3.

23. Gregersen PK, Amos CI, Lee AT, et al. REL, encoding a member of the NF-kappaB family of transcription factors, is a newly defined risk locus for rheumatoid arthritis. Nat Genet 2009;41(7):820–3.

24. Hirschhorn JN, Daly MJ. Genome-wide association studies for common diseases and complex traits. Nat Rev Genet 2005;6(2):95–108.

25. Vang T, Congia M, Macis MD, et al. Autoimmune-associated lymphoid tyrosine phosphatase is a gain-of-function variant. Nat Genet 2005;37(12):1317–9.

26. Vang T, Miletic AV, Bottini N, et al. Protein tyrosine phosphatase PTPN22 in human autoimmunity. Autoimmunity 2007;40(6):453–61.

27. Moreland L, Bate G, Kirkpatrick P. Abatacept. Nat Rev Drug Discov 2006;5(3): 185–6.

28. Gough SC, Walker LS, Sansom DM. CTLA4 gene polymorphism and autoimmunity. Immunol Rev 2005;204:102–15.

29. Ruderman EM, Pope RM. The evolving clinical profile of abatacept (CTLA4-Ig): a novel co-stimulatory modulator for the treatment of rheumatoid arthritis. Arthritis Res Ther 2005;7(Suppl 2):S21–5.

30. Ueda H, Howson JM, Esposito L, et al. Association of the T-cell regulatory gene CTLA4 with susceptibility to autoimmune disease. Nature 2003;423(6939): 506–11.

31. Raychaudhuri S, Plenge RM, Rossin EJ, et al. Identifying relationships among genomic disease regions: predicting genes at pathogenic SNP associations and rare deletions. PLoS Genet 2009;5(6):e1000534.

32. Kathiresan S, Musunuru K, Orho-Melander M. Defining the spectrum of alleles that contribute to blood lipid concentrations in humans. Curr Opin Lipidol 2008; 19(2):122–7.

33. Altshuler D, Hirschhorn JN, Klannemark M, et al. The common PPARgamma Pro12Ala polymorphism is associated with decreased risk of type 2 diabetes. Nat Genet 2000;26(1):76–80.

34. Florez JC, Burtt N, de Bakker PI, et al. Haplotype structure and genotype-phenotype correlations of the sulfonylurea receptor and the islet ATP-sensitive potassium channel gene region. Diabetes 2004;53(5):1360–8.

35. Styrkarsdottir U, Halldorsson BV, Gretarsdottir S, et al. Multiple genetic loci for bone mineral density and fractures. N Engl J Med 2008;358(22):2355–65.

36. Smith MR, Egerdie B, Hernandez Toriz N, et al. Denosumab in men receiving androgen-deprivation therapy for prostate cancer. N Engl J Med 2009;361(8): 745–55.

37. Cummings SR, San Martin J, McClung MR, et al. Denosumab for prevention of fractures in postmenopausal women with osteoporosis. N Engl J Med 2009; 361(8):756–65.

38. Davis MM. A prescription for human immunology. Immunity 2008;29(6):835–8.

39. Hayday AC, Peakman M. The habitual, diverse and surmountable obstacles to human immunology research. Nat Immunol 2008;9(6):575–80.

40. Gregersen PK. Closing the gap between genotype and phenotype. Nat Genet 2009;41(9):958–9.

41. Gregersen PK, Behrens TW. Genetics of autoimmune diseases–disorders of immune homeostasis. Nat Rev Genet 2006;7(12):917–28.

42. De Jager PL, Baecher-Allan C, Maier LM, et al. The role of the CD58 locus in multiple sclerosis. Proc Natl Acad Sci U S A 2009;106(13):5264–9.

43. Dendrou CA, Plagnol V, Fung E, et al. Cell-specific protein phenotypes for the autoimmune locus IL2RA using a genotype-selectable human bioresource. Nat Genet 2009;41(9):1011–5.

44. Takahashi K, Yamanaka S. Induction of pluripotent stem cells from mouse embryonic and adult fibroblast cultures by defined factors. Cell 2006;126(4):663–76.

45. Park IH, Arora N, Huo H, et al. Disease-specific induced pluripotent stem cells. Cell 2008;134(5):877–86.

46. Vodyanik MA, Bork JA, Thomson JA, et al. Human embryonic stem cell-derived CD34+ cells: efficient production in the coculture with OP9 stromal cells and analysis of lymphohematopoietic potential. Blood 2005;105(2):617–26.

47. Kaufman DS, Hanson ET, Lewis RL, et al. Hematopoietic colony-forming cells derived from human embryonic stem cells. Proc Natl Acad Sci U S A 2001; 98(19):10716–21.

48. Chadwick K, Wang L, Li L, et al. Cytokines and BMP-4 promote hematopoietic differentiation of human embryonic stem cells. Blood 2003;102(3):906–15.

49. Zambidis ET, Peault B, Park TS, et al. Hematopoietic differentiation of human embryonic stem cells progresses through sequential hematoendothelial, primitive, and definitive stages resembling human yolk sac development. Blood 2005;106(3):860–70.

50. Martin CH, Woll PS, Ni Z, et al. Differences in lymphocyte developmental potential between human embryonic stem cell and umbilical cord blood-derived hematopoietic progenitor cells. Blood 2008;112(7):2730–7.

51. Woll PS, Martin CH, Miller JS, et al. Human embryonic stem cell-derived NK cells acquire functional receptors and cytolytic activity. J Immunol 2005;175(8): 5095–103.

52. Galic Z, Kitchen SG, Kacena A, et al. T lineage differentiation from human embryonic stem cells. Proc Natl Acad Sci U S A 2006;103(31):11742–7.
53. Galic Z, Kitchen SG, Subramanian A, et al. Generation of T lineage cells from human embryonic stem cells in a feeder free system. Stem Cells 2009;27(1): 100–7.
54. Plenge RM, Criswell LA. Genetic variants that predict response to anti-tumor necrosis factor therapy in rheumatoid arthritis: current challenges and future directions. Curr Opin Rheumatol 2008;20(2):145–52.
55. van Ede AE, Laan RF, Blom HJ, et al. The C677 T mutation in the methylenetetrahydrofolate reductase gene: a genetic risk factor for methotrexate-related elevation of liver enzymes in rheumatoid arthritis patients. Arthritis Rheum 2001;44(11): 2525–30.
56. Urano W, Taniguchi A, Yamanaka H, et al. Polymorphisms in the methylenetetrahydrofolate reductase gene were associated with both the efficacy and the toxicity of methotrexate used for the treatment of rheumatoid arthritis, as evidenced by single locus and haplotype analyses. Pharmacogenetics 2002; 12(3):183–90.
57. Kumagai K, Hiyama K, Oyama T, et al. Polymorphisms in the thymidylate synthase and methylenetetrahydrofolate reductase genes and sensitivity to the low-dose methotrexate therapy in patients with rheumatoid arthritis. Int J Mol Med 2003;11(5):593–600.
58. Weisman MH, Furst DE, Park GS, et al. Risk genotypes in folate-dependent enzymes and their association with methotrexate-related side effects in rheumatoid arthritis. Arthritis Rheum 2006;54(2):607–12.
59. Kurzawski M, Pawlik A, Safranow K, et al. 677C>T and 1298A>C MTHFR polymorphisms affect methotrexate treatment outcome in rheumatoid arthritis. Pharmacogenomics 2007;8(11):1551–9.
60. Kooloos WM, Huizinga TW, Guchelaar HJ, et al. Pharmacogenetics in Treatment of Rheumatoid Arthritis. Curr Pharm Des 2010;16:164–75.
61. Kooloos WM, Wessels JA, van der Kooij SM, et al. Optimalization of the clinical pharmacogenetic model to predict methotrexate treatment response: the influence of the number of haplotypes of MTHFR 1298A-677C alleles on probability to respond. Ann Rheum Dis 2009;68(8):1371.
62. Kraft P, Wacholder S, Cornelis MC, et al. Beyond odds ratios–communicating disease risk based on genetic profiles. Nat Rev Genet 2009;10(4):264–9.
63. Potter C, Hyrich KL, Tracey A, et al. Association of rheumatoid factor and anti-cyclic citrullinated peptide positivity, but not carriage of shared epitope or PTPN22 susceptibility variants, with anti-tumour necrosis factor response in rheumatoid arthritis. Ann Rheum Dis 2009;68(1):69–74.
64. Bowes JD, Potter C, Gibbons LJ, et al. Investigation of genetic variants within candidate genes of the TNFRSF1B signalling pathway on the response to anti-TNF agents in a UK cohort of rheumatoid arthritis patients. Pharmacogenet Genomics 2009;19(4):319–23.
65. Collier DS, Kay J, Estey G, et al. A rheumatology-specific informatics-based application with a disease activity calculator. Arthritis Rheum 2009;61(4):488–94.
66. Hetland ML. DANBIO: a nationwide registry of biological therapies in Denmark. Clin Exp Rheumatol 2005;23(5 Suppl 39):S205–7.
67. Steinbrook R. Personally controlled online health data–the next big thing in medical care? N Engl J Med 2008;358(16):1653–6.
68. Murphy S, Churchill S, Bry L, et al. Instrumenting the health care enterprise for discovery research in the genomic era. Genome Res 2009;19(9):1675–81.

69. Kochi Y, Yamada R, Suzuki A, et al. A functional variant in FCRL3, encoding Fc receptor-like 3, is associated with rheumatoid arthritis and several autoimmunities. Nat Genet 2005;37:478–85.

70. Orozco G, Hinks A, Eyre S, et al. Combined effects of three independent SNPs greatly increase the risk estimate for RA at 6q23. Hum Mol Genet 2009;18: 2693–9.

71. Kurreeman FA, Padyukov L, Marques RB, et al. A candidate gene approach identifies the TRAF1/C5 region as a risk factor for rheumatoid arthritis. PLoS Med 2007;4:e278.

72. Kurreeman FA, Daha NA, Chang M, et al. Association of IL2RA and IL2RB with rheumatoid arthritis: a replication study in a Dutch population. Ann Rheum Dis 2009;68:1789–90.

73. Suzuki A, Yamada R, Kochi Y, et al. Functional SNPs in CD244 increase the risk of rheumatoid arthritis in a Japanese population. Nat Genet 2008;40:1224–9.

74. Stahl EA, Raychaudhuri S, Remmers EF, et al. Genome-wide association study meta-analysis identifies seven new rheumatoid arthritis risk loci. Nat Genet 2010; May 9. [Epub ahead of print].

Innate Immunity and Rheumatoid Arthritis

Angelica Gierut, MD, Harris Perlman, PhD, Richard M. Pope, MD*

KEYWORDS

• Macrophage • Fibroblast • Receptor

Although environmental insults such as smoking have been implicated in the initiation of rheumatoid arthritis (RA) in patients who express the shared epitope, the understanding of the role of innate immunity in the pathogenesis of this disease is also expanding. The clinical picture of pain, stiffness, swelling, and joint destruction seen in RA is a result of chronic inflammation of the synovium, characterized by interactions of fibroblast-like synoviocytes with cells of the innate immune system, including macrophages, dendritic cells (DCs), mast cells, and natural killer (NK) cells, as well as cells of the adaptive immune system, B and T lymphocytes.[1] Also present are immune complexes; proteins of the complement system; autocrine- and paracrine-acting cytokines; as well as chemokines that have inflammatory, homeostatic, and even antiinflammatory properties.[2] As knowledge of the complexities of RA grows, gaps in the understanding of its pathogenesis are filled and new potential therapeutic targets are uncovered.

The best-known function of the innate immune system is the initial recognition of microbial pathogens. On encounter with nonself, primarily by macrophages and DCs via membrane-bound or intracellular pattern-recognition receptors (PRRs), cells of the innate system become activated, leading to the production of inflammatory cytokines and chemokines. Effector cells and molecules of the innate system are recruited locally, and if unable to overcome the pathogen alone, macrophages and DCs travel to local lymphoid tissues where processed antigens are presented by major histocompatibility complex (MHC) molecules to naive T cells, thus initiating an adaptive response complete with lasting immunologic memory. On clearance of the organism, with the help of opposing antiinflammatory mediators, the inflammatory response is terminated.[3] In RA, however, "self" is either the primary target or an innocent bystander that then becomes the focus of attack. In RA, there is abundant evidence that the innate immune system is persistently activated, as evidenced by the continual expression of macrophage-derived cytokines, such as tumor necrosis

This work is supported by grants from the National Institutes of Health: AR050250, AI067590, AR054796 to HP and AR049217 to RMP.
Division of Rheumatology, Department of Medicine, Feinberg School of Medicine, Northwestern University, 240 East Huron Street, McGaw M300, Chicago, IL 60611, USA
* Corresponding author.
E-mail address: rmp158@northwestern.edu

Rheum Dis Clin N Am 36 (2010) 271–296
doi:10.1016/j.rdc.2010.03.004
0889-857X/10/$ – see front matter. Published by Elsevier Inc.

rheumatic.theclinics.com

factor α (TNF-α), interleukin (IL) 1, and IL-6. As the understanding of the innate immune system in RA continues to expand, enticing targets for new therapeutic interventions continue to be identified. This article focuses on cells of myelomonocytic origin, their receptors, and factors that interact with them.

MONOCYTES AND MACROPHAGES
Background and Role in RA

Macrophages, together with osteoclasts and myeloid DCs, are derived from myelo-monocytic origins and are key cellular components of the innate immune system. Macrophages differentiate from circulating monocytes and have primary roles in tissues as phagocytes of invading pathogens and as scavengers of apoptotic debris. In addition, macrophage activation results in the expression of chemokines and cyto-kines, such as TNF-α and IL-1β, that helps to attract other cells and proteins to the sites of inflammation.[3] The central role of macrophages in RA pathogenesis is sup-ported by the fact that conventional therapies, including methotrexate and cytokine inhibitors, act to decrease the production of cytokines that are produced primarily by macrophages.[4] Indeed, a correlation has been found between synovial macro-phage infiltration and subsequent radiographic joint destruction.[5] A remarkable fact is that a reduction in the number of sublining macrophages in RA synovial tissue has been shown to strongly correlate with the degree of clinical improvement, regard-less of the type of therapy chosen.[6] In addition to local effects of macrophages in the synovial tissue, systemic consequences of macrophage-mediated inflammation in RA may be manifested by damage to other areas such as the subendothelial space where macrophages become foam cells contributing to atherosclerotic plaques.[7]

Mechanisms for Increased Macrophage Number in RA Tissue

Possible mechanisms for the increased number of macrophages in diseased tissue include increased chemotaxis[8,9] and reduced emigration.[10] Some studies also suggest local proliferation of macrophages in areas of inflammation.[11–14] Decreased apoptosis may also contribute to the accumulation of macrophages in the RA joint. Several studies have shown that induction of synoviocyte apoptosis in animal models of inflammatory arthritis ameliorates joint inflammation and joint destruction.[15] In both experimental arthritis and synovial tissue from patients with RA, reduced expression of the proapoptotic Bcl-2 family member, Bim, was seen in macrophages and corre-sponded to the increased expression of IL-1β by macrophages. Furthermore, admin-istration of a Bim mimetic dramatically reduced the incidence of arthritis and successfully ameliorated established arthritis in mice.[16] This result suggests that therapies that restore the homeostasis between survival and cell death of RA macrophages may be successful in ameliorating arthritis in patients.

Heterogeneity of Monocyte and Macrophage Populations

Within monocyte and macrophage populations, there is a great deal of heterogeneity. For example, 2 human monocyte populations have been defined based on their surface marker expression: the CD14$^+$CD16$^-$ and the CD14^{low}CD16$^+$ subsets.[17] CD16 is a receptor for immunoglobulin (Ig) G, FcγIIIA, which binds to IgG-containing immune complexes (see later discussion). The number of CD14^{low}CD16$^+$ monocytes is elevated in RA peripheral blood, and CD14^{low}CD16$^+$ macrophages are enriched in RA synovial tissue.[18] CD14^{low}CD16$^+$ monocytes produce more TNF-α in response to the microbial toll-like receptor (TLR) 4 ligand lipopolysaccharide (LPS) compared with the CD14$^+$CD16$^-$ subset.[19,20] These observations suggest that the proinflammatory

CD14[low]CD16[+] monocytes migrate to the RA joint and become highly responsive macrophages. However, CD14[+]CD16[-] monocytes also express the chemokine receptor (CCR) 2, which binds monocyte chemotactic protein 1, and thereby promotes monocyte migration to the site of inflammation. Because the RA joint is rich in this chemokine, it is possible that CD14[+]CD16[-] and CCR2[+] monocytes are recruited to the joint where CD16 expression is then induced. Nonetheless, because monocytes migrate from the peripheral blood into RA synovial tissue, identification of circulating monocyte subpopulations may be an extremely useful clinical tool for tracking disease activity and for identifying additional therapeutic targets.[20–22]

In addition, diversity in activation states of macrophages has been found.[23] In general, macrophages exhibiting a more inflammatory phenotype have been named M1, or classically activated macrophages, whereas those that trend toward a more antiinflammatory and repair role are known as M2, or alternatively activated macrophages.[23] Most macrophages in the RA joint express proinflammatory cytokines and are thus most consistent with classically activated macrophages. Therapies that promote the balance in favor of an M2 phenotype may be useful in RA.[8]

Therapies Targeting Macrophages

Conventional therapies such as prednisone, methotrexate, leflunomide, sulfasalazine, and TNF-α inhibitors have been shown to decrease the number of CD68[+] macrophages in the synovial sublining.[24] Another study of synovial tissue response to rituximab found a significant reduction in the number of sublining macrophages at 16 weeks, providing evidence for synovial tissue sublining macrophage reduction after B-cell depletion therapy in RA as well.[25] Furthermore, a reduction in the number of synovial sublining macrophages correlated clinically with the improvement of the values of disease activity score (DAS) 28, suggesting an association between sublining CD68[+] macrophages and therapeutic efficacy.[24] The positive correlation between the change in RA clinical activity and CD68 expression in the synovial sublining has been independently confirmed.[26]

Specifically, targeting activated macrophages at sites of inflammation would be a way of circumventing the potential untoward effects of systemic macrophage depletion. The bisphosphonate clodronate, encapsulated within liposomes, has been used to specifically deplete macrophages. After injecting rats intraperitoneally with streptococcal cell-wall (SCW) fragments to induce arthritis, intravenous (IV) liposomal clodronate suppressed the development of chronic arthritis for up to 26 days after treatment. Treatment was also associated with the depletion of synovial and hepatic, but not splenic, macrophages, as well as a reduction in articular IL-1β, IL-6, TNF-α, and matrix metallopeptidase (MMP) 9 levels.[27] Similarly, in the K/B × N serum transfer model of arthritis, where spontaneously produced anti–glucose phosphate isomerase (GPI) antibodies from a K/B × N mouse are injected into a naive host, treatment with liposomal clodronate before serum transfer caused depletion of macrophages in the bone marrow and liver, and the treated mice were completely resistant to arthritis. Resistance to arthritis was reversed when the macrophage-depleted mice were reconstituted with macrophages from naive animals and immediately injected with K/B × N serum.[28] In rabbits with established antigen-induced arthritis (AIA), repeated intraarticular administrations of low, noncytotoxic doses of liposomal clodronate led to an early reduction of joint swelling, delay in radiographic progression, and decrease in the number of synovial lining macrophages. However, no difference was seen in pannus formation or radiographic erosions at 8 weeks.[29] In patients with RA undergoing knee replacement surgery, a single intraarticular dose of clodronate liposomes significantly reduced the number of CD68[+] cells and the expression of adhesion molecules in the synovial lining. In contrast, no immunohistologic difference was observed in the control group.[30] These observations suggest that depletion of synovial tissue macrophages may be an important therapeutic goal in RA.

Systemic depletion of all macrophages could have serious consequences in patients, and this may be avoided by specifically targeting receptors present on activated macrophages. Folate receptor β (FRβ) has been described on both activated macrophages from RA synovial fluid and animal models of arthritis but not on resting or quiescent macrophages or normal cells of the body except for the proximal tubule cells of the kidneys.[31–33] The FRβ has been used to deliver folate-conjugated imaging agents to inflamed joints in patients with RA[34] and is a target for novel therapeutic agents. Several new-generation folate antagonists are selectively taken up by the FRβ and show growth inhibition capabilities against FRβ-expressing cells, thus circumventing the systemic effects.[35] In addition, antibodies or fragments of antibodies against FRβ linked with immunotoxins have been developed and have been shown to reduce the number of macrophages and levels of IL-6 and to increase the number of apoptotic cells in RA synovial tissue engrafted into severe combined immunodeficient mice.[36,37] Another approach involved the conjugation of folate to superoxide dismutase and catalase, 2 enzymes that scavenge the damaging reactive oxygen species secreted by activated macrophages. Folate conjugation dramatically enhanced the ability of catalase and superoxide dismutase to scavenge reactive oxygen species produced by activated macrophages in cell culture experiments and the uptake of the enzyme catalase into activated macrophages.[38] Folate has also been conjugated to small molecules, or haptens such as fluorescein, and given to rodents previously immunized to the hapten after the onset of experimental arthritis. The folate-hapten conjugate selectively "decorated" and promoted immune-mediated elimination of activated macrophages and decreased paw swelling, spleen size, systemic inflammation, arthritis score, and bone erosion.[39] Thus, the presence of select folate receptors on activated macrophages offers exciting potential to target activated macrophages in the RA joint.

DENDRITIC CELLS
Background

DCs, along with macrophages and B cells, have the ability to present antigen to T cells, and therefore play a central role in the development of innate and adaptive immune responses. In the periphery, immature DCs are stimulated to undergo differentiation by an array of pathogens, mainly via the activation of TLRs by exogenous or endogenous stimuli, and also in response to cytokines or immune complexes produced during the inflammatory response. TLR signaling results in a significant change in chemokine receptors expressed by DCs, allowing for maturation of DCs and migration to the lymphoid tissue, where mature DCs display antigen on MHC molecules to naive T cells. DCs also express the critical costimulatory molecules, CD80 and CD86, which interact with CD28 on T cells, completing the necessary signal for antigen-specific effector T-cell maturation to occur. In addition to stimulation of naive T cells, DCs can process and display antigen in local tissues and contribute to the inflammatory response by the production of cytokines, such as TNF-α, IL-1β, and IL-6. Furthermore, DCs can direct the formation of distinct T helper (T_H) cells by producing key cytokines, such as IL-12 and IL-18 for T_H1 cells and IL-23 for T_H17 cells.[3] Finally, DCs are important in the development of both central and peripheral tolerance, and their depletion in animal models is associated with the onset of fatal autoimmune-type disease.[40] In the thymus, DCs present endogenous self-antigens to T cells and delete those that are strongly reactive, whereas in the periphery, interaction between autoreactive T cells and immature DCs bearing self-antigen may result in anergy, apoptosis, or differentiation into regulatory T cells.[3] Deviations in this pathway, either failed clearance of dead cells or exposure of DCs bearing self-antigens to maturation signals, can abrogate their tolerogenic ability and are implicated in the development of autoimmunity.[41]

DCs may be categorized into subtypes based on the expression of various cell-surface markers.[42,43] Functionally, however, DCs may be separated into 2 main classes: classical or conventional DCs (cDCs), which are resident in lymphoid tissues or migratory in nonlymphoid tissues, and plasmacytoid DCs (pDCs). Both types may be activated by particular TLRs that induce the molecules necessary to promote antigen presentation, T-cell stimulation, and cytokine production. cDCs express CD11c:CD18, also known as complement receptor (CR) 4, and all known TLRs, except for TLR9. cDCs are the main participants in antigen presentation and activation of naive T cells as well as the mediators of peripheral tolerance. pDCs, on the other hand, are particularly important in modifying the immune response toward viruses. They do not express high levels of CD11c and have been identified by the expression of specific markers, such as blood dendritic cell antigen 2. In addition, pDCs express TLRs 1, 7, and 9 and other TLRs to a lesser degree.[3] In response to stimuli such as viruses, pDCs are able to generate abundant amounts of type I interferons (IFNs) (IFN-α and IFN-β) and other cytokines such as TNF-α and IL-12. These cytokines increase the production of inflammatory mediators by macrophages, and in the case of IL-12, they can direct a potent T_H1 response.[44]

DCs and RA

The vast majority of studies that have examined the role of DCs in RA have relied on immunohistochemical techniques or have isolated DCs from peripheral blood and characterized their phenotype and function. In RA synovial tissue, the number of pDCs that are localized to perivascular lymphocytic infiltrates[45] correlates with anti–cyclic citrullinated peptide (anti-CCP) antibodies.[46] These pDCs produced B-cell activating factor, IL-18, and IFN-α/-β, whereas the cDCs secreted IL-12 and IL-23.[46] The total numbers of cDCs or pDCs or the number of mature DCs in RA synovial tissue were not significantly different from patients with osteoarthritis (OA) or psoriatic arthritis,[46,47] although there was a statistical increase in the ratio of pDC/cDC in RA synovial tissue.[46] These data suggest that the number of DCs in synovial tissue may not reflect their true contribution to RA pathogenesis.

Few cDCs or pDCs are detected in peripheral blood of patients with RA, and the numbers are lower compared with healthy controls. The expression of the inhibitory FcγRIIB on DCs derived from peripheral blood monocytes of patients with RA correlated with disease activity. In addition, DCs expressing higher levels of FcγRIIB inhibited T-cell proliferation and promoted the T-regulatory phenotype after TLR and Fc receptor (FcR) stimulation in coculture studies.[48] Treatment with methotrexate or infliximab dramatically affects the number, maturation, and function of the DC. DCs derived from monocytes of patients treated with infliximab displayed an antiinflammatory phenotype[49] and increased numbers of cDCs in the circulation.[50] In addition, the numbers of pDCs were increased in the peripheral blood in patients in clinical remission induced by either methotrexate or infliximab. Further, isolation of these pDCs and coculture with naive T cells led to an induction of the T-regulatory phenotype, which was capable of inhibiting autologous T-cell proliferation.[51] In contrast, there was a reduction in both circulating cDC and pDC numbers in anti–IL-6 receptor–treated patients with RA, which was not observed in anti-TNF or cytotoxic T-lymphocyte antigen (CTLA) 4 immunoglobulin–treated patients with RA.[52] These data suggest that clinically relevant information may be gleaned from examining circulating DCs in patients with RA and that there are differences related to the mode of therapy.

DCs and Murine Models of RA

The use of murine models of inflammatory arthritis has supported the human studies on the roles of DCs in RA. Follicular DCs are required for the development of the K/B × N mouse model of arthritis.[53] In contrast, selective depletion of pDCs enhanced the severity and pathology of collagen-induced arthritis (CIA).[54] These data suggest that pDCs may prevent the break of tolerance and that the follicular DC or cDC may be the central culprit that leads to the activation of autoreactive lymphocytes. Adoptive transfer of DCs from CTLA4 immunoglobulin–treated mice was sufficient to inhibit arthritis in CIA-recipient mice.[55] In addition, adoptive transfer of TLR-stimulated DCs after immunization reduced CIA.[56] Thus, similar to patients with RA, modification of the DC function by biologic therapies may lead to a skewing of T-cell development toward a T-regulatory phenotype mediated by DCs.

PATTERN-RECOGNITION RECEPTORS
Background

There are several mechanisms by which macrophages and other innate immune cells become activated. One way is via PRRs that are designed to recognize simple and regular nonself patterns of molecular structure, conserved during evolution, called pathogen-associated molecular patterns (PAMPs). Furthermore, when cells are under duress, such as in chronic inflammation, they may express danger-associated molecular patterns (DAMPs), such as uric acid, adenosine triphosphate, heat shock proteins (HSPs), or glycoprotein 96 (gp96), that may also be recognized by PRRs.[57–60] PRRs may be membrane bound or soluble plasma proteins. Examples include mannose-binding lectin (MBL) that is important in the lectin pathway of complement activation, the transmembrane PRRs composed of 10 known human TLRs that may be activated on cell surfaces or within endosomal compartments, and the cytosolic PRRs that include the nucleotide-binding oligomerization domain (NOD)–like receptors (NLRs) and the retinoic acid–inducible gene I (RIG-I)–like receptors (RLRs).

Toll-like Receptors

The cell-surface TLRs include TLR1, 2, 4, 5, and 6, with the recognition motifs outside the cell, whereas TLR3, 7, 8, and 9 are on the endosomal membrane, with the PRR recognition motifs within the endosomal compartment. The TLR system recognizes PAMPs, including LPS (TLR4), peptidoglycans (PGNs) (TLR2 together with TLR1 or 6), unmethylated CpG DNA motifs (TLR9) from bacteria, and single-stranded RNA (TLR7) and double-stranded RNA (TLR3) from viruses. The cytoplasmic domain of the TLR is called the Toll–IL-1 receptor (TIR) motif because it is also present in the IL-1 receptor. TLR signals are mediated through the TIR, which interacts with adapter molecules. All TLRs except TLR3 signal through the adapter molecule myeloid differentiation factor 88 (MyD88), whereas TLR3 signals only through the adapter molecule TIR domain-containing adapter-inducing IFN-β (TRIF), and TLR4 signals through both MyD88 and TRIF. Signaling through the MyD88 leads to the activation of nuclear factor κB (NF-κB) and the mitogen-activated protein (MAP) kinases, c-Jun N-terminal kinase and p38. Activation of NF-κB and the MAP kinases leads to the transcription of genes involved in inflammation, proliferation, and protection against apoptosis,[3,61,62] whereas activation through TRIF results in the expression of type I IFNs, IFN-α and -β.[63]

Clinically, further elucidation of TLR signaling cascades is important because they offer attractive targets for intervention.

TLR Expression in RA

TLRs are expressed in the RA joint. In RA synovial tissue, CD16$^+$ synovial lining macrophages also expressed TLR2,[64] and the expression of both TLR2 and TLR4 was significantly higher in RA tissue than in samples from patients with OA.[65] RA synovial tissues have a pronounced expression of TLR2 messenger RNA (mRNA) in the synovial lining and at sites of attachment and invasion into cartilage or bone tissue.[66] In addition, TLR3 and TLR7 were also found to be highly expressed in RA synovium,[67] and samples of tissue from patients with either early or long-standing RA showed similar levels of TLR3 and TLR4, both of which were significantly higher than those in patients with OA.[68]

In RA synovial fibroblasts, levels of baseline mRNA for TLR2 and TLR4 did not differ compared with OA tissue fibroblasts. However, compared with OA fibroblasts, RA synovial fibroblasts demonstrated a significantly increased expression of TLR2 after treatment with IL-1β, TNF-α, LPS, or synthetic bacterial lipopeptide, leading to a strong increase of NF-κB translocation into the nucleus.[66] In contrast, another study found that levels of both TLR2 and TLR4 mRNA were significantly higher in RA synovial fibroblasts compared with those from patients with OA and normal skin fibroblasts.[69] In contrast to whole synovial tissue, TLR7 mRNA expression by synovial fibroblasts was not seen, suggesting that previous TLR7 staining may have been reflecting expression by macrophages or DCs.[68]

Peripheral blood monocytes also express TLRs. Both TLR2 and TLR4 were increased on CD16$^+$ and CD16$^-$ peripheral blood monocytes from patients with RA versus healthy controls, and the TLR2 expression on the CD16$^+$ subset was higher than that on the CD16$^-$ subset.[64] Furthermore, IFN-γ increased the expression of TLR2 and TLR4 on RA peripheral blood monocytes.[65] In RA synovial fluid, CD14$^+$ macrophages demonstrated increased expression of TLR2 and TLR4 compared with peripheral blood monocytes or control macrophages differentiated in vitro from normal monocytes.[70]

Activation of Cells from the RA Joint by Microbial TLR Ligands

Isolated RA synovial fibroblasts treated with microbial TLR2 and TLR4 ligands demonstrated a marked increase in the osteoclast activator RANKL, at both the mRNA and protein levels.[69] Inflammatory cytokines IL-6 and IL-8, as well as MMP-1 and -3, were induced by stimulation of RA synovial fibroblasts with bacterial PGN.[71] Furthermore, RA synovial fibroblasts demonstrated increased expression of vascular endothelial growth factor after stimulation with bacterial PGN and increased IL-15 after stimulation by TLR2 and TLR4 ligands.[72] Stimulation of RA synovial fibroblasts with the synthetic TLR3 ligand, poly I:C, led to the production of IL-6 and TNF-α, which was significantly enhanced when the cells were preincubated with IFN-α compared with cells stimulated with poly I:C alone.[73] These observations suggest that in RA, synovial fibroblasts may be activated through the TLR pathway.

RA synovial fluid macrophages demonstrate an increased response to microbial TLR2 and TLR4 ligands compared with control macrophages differentiated in vitro from normal monocytes, macrophages from the joints of patients with other forms of inflammatory arthritis, or RA peripheral blood monocytes.[70] In addition, treatment of RA synovial fluid macrophages with a microbial TLR2 ligand significantly increased the levels of IFN-γ and IL-23 mRNA compared with in vitro–differentiated control macrophages.[74] It is possible that alterations of intracellular signaling pathways, such as those regulated by IFN-γ or IL-10, might be responsible.[75]

Endogenous TLR Ligands in RA

Because microbial ligands are not likely the cause of TLR signaling in the RA joint, studies have examined RA synovial fluids and tissues for the presence of potential endogenous TLR ligands. RA synovial fluid activated human embryonic kidney 293 cells only when these cells expressed TLR4, suggesting the presence of endogenous TLR4 ligands in RA synovial fluid.[76] In addition, the authors have demonstrated that RA synovial fluid is capable of activating normal macrophages and that this activation was mediated through TLR2 and TLR4 (Pope and colleagues, unpublished data, 2010). Together, these observations suggest that endogenous TLR ligands or DAMPs may be released in response to inflammation in early RA and result in continuous persistence of inflammatory mediators through activation of cells of the innate immune system.

Several potentially relevant endogenous TLR ligands or DAMPs have been identified in the RA joint. Ligands such as HSP22, tenascin-C, high-mobility group box chromosomal protein 1, serum amyloid A protein, and fragments of hyaluronic acid are highly expressed in the RA joint and are capable of activating monocytic cells through TLR2, or TLR4, or both. Another DAMP, gp96, was also highly expressed in RA synovial fluid and synovial tissue. The addition of gp96 in vitro to RA synovial fluid macrophages induced significantly higher levels of TNF-α, IL-8, and TLR2 compared with control macrophages.[60] Although gp96 bound to both TLR2 and TLR4, macrophage activation was mediated primarily through TLR2. The quantity of TLR2 expression on synovial fluid macrophages strongly correlated with the level of gp96 in the same synovial fluids. Further studies, using a murine model of arthritis mediated by immune complexes, demonstrated that in the normal joint, an extracellular matrix (ECM) glycoprotein, tenascin-C, was not expressed. However, tenascin-C was induced during the early phase of the arthritis, and it contributed to the progression of the arthritis, mediated through TLR4 activation of macrophages and synovial fibroblasts.[77] These observations support a potentially important role of endogenous TLR ligands in the persistent activation of macrophages and synovial fibroblasts that is observed in the joints of patients with RA.

TLR Signaling as a Target in RA

Understanding the potential role of TLRs in inflammation has led to its therapeutic exploitation. In mice with CIA, in which intradermal injections of type II collagen leads to the priming and the effector phases of inflammatory arthritis, treatment with a TLR4 antagonist both before the onset of disease and during established arthritis led to a significant reduction of arthritis.[78] Furthermore, there was decreased histologic destruction of the cartilage matrix and infiltration of inflammatory cells into the joint space. In addition, IL-1 receptor antagonist–deficient mice developed a spontaneous chronic arthritis, which was ameliorated when treated with a TLR4 antagonist.[78] The results of these animal models support the potential benefits of suppressing TLR signaling as a therapeutic approach in RA.

In ex vivo synovial tissue cultures from patients with RA, the addition of a TLR4 antagonist suppressed the spontaneous secretion of IL-1β and TNF-α, thus supporting the role of TLR4 in the production of inflammatory cytokines.[76] Currently available antirheumatic therapies that are known to have a suppressive effect on the TLR signaling pathway include hydroxychloroquine (TLR7, 8, and 9) and auranofin (TLR4). Antagonists of TLR4 are being studied for possible use in sepsis and endotoxemia. Lipid A, the innermost of the 3 regions of LPS, was created in a stable, synthetic form called E5564 (eritoran).[79] It is currently undergoing clinical trials and may become a viable agent in RA. Another TLR4 receptor antagonist, chaperonin 10 (HSP10), has been studied in a randomized, double-blind, multicenter study of 23 patients with moderate to severe active RA who received twice weekly IV therapy at different concentrations for 12 weeks. All 3 treatment groups tolerated the therapy well and had significant improvement in the primary endpoint of clinical improvement as measured by the DAS28 score. The effect seemed to be dose dependent, with 4 of 7 patients in the highest group achieving an American College of Rheumatology (ACR) 50 response and 2 of 7 achieving an ACR 70 response. The highest treatment group also had significant improvement in all secondary endpoint measures, including swollen and tender joint count, patient's assessment of pain on the visual analog scale, disability index on the health assessment questionnaire, and morning stiffness.[80] In summary, the TLR signaling pathway, which may be activated by endogenous TLR ligands or DAMPs, is a novel target for therapeutic intervention in patients with RA.

Nucleotide-binding Oligomerization Domain–like Receptors

Similar to TLRs, the NLRs are intracellular, cytosolic receptors that sense PAMPs or DAMPS and mediate an inflammatory response. Thus far, there are 22 proteins in the NLR family, including the NOD and NTPases implicated in apoptosis and multihistocompatability complex transcription leucine rich repeat protein (NALP) subfamilies, with the 14 NALPs characterizing the largest subfamily. Common features of the NLRs include a central nucleotide-binding domain, a C-terminal leucine-rich repeat domain, and N-terminal caspase-recruitment and pyrin domains.[81] The NOD proteins recognize fragments of bacterial cell-wall proteoglycans and activate the transcription factor NF-κB. Although NOD proteins are expressed in phagocytes along with TLRs, they are especially important activators of the innate response in epithelial cells, where expression of TLRs is weak or absent.[3] Members of the NALP family, including NALP1, 3, and 12, are capable of forming functional caspase-1 activation complexes, or inflammasomes, that are important in the processing and release of IL-1β and IL-18 in response to PAMPs or DAMPs.

It has been shown that the induction of SCW-driven arthritis in *NOD2* gene–deficient mice results in reduced joint swelling and decreased levels of TNF-α and IL-1β, whereas the opposite effect was seen in *NOD1*–deficient mice, suggesting an antiinflammatory role for NOD1. Moreover, the microbial ligand for NOD2, muramyl dipeptide (MDP), has been detected in RA synovium, whereas none was found in synovium from patients with OA.[82] NOD2 was expressed by both macrophages and synovial fibroblasts, as detected by immunohistochemistry, but not by lymphocytes or blood vessels. Transcription of NOD2 mRNA by RA synovial fibroblasts was induced by TNF-α, poly I:C, and LPS. Adding MDP to other inflammatory stimuli augmented RA synovial fibroblast production of inflammatory cytokines and matrix-degrading enzymes compared with the stimuli alone. These observations suggest that TLR activation may induce NOD2 expression and that TLRs and NOD2 may act synergistically in promoting inflammation and matrix destruction in the RA joint.[83] Further studies will be required to determine whether NODs may potentially become effective therapeutic targets in RA.

The Inflammasome and RA

In macrophages, the essential link between pro-IL-1β and pro-IL-18 and their bioactive counterparts is the protease caspase 1, which cleaves these molecules and generates the active cytokines that are then released from the cell.[84] Activation of caspase 1 depends on the formation of inflammasomes, which are multiprotein complexes consisting of an NLR protein such as an NALP, the adapter molecule apoptosis-associated speck-like protein containing a caspase recruitment domain (ASC), and caspase 1, and which are assembled in response to cellular recognition of DAMPs or PAMPs.[85] Inflammasomes are implicated in diseases such as systemic onset juvenile idiopathic arthritis and familial Mediterranean fever.[86,87] In addition, mutations in NALP3 are responsible for cryopyrin-associated periodic syndromes,[88] and NALP3-containing inflammasomes are activated by monosodium urate (MSU) and calcium pyrophosphate dihydrate (CPPD) crystals in gout and pseudogout, respectively.[89] In addition to MSU and CPPD crystals, other ligands of the NALP3 inflammasome include Alzheimer disease–associated amyloid deposits (amyloid-β) and the ECM components, biglycan and hyaluronan.[90]

NALP3 is expressed in the RA joint. Using real-time PCR, it has been shown that NALP3 mRNA levels were increased in RA synovium compared with OA and that monocyte-derived macrophages from healthy donors differentiated in vitro increased NALP3 expression when stimulated by TNF-α.[91] Another study did not find any differences between RA and OA synovial expression of NALP1, NALP3, NALP12, or ASC using densitometric analysis of Western blots. However, using enzyme-linked immunosorbent assay, caspase-1 levels were significantly enhanced in RA synovial tissues, even though there was no difference in concentrations of IL-1β.[92] Thus, further studies are needed to clarify the role of the inflammasome in RA pathogenesis.

Caspase 1 is not the only IL-1β converting enzyme (ICE) involved in IL-1β processing, which is likely the reason why inhibition of caspase 1 only partially inhibits experimental models of RA, whereas deficiency of IL-1β completely ameliorates the arthritis.[85] Alternative ICEs, such as elastase or proteinase 3 in neutrophils or chymase in mast cells, may be involved in the early stages of inflammatory arthritis by contributing to the processing of IL-1, whereas caspase 1 may play more of a role in the chronic stage of the arthritis.[93,94]

Retinoic Acid–inducible Gene I–like Receptors

Three genes encode RLRs in human and mouse genomes.[95] One of these genes, *RIG-I*, encodes an RNA helicase protein whose expression is induced by IFN-γ and which is found in cells such as endothelial cells, bronchial epithelial cells, smooth muscle cells, and macrophages.[96–98] It is a sensor of viral RNAs and activates cells of the innate immune system.[99] It is also associated with various chronic inflammatory diseases, including lupus nephritis, and is considered important in mediating reactions induced by IFN-γ.[100] Recently, high levels of RIG-I expression have been found in RA synovial tissues compared with OA controls. Treatment of RA synovial fibroblasts with IFN-γ significantly induced the expression of RIG-I, and knockdown of RIG-I in RA synovial fibroblasts with small interfering RNA (siRNA) resulted in the inhibition of the expression of the chemokine CXCL10.[101] In addition, RIG-I was expressed in RA synovial fibroblasts stimulated with TNF-α and knockdown of RIG-I with siRNA suppressed TNF-α–induced RANTES (chemokine (C-C motif) ligand 5 [CCL5]) expression, suggesting a possible role for the TNF-α/RIG-I/CCL5 pathway in RA pathogenesis.[102] Further studies are needed to show whether RIG-I is a plausible target for therapy in RA.

COMPLEMENT PATHWAYS
Background

The complement system is a key mediator of inflammation in the effector phase of RA. It is composed of a family of plasma proteins that act alone or in concert with antibodies to opsonize pathogens and dying cells of the host, to enhance phagocytosis, and to recruit effector cells to areas of inflammation. In addition, the coating of antigens with complement facilitates uptake by antigen-presenting cells, and thus enhances the presentation of antigen to the adaptive immune system. Several complement proteins, including C3 and C5, are present in inactive states called zymogens. A cleaved zymogen yields 2 fragments. The larger fragment is a serine protease that remains covalently bound to the immune complex or pathogen surface (eg, C3b), whereas the smaller peptide fragment acts locally as a mediator of inflammation (eg, C3a). On activation, the proteases cleave other complement proteins into their active forms, thus amplifying the response.

There are 3 pathways of complement activation. The classical pathway is initiated by the binding of C1 to antigen:antibody complexes, either circulating or tissue bound or on pathogen surfaces, or directly to the surface components of some bacteria. Once activated, C1 cleaves C2 and C4, which together forms C4b2a, the C3 convertase of the classical pathway. The lectin pathway is initiated by the binding of carbohydrate-binding proteins, such as MBL, to arrays of carbohydrates on the surface of pathogens. This pathway also leads to the creation of the C3 convertase formed by C4b2a. The alternative pathway primarily amplifies activation that is initiated by the other 2 pathways. C3b generated by the cleavage of C3 by the classical or lectin pathways is able to bind factor B that is cleaved by factor D, ultimately forming the alternative pathway C3 convertase, C3bBb. The most important activity of the C3 convertase is to cleave large numbers of C3 molecules into C3b fragments that opsonize pathogens, dying cells, and immune complexes and amplify the complement cascade. Surfaces opsonized by C3b and its derivatives are recognized by effector cells bearing CRs and can stimulate phagocytosis augment inflammatory signals in innate and adaptive cells.

Formation of the C3 convertases is the merging point of the 3-complement pathways. The next step involves the formation of the C5 convertase, which is capable of generating the most potent inflammatory peptide, C5a. Finally, the terminal complement proteins, C5b-C9, form the membrane attack complex, which constructs pores in the cell membranes of some pathogens, thus causing death. The enzymatic complement cascade is balanced by membrane and plasma proteins, such as decay-accelerating factor (DAF) or factor I, that inhibit the formation of the C3 convertase or promote its dissociation, thus preventing complement activation on normal host cells. Deficiencies in these proteins may lead to excessive complement activation and inflammation, as well as complement depletion and susceptibility to recurrent bacterial infections.[3]

Evidence of Complement Activation in Murine Models of RA

Findings from experimental models suggest roles for the alternative and classical pathways in the development of arthritis. In the CIA model, mice deficient in C3 demonstrate a significantly lower arthritis score than controls, whereas the arthritis was intermediate in mice deficient in the factor B, suggesting that C3 activation occurs via classical and alternative C3 pathways in CIA.[103] In contrast, another study found no resistance to CIA in C4-deficient mice, suggesting a more important role for the alternative pathway in this model.[104] Intriguingly, however, both CIA and a passive serum transfer model showed that injection of C4-binding protein was effective at delaying the onset of arthritis and reducing the severity of already established disease by inhibiting activity of both the classical and the alternative pathways.[105] Mice with C5 deficiency were highly resistant to CIA despite evidence of normal cellular and humoral immune responses to type II collagen and intra-articular deposition of IgG antibodies.[106] In the K/B × N serum transfer model, anti-GPI antibodies were effective at causing arthritis in mice deficient in C4, whereas no arthritis was seen in C3- or C5-deficient mice, suggesting that the pathogenesis of K/B × N serum–induced arthritis relies on activation of the alternative pathway.[107,108] Together, these observations support a major role for the alternative pathway in CIA and anti-GPI–mediated arthritis.

Evidence of Complement Activation in RA

Complement-activating immune complexes are abundant in the joints of patients with RA and seem to be the crucial mediators of the effector phase of inflammation in the pathogenesis of RA.[109–111] In RA synovial fluid, a decrease in C3 and C4 along with increased cleavage products of C3 suggests increased complement consumption within the joint.[112,113]

The concentration of C5a in plasma and synovial fluid of patients with RA is significantly higher than that in patients with OA,[114] and levels of C5a in RA synovial fluid are sufficient to induce both neutrophil chemotaxis and microvascular plasma protein leakage, 2 important features of inflammation in RA.[115] Neutrophils that migrate into inflamed joints demonstrate upregulated expression of CRs that enhance phagocytosis of material opsonized by C3b.[116] The terminal complement proteins, C5b-C9 have also been implicated in RA. Plasma levels of C5b-C9 are significantly higher in RA than in controls.[117] Compared with crystal-induced arthritis and OA, RA had significantly higher synovial fluid levels of the C5b-9 complex and were positively correlated with synovial fluid C3a and Bb levels.[118]

Further supporting the importance of the classical pathway, microparticles from RA synovial fibroblasts were found to contain abundant quantities of bound C1q, C4, and C3, as well as IgM and IgG antibodies.[119] Components of the ECM exposed during cartilage damage can also activate the classical pathway. ECM-stabilizing proteins, fibromodulin and osteoadherin, are able to bind to and activate C1q by its globular head domain, resulting in a significant deposition of C3b and C4b.[120] In addition, new activation products have recently been described in the classical complement pathway. One such molecule is a covalent complex between C1q and activated C4. The plasma levels of C1q-C4 complex were found to be significantly higher in patients with active RA compared with patients with RA in clinical remission.[121] Finally, it has been shown that human anti-CCP antibodies activate both the classical and the alternative pathways of complement in vitro.[122]

In addition to plasma and RA synovial fluid, complement-mediated inflammation is evident in RA synovial tissue. On RA synovial fibroblasts and macrophages, the cell-surface expression of the C5a receptor (C5aR) was elevated and positively correlated with joint swelling, erythrocyte sedimentation rate, and C-reactive protein levels.[123] Furthermore, aside from the classic role of the C5b-C9 complex in cell lysis, it has been shown that synovial fibroblasts are activated when exposed to sublytic concentrations of C5b-C9 in vitro. Thus, enhanced activation of synovial fibroblasts provides an additional mechanism by which complement promotes inflammation in RA.[124] Together, these observations support an important role for the classical and the alternative pathways of complement activation in the pathogenesis of RA.

Therapeutic Strategies Targeting Complement in RA

Therapies that target complement activation may be effective in ameliorating disease given that it is one of the key mediators of inflammation in the effector phase of RA. In mice, it was previously shown that inhibition of C5 with a monoclonal antibody was successful at preventing the onset of CIA and was also effective at ameliorating established disease.[125] This led to the development of eculizumab, which prevents the release of C5a and the formation of C5b-C9 complexes by inhibiting cleavage of C5 into C5a and C5b.[126] Eculizumab has been most beneficial for patients suffering with paroxysmal nocturnal hemoglobinuria. In phase 2 trials, published only in abstract form, significant improvement in RA clinical score was seen after 3 months of treatment with eculizumab, and the best responders were those patients who had high baseline levels of C5b-9 complexes in the serum.[127,128] Another approach used soluble CR1 (sCR1) derivatives that act as cofactors for complement inhibitory proteins, DAF and factor I.[129] In mice with established CIA, gene therapy with sCR inhibited the progression of CIA, reduced anticollagen antibody levels, and inhibited T-cell response to type II collagen in vitro.[130] In addition, rats with AIA were concomitantly treated with a single intra-articular dose of a membrane-targeting complement regulator derived from human CR1 (APT070) or vehicle buffer only. Animals treated with APT070 demonstrated significantly less clinical and histologic disease compared with controls after 14 days.[131] APT070 is a truncated version of sCR1 with the addition of a membrane-targeting moiety that improves protein retention at the site of inflammation, and it is currently undergoing phase 1/2 clinical trials in RA. Other potential therapies targeting complement activation have shown positive results in animal studies and include serine protease inhibitors, C3a and C5a receptor antagonists, and synthetic regulatory proteins involved in complement inhibition.[132]

FC RECEPTORS
Background

FcRs are surface molecules on myeloid cells and B cells that are capable of interacting with the Fc portion of immunoglobulin molecules. FcRs help to bridge the adaptive and innate immune responses and function as mediators of effector cell activation and inhibition, antibody-dependent cellular cytotoxicity (ADCC), and release of inflammatory mediators. For human IgG, there are 3 known activating receptors: FcγRI (CD64); FcγRIIA (CD32a); and FcγRIIIA (CD16); and 1 inhibitory receptor, FcγRIIB (CD32b). The activation receptors are distinguished by the presence of a cytoplasmic immunoreceptor tyrosine-based activation motif (ITAM), whereas the inhibitory receptor possesses an immunoreceptor tyrosine-based inhibitory motif (ITIM). Initiation of the activation pathway leads to phosphorylation of ITAM sequences by Src family kinases and recruitment and activation of spleen tyrosine kinase (Syk), ultimately resulting in activation of downstream signaling pathways such as MAP kinases that are important for cellular proliferation. On the other hand, engagement of the inhibitory pathway and phosphorylation of ITIM sequences leads to the prevention of calcium influx and thus blocks calcium-dependent processes such as degranulation, phagocytosis, ADCC, cytokine release, and proinflammatory activation. The critical step in effector cell activation by FcRs occurs via the cross-linking of the receptors by immunoglobulin. Thus, the cross-linking of 2 ITAM-bearing FcRs leads to an activation signal, whereas cross-linking of ITIM-bearing FcRs results in the arrest of effector responses. In general, both the activating and inhibitory receptors are coexpressed on myeloid cells and are engaged at the same time by circulating immune complexes or cells that have been opsonized by immunoglobulin. The threshold of effector cell activation is determined by the levels of expression of each receptor class on effector cells, as well as the ratio of an antibody's binding affinity for an activating receptor to an inhibitory receptor (A/I ratio). Therefore, either increased expression of FcγIIB or higher avidity of immunoglobulin subclass for FcγIIB results in a higher threshold for effector cell activation. Activating and inhibitory receptors may be up- and downregulated by inflammatory or inhibitory cytokines. In addition, polymorphisms of FcγRs have been described, which affect the binding affinities for specific

IgG subclasses and result in greater or lesser activation of effector cells when stimulated. Disequilibrium between activating and inhibitory FcR pathways can result in pathologic responses, and further understanding of perturbations in the FcR system that contribute to RA will aid in the development of new therapeutic strategies that target this system.[133]

FcRs in Murine Models of RA

Studying mice that are deficient in various FcRs has led to better understanding of how these receptors contribute to experimental arthritis. A role for the FcγRIIB receptor in preventing arthritis has been demonstrated using several models of arthritis. Mice with a haplotype that confers resistance to CIA were rendered susceptible to arthritis when they were made FcγRIIB deficient.[134] Similarly, FcγRIIB-deficient mice developed accelerated arthritis when they were administered anti-GPI antibody from K/B × N mice.[135] In contrast, deficiencies in activating receptors have been shown to reduce the severity of arthritis. Mice deficient in the common activating FcRγ chain were protected from CIA.[136,137] Another study showed that, although FcγRIII was critical in early development of CIA, both FcγRIII and FcγRI were dispensable for the progression to destructive joint disease, whereas the FcRγ chain was not, implying a likely role for FcγRIV, which is not expressed in humans but in mice.[138] Finally, studies using the K/B × N serum transfer model of arthritis showed absence of clinical arthritis in Fcγ chain–deficient mice, but erosive lesions in the bone still developed, suggesting separate mechanisms for inflammation and bony erosions.[135] Together, these observations support an important role for the FcγR signaling pathway in the pathogenesis of experimental models of RA.

FcRs in Patients with RA

FcRs are found on cells from patients with RA and may be associated with activation or inhibition of innate effector cells. Levels of activating receptors in plasma shed from macrophages and NK cells, as well as membrane-bound activating receptors on peripheral blood monocytes, were increased in patients with RA compared with healthy controls.[139,140] In addition, increases in the expression of activating FcRs on RA peripheral blood monocytes correlated with higher sedimentation rates, and disease-modifying antirheumatic drug (DMARD)–naive patients had significantly higher levels of activating FcγRIIA compared with patients with RA taking DMARDs, supporting an association between expression of activating FcRs and disease activity.[140] The stimulation of activating receptors on macrophages with immune complexes results in the expression of proinflammatory molecules. In vitro stimulation of healthy peripheral blood monocyte–derived macrophages with immune complexes formed by anti–citrullinated protein antibodies in sera from patients with RA resulted in significantly increased TNF-α secretion via engagement of FcγRIIA. Similar findings were seen when such cells were stimulated in vitro with immune complexes derived from RA synovial fluid.[141,142] In RA synovial tissue, significantly increased levels of activating FcRs were found to correlate with the number of synovial macrophages as well as the expression of TNF-α and matrix metalloproteinases.[143] No difference was seen between levels of inhibitory FcγRIIB expression on peripheral blood monocytes from patients and controls with RA,[144] whereas in the synovial tissue, the expression of all FcγRs, including FcγRIIB, was found to be significantly elevated in patients with RA compared with biopsies from healthy volunteers.[145] Thus, upregulation of activating receptors, rather than a paucity of inhibitory receptors, seems to contribute to the increased activation of monocytes and macrophages in RA. In addition, C-reactive protein, which is increased in RA, is capable of binding FcRs

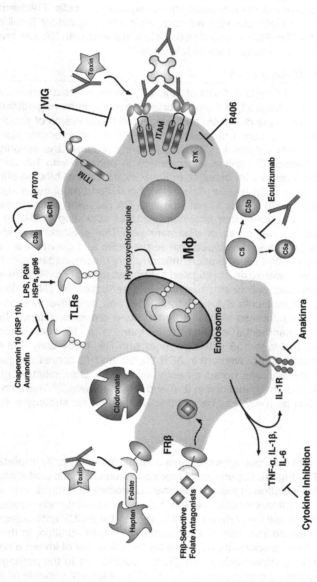

Fig. 1. Various current and novel innate immunity–directed therapeutics and their targets. IL-1R, interleukin 1 receptor; IVIG, intravenous immunoglobulin; Mφ, macrophage; sCR1, soluble complement receptor 1.

promoting the expression of proinflammatory cytokines, possibly contributing to the persistent expression of macrophage cytokines in RA.[146,147]

It has been demonstrated that FcγRIIB was selectively upregulated on monocyte-derived DCs from patients with RA with low disease activity. In vitro incubation of FcγRIIB-bearing DCs with a TLR4 agonist and immune complexes inhibited T-cell proliferation and promoted the development of regulatory T cells. Furthermore, the addition of FcγRIIB-specific blocking antibody abrogated regulatory T-cell development, suggesting that FcγRIIB expression on DCs in patients with RA with low activity may be important in the maintenance of tolerance.[48]

FcRs as Targets for Therapy in RA

Altering the balance of FcγRs in favor of inhibitory pathways is an attractive therapeutic strategy in RA. Pooled IgG from multiple donors (IV immunoglobulin) is used to treat various autoimmune diseases, and suggested mechanisms of action include blockade of activating FcRs and upregulation of FcγRIIB on effector macrophages.[148] In mice, treatment with soluble FcγRIIB significantly reduced the severity of CIA compared with controls.[149] Clinical improvement in patients with RA on DMARD therapy may be associated with changes in FcγR expression or binding affinities. In one study, the levels of activating FcγRs on peripheral blood monocytes were significantly decreased after 16 weeks in patients with RA receiving methotrexate.[150] In addition, recent data suggest that polymorphisms of activating FcγRs in patients with RA may influence outcomes of treatment with TNF-α blocking agents.[151,152] Novel approaches are being developed that target FcRs and downstream signaling pathways associated with FcR activation. Inflammatory macrophages from RA synovial fluid treated in vitro with toxin-conjugated antibodies against FcγRI were efficiently eliminated via apoptotic cell death, resulting in a reduction in TNF-α level.[153,154] Finally, a novel small molecule Syk inhibitor, R788, and its active metabolite R406 have been shown to suppress clinical arthritis, bone erosions, pannus formation, and synovitis in experimental arthritis.[155] Further, in a 12-week, randomized, placebo-controlled trial with 158 active patients with RA, twice-daily oral doses of R788 showed significant improvement in ACR 20, 50, and 70 scores compared with controls. Clinical efficacy was noted as early as 1 week after initiation of therapy and correlated with serum reductions in IL-6 and MMP-3 levels.[156] Therefore, targeting the FcR signaling pathway may be an effective therapeutic strategy in RA.

SUMMARY

Innate immunity, with macrophages playing a central role, is critically important in the pathogenesis of RA (**Fig. 1**). Experimental models document the importance in innate immune cells in the initiation of many experimental models of arthritis, promoting the development of adaptive immunity, which results in autoantibody production. In patients with RA, the presence of rheumatoid factors and anti-CCP antibodies supports the importance of innate immunity in the initiation of RA. In addition, in the joints of patients with RA, there is abundant evidence for the presence of immune complexes and the activation of complement, which directly contributes to the pathogenesis of disease. Further, immune complexes bind to FcγRs, which are capable of activating macrophages and DCs. The importance of this process is supported by the preliminary observations demonstrating that suppression of the FcγR activation pathway may be effective in treating patients with RA. Finally, synovial macrophages have clearly been demonstrated to be critically important in the pathogenesis of RA, and effective therapies result in a reduction in the number of synovial macrophages, regardless of the biologic pathway targeted. The mechanisms contributing to the persistent activation of macrophages may be a result of the expression of endogenous TLR ligands, such as gp96 and tenascin-C, which are upregulated in RA and are capable of activating macrophages through TLR signaling, thus creating a self-perpetuating, progressive chronic inflammatory process. Thus, targeting innate immunity has already proved beneficial in RA, and targeting additional pathways such as complement, the FcGR, and TLR signaling pathways holds promise for further therapeutic advances.

REFERENCES

1. Tak PP, Bresnihan B. The pathogenesis and prevention of joint damage in rheumatoid arthritis: advances from synovial biopsy and tissue analysis. Arthritis Rheum 2000;43(12):2619–33.
2. Charo IF, Ransohoff RM. The many roles of chemokines and chemokine receptors in inflammation. N Engl J Med 2006;354(6):610–21.
3. Murphy KP, Travers P, Walport M, et al. Janeway's immunobiology. 7th edition. New York: Garland Science; 2008.
4. Lavagno L, Gunella G, Bardelli C, et al. Anti-inflammatory drugs and tumor necrosis factor-alpha production from monocytes: role of transcription factor NF-kappa B and implication for rheumatoid arthritis therapy. Eur J Pharmacol 2004;501(1–3):199–208.
5. Mulherin D, Fitzgerald O, Bresnihan B. Synovial tissue macrophage populations and articular damage in rheumatoid arthritis. Arthritis Rheum 1996;39(1): 115–24.
6. Wijbrandts CA, Vergunst CE, Haringman JJ, et al. Absence of changes in the number of synovial sublining macrophages after ineffective treatment for rheumatoid arthritis: implications for use of synovial sublining macrophages as a biomarker. Arthritis Rheum 2007;56(11):3869–71.
7. Sattar N, McCarey DW, Capell H, et al. Explaining how "high-grade" systemic inflammation accelerates vascular risk in rheumatoid arthritis. Circulation 2003;108(24):2957–63.
8. Mantovani A, Sozzani S, Locati M, et al. Macrophage polarization: tumor-associated macrophages as a paradigm for polarized M2 mononuclear phagocytes. Trends Immunol 2002;23(11):549–55.
9. Vergunst CE, van de Sande MG, Lebre MC, et al. The role of chemokines in rheumatoid arthritis and osteoarthritis. Scand J Rheumatol 2005;34(6):415–25.
10. Polzer K, Baeten D, Soleiman A, et al. Tumour necrosis factor blockade increases lymphangiogenesis in murine and human arthritic joints. Ann Rheum Dis 2008;67(11):1610–6.
11. Jutila MA, Banks KL. Locally dividing macrophages in normal and inflamed mammary glands. Clin Exp Immunol 1986;66(3):615–24.
12. Ceponis A, Konttinen YT, Imai S, et al. Synovial lining, endothelial and inflammatory mononuclear cell proliferation in synovial membranes in psoriatic and reactive arthritis: a comparative quantitative morphometric study. Br J Rheumatol 1998;37(2):170–8.
13. Liva SM, Kahn MA, Dopp JM, et al. Signal transduction pathways induced by GM-CSF in microglia: significance in the control of proliferation. Glia 1999; 26(4):344–52.
14. Rekhter MD, Gordon D. Active proliferation of different cell types, including lymphocytes, in human atherosclerotic plaques. Am J Pathol 1995;147(3): 668–77.

15. Liu H, Pope RM. Apoptosis in rheumatoid arthritis: friend or foe. Rheum Dis Clin North Am 2004;30(3):603–25, x.

16. Scatizzi JC, Hutcheson J, Pope RM, et al. Bim-Bcl-2 homology 3 mimetic therapy is effective at suppressing inflammatory arthritis through the activation of myeloid cell apoptosis. Arthritis Rheum 2010;62(2):441–51.

17. Geissmann F, Auffray C, Palframan R, et al. Blood monocytes: distinct subsets, how they relate to dendritic cells, and their possible roles in the regulation of T-cell responses. Immunol Cell Biol 2008;86(5):398–408.

18. Baeten D, Boots AM, Steenbakkers PG, et al. Human cartilage gp-39+, CD16+ monocytes in peripheral blood and synovium: correlation with joint destruction in rheumatoid arthritis. Arthritis Rheum 2000;43(6):1233–43.

19. Belge KU, Dayyani F, Horelt A, et al. The proinflammatory CD14+CD16+DR++ monocytes are a major source of TNF. J Immunol 2002;168(7):3536–42.

20. Ziegler-Heitbrock L. The CD14+ CD16+ blood monocytes: their role in infection and inflammation. J Leukoc Biol 2007;81(3):584–92.

21. Geissmann F, Jung S, Littman DR. Blood monocytes consist of two principal subsets with distinct migratory properties. Immunity 2003;19(1):71–82.

22. Sunderkotter C, Nikolic T, Dillon MJ, et al. Subpopulations of mouse blood monocytes differ in maturation stage and inflammatory response. J Immunol 2004;172(7):4410–7.

23. Gordon S, Taylor PR. Monocyte and macrophage heterogeneity. Nat Rev Immunol 2005;5(12):953–64.

24. Haringman JJ, Gerlag DM, Zwinderman AH, et al. Synovial tissue macrophages: a sensitive biomarker for response to treatment in patients with rheumatoid arthritis. Ann Rheum Dis 2005;64(6):834–8.

25. Thurlings RM, Vos K, Wijbrandts CA, et al. Synovial tissue response to rituximab: mechanism of action and identification of biomarkers of response. Ann Rheum Dis 2008;67(7):917–25.

26. Bresnihan B, Pontifex E, Thurlings RM, et al. Synovial tissue sublining CD68 expression is a biomarker of therapeutic response in rheumatoid arthritis clinical trials: consistency across centers. J Rheumatol 2009;36(8):1800–2.

27. Richards PJ, Williams BD, Williams AS. Suppression of chronic streptococcal cell wall-induced arthritis in Lewis rats by liposomal clodronate. Rheumatology (Oxford) 2001;40(9):978–87.

28. Solomon S, Rajasekaran N, Jeisy-Walder E, et al. A crucial role for macrophages in the pathology of K/B × N serum-induced arthritis. Eur J Immunol 2005;35(10): 3064–73.

29. Ceponis A, Waris E, Monkkonen J, et al. Effects of low-dose, noncytotoxic, intra-articular liposomal clodronate on development of erosions and proteoglycan loss in established antigen-induced arthritis in rabbits. Arthritis Rheum 2001; 44(8):1908–16.

30. Barrera P, Blom A, van Lent PL, et al. Synovial macrophage depletion with clodronate-containing liposomes in rheumatoid arthritis. Arthritis Rheum 2000;43(9): 1951–9.

31. Nakashima-Matsushita N, Homma T, Yu S, et al. Selective expression of folate receptor beta and its possible role in methotrexate transport in synovial macrophages from patients with rheumatoid arthritis. Arthritis Rheum 1999;42(8): 1609–16.

32. Paulos CM, Turk MJ, Breur GJ, et al. Folate receptor-mediated targeting of therapeutic and imaging agents to activated macrophages in rheumatoid arthritis. Adv Drug Deliv Rev 2004;56(8):1205–17.

33. Turk MJ, Breur GJ, Widmer WR, et al. Folate-targeted imaging of activated macrophages in rats with adjuvant-induced arthritis. Arthritis Rheum 2002; 46(7):1947–55.
34. Xia W, Hilgenbrink AR, Matteson EL, et al. A functional folate receptor is induced during macrophage activation and can be used to target drugs to activated macrophages. Blood 2009;113(2):438–46.
35. van der Heijden JW, Oerlemans R, Dijkmans BA, et al. Folate receptor beta as a potential delivery route for novel folate antagonists to macrophages in the synovial tissue of rheumatoid arthritis patients. Arthritis Rheum 2009;60(1): 12–21.
36. Nagayoshi R, Nagai T, Matsushita K, et al. Effectiveness of anti-folate receptor beta antibody conjugated with truncated Pseudomonas exotoxin in the targeting of rheumatoid arthritis synovial macrophages. Arthritis Rheum 2005;52(9): 2666–75.
37. Nagai T, Tanaka M, Tsuneyoshi Y, et al. In vitro and in vivo efficacy of a recombinant immunotoxin against folate receptor beta on the activation and proliferation of rheumatoid arthritis synovial cells. Arthritis Rheum 2006;54(10):3126–34.
38. Lee S, Murthy N. Targeted delivery of catalase and superoxide dismutase to macrophages using folate. Biochem Biophys Res Commun 2007;360(1):275–9.
39. Paulos CM, Varghese B, Widmer WR, et al. Folate-targeted immunotherapy effectively treats established adjuvant and collagen-induced arthritis. Arthritis Res Ther 2006;8(3):R77.
40. Ohnmacht C, Pullner A, King SB, et al. Constitutive ablation of dendritic cells breaks self-tolerance of CD4 T cells and results in spontaneous fatal autoimmunity. J Exp Med 2009;206(3):549–59.
41. Skoberne M, Beignon AS, Larsson M, et al. Apoptotic cells at the crossroads of tolerance and immunity. Curr Top Microbiol Immunol 2005;289:259–92.
42. Ju XS, Zenke M. Differentiation of human antigen-presenting dendritic cells from CD34+ hematopoietic stem cells in vitro. Methods Mol Biol 2003;215:399–407.
43. Miloud T, Hammerling GJ, Garbi N. Review of murine dendritic cells: types, location, and development. Methods Mol Biol 2010;595:21–42.
44. Krug A, Towarowski A, Britsch S, et al. Toll-like receptor expression reveals CpG DNA as a unique microbial stimulus for plasmacytoid dendritic cells which synergizes with CD40 ligand to induce high amounts of IL-12. Eur J Immunol 2001; 31(10):3026–37.
45. Miossec P. Dynamic interactions between T cells and dendritic cells and their derived cytokines/chemokines in the rheumatoid synovium. Arthritis Res Ther 2008;10(Suppl 1):S2.
46. Lebre MC, Jongbloed SL, Tas SW, et al. Rheumatoid arthritis synovium contains two subsets of CD83-DC-LAMP- dendritic cells with distinct cytokine profiles. Am J Pathol 2008;172(4):940–50.
47. Takakubo Y, Takagi M, Maeda K, et al. Distribution of myeloid dendritic cells and plasmacytoid dendritic cells in the synovial tissues of rheumatoid arthritis. J Rheumatol 2008;35(10):1919–31.
48. Wenink MH, Santegoets KC, Roelofs MF, et al. The inhibitory Fc gamma IIb receptor dampens TLR4-mediated immune responses and is selectively up-regulated on dendritic cells from rheumatoid arthritis patients with quiescent disease. J Immunol 2009;183(7):4509–20.
49. Baldwin HM, Ito-Ihara T, Isaacs JD, et al. TNF{alpha} blockade impairs dendritic cell survival and function in rheumatoid arthritis. Ann Rheum Dis 2009. [Epub ahead of print].

50. Richez C, Schaeverbeke T, Dumoulin C, et al. Myeloid dendritic cells correlate with clinical response whereas plasmacytoid dendritic cells impact autoanti-body development in rheumatoid arthritis patients treated with infliximab. Arthritis Res Ther 2009;11(3):R100.

51. Kavousanaki M, Makrigiannakis A, Boumpas D, et al. Novel role of plasmacytoid dendritic cells in humans: induction of interleukin-10-producing Treg cells by plasmacytoid dendritic cells in patients with rheumatoid arthritis responding to therapy. Arthritis Rheum 2010;62(1):53–63.

52. Marti L, Golmia R, Golmia AP, et al. Alterations in cytokine profile and dendritic cells subsets in peripheral blood of rheumatoid arthritis patients before and after biologic therapy. Ann N Y Acad Sci 2009;1173:334–42.

53. Victoratos P, Kollias G. Induction of autoantibody-mediated spontaneous arthritis critically depends on follicular dendritic cells. Immunity 2009;30(1): 130–42.

54. Jongbloed SL, Benson RA, Nickdel MB, et al. Plasmacytoid dendritic cells regulate breach of self-tolerance in autoimmune arthritis. J Immunol 2009;182(2):963–8.

55. Ko HJ, Cho ML, Lee SY, et al. CTLA4-Ig modifies dendritic cells from mice with collagen-induced arthritis to increase the CD4+ CD25+ Foxp3+ regulatory T cell population. J Autoimmun 2010;34(2):111–20.

56. Jaen O, Rulle S, Bessis N, et al. Dendritic cells modulated by innate immunity improve collagen-induced arthritis and induce regulatory T cells in vivo. Immunology 2009;126(1):35–44.

57. Ohashi K, Burkart V, Flohe S, et al. Cutting edge: heat shock protein 60 is a putative endogenous ligand of the toll-like receptor-4 complex. J Immunol 2000; 164(2):558–61.

58. Okamura Y, Watari M, Jerud ES, et al. The extra domain A of fibronectin activates toll-like receptor 4. J Biol Chem 2001;276(13):10229–33.

59. Termeer C, Benedix F, Sleeman J, et al. Oligosaccharides of hyaluronan activate dendritic cells via toll-like receptor 4. J Exp Med 2002;195(1):99–111.

60. Huang QQ, Sobkoviak R, Jockheck-Clark AR, et al. Heat shock protein 96 is elevated in rheumatoid arthritis and activates macrophages primarily via TLR2 signaling. J Immunol 2009;182(8):4965–73.

61. Janssens S, Beyaert R. A universal role for MyD88 in TLR/IL-1R-mediated signaling. Trends Biochem Sci 2002;27(9):474–82.

62. Clark AR, Dean JL, Saklatvala J. Post-transcriptional regulation of gene expression by mitogen-activated protein kinase p38. FEBS Lett 2003;546(1):37–44.

63. Yamamoto M, Sato S, Hemmi H, et al. Role of adaptor TRIF in the MyD88-independent toll-like receptor signaling pathway. Science 2003;301(5633):640–3.

64. Iwahashi M, Yamamura M, Aita T, et al. Expression of Toll-like receptor 2 on CD16+ blood monocytes and synovial tissue macrophages in rheumatoid arthritis. Arthritis Rheum 2004;50(5):1457–67.

65. Radstake TR, Roelofs MF, Jenniskens YM, et al. Expression of toll-like receptors 2 and 4 in rheumatoid synovial tissue and regulation by proinflammatory cytokines interleukin-12 and interleukin-18 via interferon-gamma. Arthritis Rheum 2004;50(12):3856–65.

66. Seibl R, Birchler T, Loeliger S, et al. Expression and regulation of toll-like receptor 2 in rheumatoid arthritis synovium. Am J Pathol 2003;162(4):1221–7.

67. Roelofs MF, Joosten LA, Abdollahi-Roodsaz S, et al. The expression of toll-like receptors 3 and 7 in rheumatoid arthritis synovium is increased and costimulation of toll-like receptors 3, 4, and 7/8 results in synergistic cytokine production by dendritic cells. Arthritis Rheum 2005;52(8):2313–22.

68. Ospelt C, Brentano F, Rengel Y, et al. Overexpression of toll-like receptors 3 and 4 in synovial tissue from patients with early rheumatoid arthritis: toll-like receptor expression in early and longstanding arthritis. Arthritis Rheum 2008;58(12): 3684–92.
69. Kim KW, Cho ML, Lee SH, et al. Human rheumatoid synovial fibroblasts promote osteoclastogenic activity by activating RANKL via TLR-2 and TLR-4 activation. Immunol Lett 2007;110(1):54–64.
70. Huang Q, Ma Y, Adebayo A, et al. Increased macrophage activation mediated through toll-like receptors in rheumatoid arthritis. Arthritis Rheum 2007;56(7): 2192–201.
71. Kyburz D, Rethage J, Seibl R, et al. Bacterial peptidoglycans but not CpG oligodeoxynucleotides activate synovial fibroblasts by toll-like receptor signaling. Arthritis Rheum 2003;48(3):642–50.
72. Jung YO, Cho ML, Kang CM, et al. Toll-like receptor 2 and 4 combination engagement upregulate IL-15 synergistically in human rheumatoid synovial fibroblasts. Immunol Lett 2007;109(1):21–7.
73. Roelofs MF, Wenink MH, Brentano F, et al. Type I interferons might form the link between toll-like receptor (TLR) 3/7 and TLR4-mediated synovial inflammation in rheumatoid arthritis (RA). Ann Rheum Dis 2009;68(9):1486–93.
74. Shahrara S, Huang Q, Mandelin AM 2nd, et al. TH-17 cells in rheumatoid arthritis. Arthritis Res Ther 2008;10(4):R93.
75. Ivashkiv LB. Cross-regulation of signaling by ITAM-associated receptors. Nat Immunol 2009;10(4):340–7.
76. Abdollahi-Roodsaz S, Joosten LA, Koenders MI, et al. Stimulation of TLR2 and TLR4 differentially skews the balance of T cells in a mouse model of arthritis. J Clin Invest 2008;118(1):205–16.
77. Midwood K, Sacre S, Piccinini AM, et al. Tenascin-C is an endogenous activator of Toll-like receptor 4 that is essential for maintaining inflammation in arthritic joint disease. Nat Med 2009;15(7):774–80.
78. Abdollahi-Roodsaz S, Joosten LA, Roelofs MF, et al. Inhibition of toll-like receptor 4 breaks the inflammatory loop in autoimmune destructive arthritis. Arthritis Rheum 2007;56(9):2957–67.
79. Tidswell M, Tillis W, Larosa SP, et al. Phase 2 trial of eritoran tetrasodium (E5564), a toll-like receptor 4 antagonist, in patients with severe sepsis. Crit Care Med 2010;38(1):72–83.
80. Vanags D, Williams B, Johnson B, et al. Therapeutic efficacy and safety of chaperonin 10 in patients with rheumatoid arthritis: a double-blind randomised trial. Lancet 2006;368(9538):855–63.
81. Tschopp J, Martinon F, Burns K. NALPs: a novel protein family involved in inflammation. Nat Rev Mol Cell Biol 2003;4(2):95–104.
82. Joosten LA, Heinhuis B, Abdollahi-Roodsaz S, et al. Differential function of the NACHT-LRR (NLR) members Nod1 and Nod2 in arthritis. Proc Natl Acad Sci U S A 2008;105(26):9017–22.
83. Ospelt C, Brentano F, Jungel A, et al. Expression, regulation, and signaling of the pattern-recognition receptor nucleotide-binding oligomerization domain 2 in rheumatoid arthritis synovial fibroblasts. Arthritis Rheum 2009;60(2):355–63.
84. Martinon F, Burns K, Tschopp J. The inflammasome: a molecular platform triggering activation of inflammatory caspases and processing of proIL-[beta]. Mol Cell 2002;10(2):417–26.
85. Stehlik C. Multiple interleukin-1beta-converting enzymes contribute to inflammatory arthritis. Arthritis Rheum 2009;60(12):3524–30.

86. Pascual V, Allantaz F, Arce E, et al. Role of interleukin-1 (IL-1) in the pathogenesis of systemic onset juvenile idiopathic arthritis and clinical response to IL-1 blockade. J Exp Med 2005;201(9):1479–86.

87. Chae JJ, Wood G, Masters SL, et al. The B30.2 domain of pyrin, the familial Mediterranean fever protein, interacts directly with caspase-1 to modulate IL-1beta production. Proc Natl Acad Sci U S A 2006;103(26): 9982–7.

88. Lachmann HJ, Kone-Paut I, Kuemmerle-Deschner JB, et al. Use of canakinumab in the cryopyrin-associated periodic syndrome. N Engl J Med 2009; 360(23):2416–25.

89. Martinon F, Petrilli V, Mayor A, et al. Gout-associated uric acid crystals activate the NALP3 inflammasome. Nature 2006;440(7081):237–41.

90. Schaefer L. Extracellular matrix molecules: endogenous danger signals as new drug targets in kidney diseases. Curr Opin Pharmacol 2010;10(2):185–90.

91. Rosengren S, Hoffman HM, Bugbee W, et al. Expression and regulation of cryopyrin and related proteins in rheumatoid arthritis synovium. Ann Rheum Dis 2005;64(5):708–14.

92. Kolly L, Busso N, Palmer G, et al. Expression and function of the NALP3 inflammasome in rheumatoid synovium. Immunology 2010;129(2):178–85.

93. Joosten LA, Netea MG, Fantuzzi G, et al. Inflammatory arthritis in caspase 1 gene-deficient mice: contribution of proteinase 3 to caspase 1-independent production of bioactive interleukin-1beta. Arthritis Rheum 2009;60(12): 3651–62.

94. Guma M, Ronacher L, Liu-Bryan R, et al. Caspase 1-independent activation of interleukin-1beta in neutrophil-predominant inflammation. Arthritis Rheum 2009; 60(12):3642–50.

95. Yoneyama M, Kikuchi M, Matsumoto K, et al. Shared and unique functions of the DExD/H-box helicases RIG-I, MDA5, and LGP2 in antiviral innate immunity. J Immunol 2005;175(5):2851–8.

96. Imaizumi T, Aratani S, Nakajima T, et al. Retinoic acid-inducible gene-I is induced in endothelial cells by LPS and regulates expression of COX-2. Biochem Biophys Res Commun 2002;292(1):274–9.

97. Imaizumi T, Yagihashi N, Hatakeyama M, et al. Expression of retinoic acid-inducible gene-I in vascular smooth muscle cells stimulated with interferon-gamma. Life Sci 2004;75(10):1171–80.

98. Imaizumi T, Yagihashi N, Kubota K, et al. Expression of retinoic acid-inducible gene-I (RIG-I) in macrophages: possible involvement of RIG-I in atherosclerosis. J Atheroscler Thromb 2007;14(2):51–5.

99. Yoneyama M, Kikuchi M, Natsukawa T, et al. The RNA helicase RIG-I has an essential function in double-stranded RNA-induced innate antiviral responses. Nat Immunol 2004;5(7):730–7.

100. Suzuki K, Imaizumi T, Tsugawa K, et al. Expression of retinoic acid-inducible gene-I in lupus nephritis. Nephrol Dial Transplant 2007;22(8):2407–9.

101. Imaizumi T, Arikawa T, Sato T, et al. Involvement of retinoic acid-inducible gene-I in inflammation of rheumatoid fibroblast-like synoviocytes. Clin Exp Immunol 2008;153(2):240–4.

102. Imaizumi T, Matsumiya T, Yoshida H, et al. Tumor-necrosis factor-alpha induces retinoic acid-inducible gene-I in rheumatoid fibroblast-like synoviocytes. Immunol Lett 2009;122(1):89–93.

103. Hietala MA, Jonsson IM, Tarkowski A, et al. Complement deficiency ameliorates collagen-induced arthritis in mice. J Immunol 2002;169(1):454–9.

104. Banda NK, Thurman JM, Kraus D, et al. Alternative complement pathway activation is essential for inflammation and joint destruction in the passive transfer model of collagen-induced arthritis. J Immunol 2006;177(3):1904–12.

105. Blom AM, Nandakumar KS, Holmdahl R. C4b-binding protein (C4BP) inhibits development of experimental arthritis in mice. Ann Rheum Dis 2009;68(1):136–42.

106. Wang Y, Kristan J, Hao L, et al. A role for complement in antibody-mediated inflammation: C5-deficient DBA/1 mice are resistant to collagen-induced arthritis. J Immunol 2000;164(8):4340–7.

107. Solomon S, Kolb C, Mohanty S, et al. Transmission of antibody-induced arthritis is independent of complement component 4 (C4) and the complement receptors 1 and 2 (CD21/35). Eur J Immunol 2002;32(3):644–51.

108. Ji H, Ohmura K, Mahmood U, et al. Arthritis critically dependent on innate immune system players. Immunity 2002;16(2):157–68.

109. Aho K, Palosuo T, Raunio V, et al. When does rheumatoid disease start? Arthritis Rheum 1985;28(5):485–9.

110. Rantapaa-Dahlqvist S, de Jong BA, Berglin E, et al. Antibodies against cyclic citrullinated peptide and IgA rheumatoid factor predict the development of rheumatoid arthritis. Arthritis Rheum 2003;48(10):2741–9.

111. Mewar D, Wilson AG. Autoantibodies in rheumatoid arthritis: a review. Biomed Pharmacother 2006;60(10):648–55.

112. Moxley G, Ruddy S. Elevated C3 anaphylatoxin levels in synovial fluids from patients with rheumatoid arthritis. Arthritis Rheum 1985;28(10):1089–95.

113. Swaak AJ, Van Rooyen A, Planten O, et al. An analysis of the levels of complement components in the synovial fluid in rheumatic diseases. Clin Rheumatol 1987;6(3):350–7.

114. Hogasen K, Mollnes TE, Harboe M, et al. Terminal complement pathway activation and low lysis inhibitors in rheumatoid arthritis synovial fluid. J Rheumatol 1995;22(1):24–8.

115. Jose PJ, Moss IK, Maini RN, et al. Measurement of the chemotactic complement fragment C5a in rheumatoid synovial fluids by radioimmunoassay: role of C5a in the acute inflammatory phase. Ann Rheum Dis 1990;49(10):747–52.

116. Crockard AD, Thompson JM, McBride SJ, et al. Markers of inflammatory activation: upregulation of complement receptors CR1 and CR3 on synovial fluid neutrophils from patients with inflammatory joint disease. Clin Immunol Immunopathol 1992;65(2):135–42.

117. Corvetta A, Pomponio G, Rinaldi N, et al. Terminal complement complex in synovial tissue from patients affected by rheumatoid arthritis, osteoarthritis and acute joint trauma. Clin Exp Rheumatol 1992;10(5):433–8.

118. Brodeur JP, Ruddy S, Schwartz LB, et al. Synovial fluid levels of complement SC5b-9 and fragment Bb are elevated in patients with rheumatoid arthritis. Arthritis Rheum 1991;34(12):1531–7.

119. Biro E, Nieuwland R, Tak PP, et al. Activated complement components and complement activator molecules on the surface of cell-derived microparticles in patients with rheumatoid arthritis and healthy individuals. Ann Rheum Dis 2007;66(8):1085–92.

120. Sjoberg AP, Manderson GA, Morgelin M, et al. Short leucine-rich glycoproteins of the extracellular matrix display diverse patterns of complement interaction and activation. Mol Immunol 2009;46(5):830–9.

121. Wouters D, Voskuyl AE, Molenaar ET, et al. Evaluation of classical complement pathway activation in rheumatoid arthritis: measurement of C1q-C4 complexes as novel activation products. Arthritis Rheum 2006;54(4):1143–50.

122. Trouw LA, Haisma EM, Levarht EW, et al. Anti-cyclic citrullinated peptide antibodies from rheumatoid arthritis patients activate complement via both the classical and alternative pathways. Arthritis Rheum 2009;60(7): 1923–31.

123. Yuan G, Wei J, Zhou J, et al. Expression of C5aR (CD88) of synoviocytes isolated from patients with rheumatoid arthritis and osteoarthritis. Chin Med J (Engl) 2003;116(9):1408–12.

124. Jahn B, Von Kempis J, Kramer KL, et al. Interaction of the terminal complement components C5b-9 with synovial fibroblasts: binding to the membrane surface leads to increased levels in collagenase-specific mRNA. Immunology 1993; 78(2):329–34.

125. Wang Y, Rollins SA, Madri JA, et al. Anti-C5 monoclonal antibody therapy prevents collagen-induced arthritis and ameliorates established disease. Proc Natl Acad Sci U S A 1995;92(19):8955–9.

126. Thomas TC, Rollins SA, Rother RP, et al. Inhibition of complement activity by humanized anti-C5 antibody and single-chain Fv. Mol Immunol 1996; 33(17–18):1389–401.

127. Tesser J, Kivitz A, Fleischmann R, et al. Safety and efficacy of the humanized anti-C5 antibody h5G1.1 in patients with rheumatoid arthritis. Arthritis Rheum 2001;44(9):S274.

128. Burch F, Tesser J, Bell L, et al. Baseline C5b-9 level correlates with CRP and ACR 20 response to the humanized anti-C5 antibody h5G1.1 in patients with rheumatoid arthritis. Arthritis Rheum 2001;44(9):S214.

129. Krych-Goldberg M, Atkinson JP. Structure-function relationships of complement receptor type 1. Immunol Rev 2001;180:112–22.

130. Dreja H, Annenkov A, Chernajovsky Y. Soluble complement receptor 1 (CD35) delivered by retrovirally infected syngeneic cells or by naked DNA injection prevents the progression of collagen-induced arthritis. Arthritis Rheum 2000; 43(8):1698–709.

131. Linton SM, Williams AS, Dodd I, et al. Therapeutic efficacy of a novel membrane-targeted complement regulator in antigen-induced arthritis in the rat. Arthritis Rheum 2000;43(11):2590–7.

132. Mizuno M. A review of current knowledge of the complement system and the therapeutic opportunities in inflammatory arthritis. Curr Med Chem 2006; 13(14):1707–17.

133. Paul WE. Fundamental immunology. 6th edition. Philadelphia: Wolters Kluwer/Lippincott Williams & Wilkins; 2008.

134. Yuasa T, Kubo S, Yoshino T, et al. Deletion of fcgamma receptor IIB renders H-2(b) mice susceptible to collagen-induced arthritis. J Exp Med 1999;189(1): 187–94.

135. Corr M, Crain B. The role of FcgammaR signaling in the K/B x N serum transfer model of arthritis. J Immunol 2002;169(11):6604–9.

136. Kleinau S, Martinsson P, Heyman B. Induction and suppression of collagen-induced arthritis is dependent on distinct fcgamma receptors. J Exp Med 2000;191(9):1611–6.

137. Kagari T, Tanaka D, Doi H, et al. Essential role of Fc gamma receptors in anti-type II collagen antibody-induced arthritis. J Immunol 2003;170(8): 4318–24.

138. Boross P, van Lent PL, Martin-Ramirez J, et al. Destructive arthritis in the absence of both FcgammaRI and FcgammaRIII. J Immunol 2008;180(7): 5083–91.

139. Masuda M, Morimoto T, De Haas M, et al. Increase of soluble FcgRIIIa derived from natural killer cells and macrophages in plasma from patients with rheumatoid arthritis. J Rheumatol 2003;30(9):1911–7.

140. Wijngaarden S, van Roon JA, Bijlsma JW, et al. Fcgamma receptor expression levels on monocytes are elevated in rheumatoid arthritis patients with high erythrocyte sedimentation rate who do not use anti-rheumatic drugs. Rheumatology (Oxford) 2003;42(5):681–8.

141. Clavel C, Nogueira L, Laurent L, et al. Induction of macrophage secretion of tumor necrosis factor alpha through Fcgamma receptor IIa engagement by rheumatoid arthritis-specific autoantibodies to citrullinated proteins complexed with fibrinogen. Arthritis Rheum 2008;58(3):678–88.

142. Mathsson L, Lampa J, Mullazehi M, et al. Immune complexes from rheumatoid arthritis synovial fluid induce FcgammaRIIa dependent and rheumatoid factor correlated production of tumour necrosis factor-alpha by peripheral blood mononuclear cells. Arthritis Res Ther 2006;8(3):R64.

143. Blom AB, Radstake TR, Holthuysen AE, et al. Increased expression of Fcgamma receptors II and III on macrophages of rheumatoid arthritis patients results in higher production of tumor necrosis factor alpha and matrix metalloproteinase. Arthritis Rheum 2003;48(4):1002–14.

144. Wijngaarden S, van de Winkel JG, Jacobs KM, et al. A shift in the balance of inhibitory and activating Fcgamma receptors on monocytes toward the inhibitory Fcgamma receptor IIb is associated with prevention of monocyte activation in rheumatoid arthritis. Arthritis Rheum 2004;50(12):3878–87.

145. Magnusson SE, Engstrom M, Jacob U, et al. High synovial expression of the inhibitory FcgammaRIIb in rheumatoid arthritis. Arthritis Res Ther 2007;9(3):R51.

146. Du Clos TW. C-reactive protein as a regulator of autoimmunity and inflammation. Arthritis Rheum 2003;48(6):1475–7.

147. Bharadwaj D, Stein MP, Volzer M, et al. The major receptor for C-reactive protein on leukocytes is fcgamma receptor II. J Exp Med 1999;190(4):585–90.

148. Nimmerjahn F, Ravetch JV. Anti-inflammatory actions of intravenous immunoglobulin. Annu Rev Immunol 2008;26:513–33.

149. Magnusson SE, Andren M, Nilsson KE, et al. Amelioration of collagen-induced arthritis by human recombinant soluble FcgammaRIIb. Clin Immunol 2008; 127(2):225–33.

150. Wijngaarden S, van Roon JA, van de Winkel JG, et al. Down-regulation of activating Fcgamma receptors on monocytes of patients with rheumatoid arthritis upon methotrexate treatment. Rheumatology (Oxford) 2005;44(6):729–34.

151. Tutuncu Z, Kavanaugh A, Zvaifler N, et al. Fcgamma receptor type IIIA polymorphisms influence treatment outcomes in patients with inflammatory arthritis treated with tumor necrosis factor alpha-blocking agents. Arthritis Rheum 2005;52(9):2693–6.

152. Canete JD, Suarez B, Hernandez MV, et al. Influence of variants of Fc gamma receptors IIA and IIIA on the American College of Rheumatology and European League Against Rheumatism responses to anti-tumour necrosis factor alpha therapy in rheumatoid arthritis. Ann Rheum Dis 2009;68(10):1547–52.

153. van Roon JA, van Vuuren AJ, Wijngaarden S, et al. Selective elimination of synovial inflammatory macrophages in rheumatoid arthritis by an Fcgamma receptor I-directed immunotoxin. Arthritis Rheum 2003;48(5):1229–38.

154. van Roon JA, Bijlsma JW, van de Winkel JG, et al. Depletion of synovial macrophages in rheumatoid arthritis by an anti-FcgammaRI-calicheamicin immunoconjugate. Ann Rheum Dis 2005;64(6):865–70.

155. Pine PR, Chang B, Schoettler N, et al. Inflammation and bone erosion are suppressed in models of rheumatoid arthritis following treatment with a novel Syk inhibitor. Clin Immunol 2007;124(3):244–57.
156. Weinblatt ME, Kavanaugh A, Burgos-Vargas R, et al. Treatment of rheumatoid arthritis with a Syk kinase inhibitor: a twelve-week, randomized, placebo-controlled trial. Arthritis Rheum 2008;58(11):3309–18.

Immune Aging and Rheumatoid Arthritis

Jorg J. Goronzy, MD, Lan Shao, PhD, Cornelia M. Weyand, MD*

KEYWORDS

- Immunosenescence • Aging • Autoimmunity
- Rheumatoid arthritis • Telomere

Rheumatoid arthritis (RA) is a chronic inflammatory disease that manifests predominantly as synovial inflammation leading to cartilage damage and destruction of the joint infrastructure. Although the joint symptomatology is eventually dominant, the disease is preceded by immune abnormalities that are not joint-specific, but systemic and already apparent many years before onset of the disease.[1] The best defined autoimmune phenomena are antibody responses against immunoglobulin (Ig)G and against citrullinated peptides, self-antigens, or neoantigens that are ubiquitously expressed. Although the focus of research in the 1990s was on identifying a tolerance defect to a joint-specific antigen,[2] the last decade has seen a shift to the model that patients with RA have a fundamental breakdown in self-tolerance and that patients are not able to induce or maintain tolerance to neoantigens.[3] This breakdown in tolerance occurs in the second half of life, suggesting that it is acquired.[4] Most patients who develop disease are postmenopausal women; indeed the incidence of the disease continues to rise at least into the seventh decade of life and possibly even beyond that.[4,5] The relationship between RA incidence and age is inverse to that of immunocompetence and age as illustrated in **Fig. 1** for thymic epithelial space (TES) and frequency of recent thymic emigrants.

AGING AS A RISK FACTOR FOR AUTOIMMUNITY

The age relationship of RA is different from that of organ-specific autoimmune diseases, such as diabetes mellitus or systemic lupus erythematosus that peak earlier in life. RA does not stand alone in this aspect, however; age is a major risk factor in many other chronic inflammatory diseases, most notable in giant cell arteritis.[6–8] This important role of age in the development of selected autoimmune diseases raises questions whether immune aging is a contributing factor and tolerance defects are

This work was supported by grant R01 AR 41974, R01 AR 42527, R01 EY 11916, R01 AG 15043, R01 AI 44142, U19 AI 57266, and P01 HL58000 from the National Institutes of Health.
Division of Immunology and Rheumatology, Department of Medicine, Stanford University, 269 West Campus Drive, Stanford, CA 94305-5166, USA
* Corresponding author.
E-mail address: jgoronzy@stanford.edu

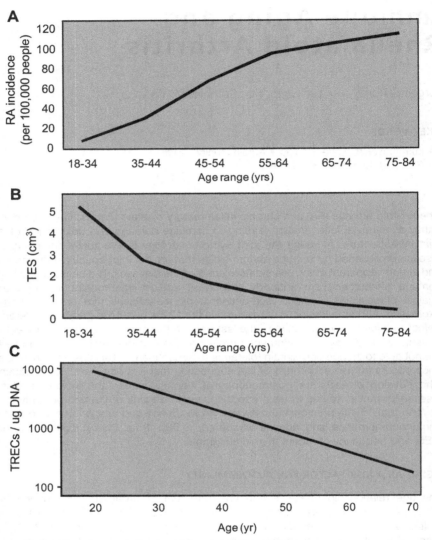

Fig. 1. Thymic function and rheumatoid arthritis (RA) incidence—an inverse relationship. The incidence of RA (*A*) is low before menopause and peaks in the seventh to eighth decades of life. Thymic function rapidly declines with age and is minimal after the age of 40 years. Shown are the involution of thymic epithelial space (TES) (*B*) and the frequencies of recent thymic emigrants as estimated by the concentrations of peripheral T-cells with T-cell receptor excision circles (TREC) (*C*). (*From* Goronzy JJ, Weyand CM. Rheumatoid arthritis. Immunol Rev 2005;204:62; with permission.)

part of the degenerative process of the immune system. Indeed, autoantibodies are a common finding in healthy elderly.[9] Of interest, many of these autoantibodies are specific for common autoantigens, such as rheumatoid factor and antinuclear antibodies, while tissue-specific antibodies do not appear to be a normal by-product of immune aging. Studies on the frequency of anti-cyclic citrullinated peptide (CCP) antibodies with age are not yet available. In general, the age-related rheumatoid factors are low titered, but otherwise not different from the autoantibodies in autoimmune diseases.

The concept that autoimmune disease is a consequence of immune aging is counterintuitive. In general, the aged immune system is less responsive to antigenic challenges; it is more difficult in the elderly to elicit an immune response to an antigen than in young adult.[10,11] As a consequence, vaccine responses decline with age.[12–14] Autoantigens, perhaps with the exception of neoantigens, are by definition low-affinity antigens, because high affinity receptors have been purged from the repertoire by negative selection. How, therefore, can an immune system that is insufficient to generate an adaptive immune response to an exogenous antigen, such as a vaccine, be able to overcome tolerance and generate immune responses to auto- or neoantigens? As always in science, identifying an obvious paradox and overcoming its conundrum provide an opportunity to take a qualitative pivotal step in understanding the mechanisms of a disease.

IMMUNE AGING—WHAT DO WE KNOW?

The immunologic evidence of immune aging is illustrated best by the increasing incidence and morbidity of infections, the failure to mount vaccine responses and the reactivation of chronic viral infections with age. Epidemiologic data suggest that clinical evidence of immune aging is already present, albeit subtle, in the middle-aged adult. Examples include the incidence of herpes zoster reactivation that starts to increase after the age of 50 years,[15,16] the increased hospitalization and mortality rates of influenza infections that also increase after the age of 50,[17] and also vaccine responses such as the response to hepatitis B vaccination, which already starts to decline after the age of 40 years.[18] Thus, immune aging is not only a feature of the very elderly, but emerges as a clinical complication already in the middle-aged adult, approximately at the same age when the susceptibility to develop RA increases.[4,6] Immune failure becomes severe in the eighth decade of life in healthy individuals.[19,20] If autoimmunity is a consequence of immune aging, but still requires a functional immune system, one would predict that the incidence of autoimmune diseases will start to dip again in the very elderly.

Immune aging affects both the innate and the adaptive immune systems. The innate immune system is constitutively activated in the elderly and the concentration of inflammatory cytokines, in particular interleukin (IL)-6, increases.[21] This proinflammatory environment accelerates and complicates numerous degenerative diseases; the classical example is the inflammation in the atherosclerotic plaque that leads to plaque rupture and acute coronary syndromes.[22,23] The mechanisms underlying this innate immune activation are not clear, but possibly are a consequence of the declining adaptive immune response. Most studies of immune senescence have focused on the adaptive system, and several defects have been described. It has been hypothesized that the defect in T-cell immunity is causatively related to the declining thymic generation of new naïve cells.[24] By the age of 40 to 50 years, thymic activity is severely limited, and the homeostasis of the T-cell compartment entirely depends on peripheral mechanisms that regulate the proliferation and survival of naïve and memory T-cells. As a consequence, the frequency of naïve T-cells declines with age, a phenomenon that is markedly more pronounced in the CD8 than the CD4 compartment.[25] The replicative stress associated with immune responses to exogenous antigen, but also due to the homeostatic proliferation to maintain a full peripheral T-cell compartment in the absence of thymic production, is associated with decline in telomere lengths, and epigenetic changes, and accumulation of effector subpopulations, in particular in the CD8 compartment.[25–27] Individual T-cells are still responsive to stimulation by exogenous antigen. Although signaling defects have been described in elderly T-cells, they alone are usually not sufficient to suppress an immune response. It is this environment in which RA and its autoimmune manifestations develop.

ACCELERATED IMMUNE AGING IN RA

The epidemiologic data clearly show that age is an important risk factor for developing RA. The obvious next question then is what the biologic age of a patient with RA is. Is the aging of the adaptive immune system age-appropriate? Is it decelerated, leading to better-preserved T-cell immune responsiveness in an otherwise aging host? Or is it accelerated such that immune responses already have declined beyond the actual age of the individual? Early evidence from T-cell depletion studies already suggested that RA patients have difficulty in regenerating the immune system.[28] In general, therapeutic T-cell depletion yielded only moderate benefits, but significant adverse effects. This was most evident for patients treated with an anti-CD52 antibody (alemtuzumab) that very effectively depletes T-cells. Many of these treated patients stayed lymphopenic for a long period of time after treatment, and in those patients who had a sizable recovery of T-cells, the population was highly oligoclonal, suggesting that the T-cells were derived from a few progenitor cells.[28,29] The same clonally expanded populations that were present in the peripheral blood also were found in the synovial tissue of RA patients who maintained disease activity.[30] Longitudinal studies in these patients showed that the lymphopenia in these patients persisted over decades. Of interest, other autoimmune phenomena developed in some of the anti-CD52-treated patients, consistent with the view that tolerance is more difficult to maintain in a lymphopenic host.[31]

Subsequent studies have shown that impaired T-cell regenerative capacity and evidence for replicative stress in the peripheral T-cell compartment are already features in RA patients who have not undergone T-cell depletion.[32] The frequency of T-cell receptor excision circles (TRECs), frequently used as a surrogate measurement for thymic activity, declines in normal healthy individuals between the age of 20 and 65 by about 95%.[33,34] TRECs are episomes generated during T-cell receptor rearrangements and are likely to persist in nonproliferating cells, but are not transmitted to all daughter cells during division. TREC frequencies are therefore the net result of two events: generation of new TREC-positive cells from the thymus and loss of TREC-positive T-cells by peripheral proliferation or cell loss.[35] RA patients have an age-inappropriate decrease in TREC frequencies, suggesting that they either have reduced thymic output, increased peripheral T-cell apoptosis and proliferation, or a combination of both.[32,36] Obviously, these two processes do not need to be independent, because decreased thymic production has to be compensated with increased peripheral proliferation to maintain the size of the compartment.[37,38] Indeed, the peripheral T-cell compartment in RA patients exhibits evidence for replicative stress. T-cells, like other cells that proliferate, lose sequence stretches at their chromosomal ends, called telomeres, with each division.[39] They also change their phenotype and function; in particular, they lose the expression of the costimulatory molecule CD28.[40,41] When assessed using any or all of these senescence markers, the repertoire of T-cells in patients with RA is pre-aged by approximately 20 years. Telomeric ends are shortened; frequencies of CD28-negative T-cells are increased, and T-cell repertoire diversity is contracted, consistent with excessive T-cell loss and oligoclonal expansion.[32,42–44] Similar evidence for accelerated immune aging also has been shown for some, but not all, other autoimmune diseases. Most notable is multiple sclerosis, which is also associated with reduced TREC numbers and increased frequency of CD28-negative cells. Other chronic inflammatory diseases, such as the spondylarthropathies (which often begin in early adulthood), do not show any evidence for accelerated immune aging.[45]

ACCELERATED IMMUNE AGING—A PRIMARY OR SECONDARY EVENT?

In any inflammatory disease, the question arises whether observed findings are a primary event involved in the pathogenesis of the disease or a secondary event caused by disease-induced inflammation. Several studies have shown that accelerated immune aging is a phenomenon found in patients with early RA and is not influenced by disease duration or treatment.[32,43,46,47] Also, in longitudinal studies, the frequency of CD28-negative T-cells early in the disease is predictive of severity in joint erosion on follow-up and the frequency of extra-articular disease manifestations in cross-sectional studies.[48,49] These observations have been interpreted in favor of immune aging as a primary event involved in disease pathogenesis and not as a consequence of the presence of inflammatory cytokines. Exceptions to this interpretation do exist (eg, transcription of the CD28 gene in young T-cells can be significantly down-regulated by TNF-α).[50,51] The mechanism of TNF-mediated gene repression is the same as that which occurs with replicative T-cell aging. Under the influence of TNF, naïve T-cells lose the expression of an initiation factor that is necessary to induce CD28 transcription. However, the TNF-mediated CD28 repression is not complete and is readily reversible, which is in contrast to the CD28 loss that is seen with replicative senescence or in RA patients. All T-cells from patients with RA have reduced cell surface expression of CD28 when measured by flow cytometry, while only few have a complete CD28 loss. Full CD28 expression recovers in CD28-low T-cells with short-term cultures in vitro or with anti-TNF treatment in vivo. In contrast, CD28 loss in most cases is not reversible with anti-TNF-α. On the contrary, CD28 expression in at least some cells can be restored by another inflammatory cytokine, IL-12.[52]

The most convincing evidence that accelerated immune aging is primary (or at least not exclusively secondary) comes from genetic studies. Increased loss of CD28 on peripheral T-cells has been found to be associated with the HLA-DRB1*04 genotype, which also predisposes to RA.[5,46,48,53,54] In healthy individuals, the frequencies of CD28-negative cells have been found to be correlated to cytomegalovirus (CMV) infection.[55] This correlation is maintained in patients with RA, suggesting that CMV infection and accelerated aging rather than activity of the rheumatic disease are key risk factors that lead to senescence of the cell population.[45] HLA-DRB1*04 also is associated with accelerated telomeric shortening in healthy controls. Schönland and colleagues[46] have shown that HLA-DRB1*04-positive individuals have shorter telomeres in several hematopoietic stem cell-derived populations including neutrophils and naïve and memory T-cells. This telomeric shortening was cell-specific for hematopoietic lineages and not found in sperm cells of HLA-DRB1*04-positive donors. The difference in telomere lengths is acquired, since no HLA-related difference was seen in cord blood T-cells. These studies led to the interpretation that the major disease risk gene for RA, HLA-DRB1*04, predisposes for at least two aging features in normal individuals, telomere shortening in hematopoietic stem cell lineages and loss of CD28 in peripheral T-cell memory cell populations. In contrast, the HLA-DR4 haplotype was not associated with reduced frequency of TRECs as a marker of thymic activity or peripheral cell death, suggesting that the features of accelerated aging observed in RA patients are at least partially independent and may be additive or even synergistic.

MECHANISM OF ACCELERATED IMMUNE AGING IN RA

One of the most striking markers of aging in a highly proliferative compartment is telomeric erosion. Telomeres are protein-DNA complexes at the end of eukaryotic chromosomes that protect from fusion and degradation. Telomeric DNA is composed of repeats of G-rich sequences that are packed with a number of DNA-binding proteins involved in protection and repair.[56] In the absence of the enzyme telomerase, telomeric sequences are duplicated incompletely, with loss of 40 to 200 base pairs during each cell division. Telomeric lengths therefore can be taken as a marker of the replicative history of individual cells or a population of cells. Critically short telomeres become uncapped and recruit components of the DNA damage repair machinery, such that cells enter replicative senescence or apoptosis. Telomeric erosion is counteracted by an enzyme, telomerase, that only is expressed in selected cell types, including stem cells, sperms, and lymphocytes.[27] Even in stem cells, and certainly in lymphocytes, telomeric repair is incomplete, and telomeric erosion occurs progressively with age.[46]

The age-inappropriate accelerated telomeric erosion found in lymphocytes of patients with RA could be caused by several mechanisms, either acting alone or in concert. Telomeric erosion could reflect an increased proliferative history of lymphocytes or their precursor cells,[32] or be caused by defective telomerase expression or activity.[57,58] Alternatively, telomeric shortening could be the result of excessive DNA damage rather than replication-induced telomeric loss[47,57] (**Fig. 2**). Data on patients with RA indicate that all three of these different mechanisms play a role. Frequencies of hematopoietic stem cells in RA patients are age-inappropriately reduced, and their telomeres are already shortened, indicating that the hematopoietic stem cell system is under replicative stress.[59] Increased proliferation of peripheral naïve and memory T-cells may aggravate this defect. In support of this interpretation, the reduced frequency of TREC-positive cells either indicates reduced thymic activity or accelerated peripheral death of TREC-positive cells; both would increase homeostatic proliferation to maintain the compartment size.[19] It is of interest to note that telomeric erosion in hematopoietic stem cells, but not a reduced number of TRECs, is also found in healthy HLA-DRB1*04-positive individuals,[32] suggesting that two independent age-related mechanisms contribute to the accelerated immune aging in RA patients, one of them influenced by the disease-associated major histocompatability complex (MHC) region.

Telomerase is a reverse transcriptase composed of a catalytic protein encoded by the hTERT gene and an RNA component encoded by hTERC that contains a sequence complementary to the G-rich telomeric strands. hTERC serves as a template for the addition of telomeric repeats at the ends of chromosomes. The telomerase activity appears to be limited primarily by the expression of the catalytic subunit, hTERT. The gene is silent in most somatic cells. Transcriptional regulation and post-transcriptional regulation of hTERT expression are complex and involves epigenetic modifications, overcoming of negative regulatory factors such as tumor suppressors and inhibitory cytokines and hormones, and hTERT phosphorylation and NFκB-mediated nuclear translocation. hTERT transcription is induced in naïve, and to a much lesser degree in memory T-cells upon T-cell receptor-mediated activation.[39]

Fujii and colleagues[58] examined telomeric repair mechanisms in naïve CD4 T-cells from patients with RA. The authors found a blunted induction of telomerase activity

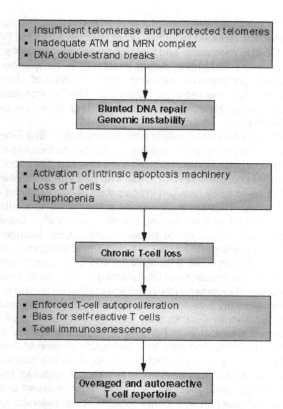

- Insufficient telomerase and unprotected telomeres
- Inadequate ATM and MRN complex
- DNA double-strand breaks

↓

**Blunted DNA repair
Genomic instability**

↓

- Activation of intrinsic apoptosis machinery
- Loss of T cells
- Lymphopenia

↓

Chronic T-cell loss

↓

- Enforced T-cell autoproliferation
- Bias for self-reactive T cells
- T-cell immunosenescence

↓

**Overaged and autoreactive
T cell repertoire**

Fig. 2. DNA instability and autoreactivity in RA. Stability and intactness of DNA and its telomeric ends are critically involved in regulating vitality, proliferative capacity, and longevity of lymphocytes. In RA, T-cell telomerase is insufficiently produced, and DNA double-strand breaks are left unrepaired, causing chronic stimulation of cellular checkpoint pathways and DNA repair activity. As a consequence, RA T-cells are highly apoptosis-sensitive, and the T-cell pool is inadequately replenished. In the absence of thymic T-cell generation, lymphopenia initiates T-cell autoproliferation. Chronic replicative stress exhausts the T-cells' replicative reserve, rendering them senescent. As T-cell renewal depends on tickling of the T-cell receptor, T-cells that recognize autoantigens are preferentially expanded. *Abbreviations:* ATM, ataxia telangiectasia mutated; MRN, MRE11-RAD50-NBS1. (*From* Weyand CM, Fujii H, Shao L, et al. Rejuvenating the immune system in rheumatoid arthritis. Nat Rev Rheumatol 2009;5:587; with permission.)

caused by reduced hTERT transcription, to about half the level that is seen healthy age-matched controls. This reduced telomerase activity in conjunction with homeostatic proliferation could be responsible for the telomeric erosion that is seen in patients with RA.[58] The authors, however, describe a function of telomerase that goes beyond preventing telomeric erosion. Although telomeres in naïve T-cells, either in healthy controls or in RA patients, are not critically short, the insufficient telomerase induction in RA T-cells after activation was closely correlated with increased cell death during cellular expansion. Mechanistic studies confirmed the interpretation that telomerase supports cell survival independent of telomeric erosion. Knockdown of hTERT expression in healthy T-cells resulted in increased apoptotic cell death through the internal pathway; in contrast, overexpression of hTERT in RA T-cells improved their survival. In summary, the reduced induction of telomerase activity in RA patients influences peripheral T-cell homeostasis and function by two mechanisms, first, increased susceptibility to undergo apoptosis during proliferation independent of telomeric lengths, and second, progressive telomeric erosion with cell division. Increased apoptosis, consistent with the reduced number of TRECs, increases the need for compensatory replication, initiating a self-perpetuating strain on peripheral T-cell homeostatic mechanisms.

The finding that T-cells from RA patients and, in particular, naïve T-cells, are susceptible to undergo apoptosis through the intrinsic pathway and that this defect can be, in part, repaired by overexpressing telomerase raises the question about the overall efficacy of DNA repair mechanisms in RA T-cells. The genome is constantly exposed to injurious insults that need to be repaired immediately. It can easily be envisioned that cumulative DNA damage contributes to cellular aging, resulting in either senescence or apoptosis. The most lethal DNA lesions are double-stranded breaks that activate the DNA repair complex, including the protein kinase ataxia telangiectasia mutated (ATM).[60] A sensitive screening assay for DNA damage is the comet assay, DNA electrophoresis at the single cell level. (**Fig. 3**) Shao and colleagues[47] compared the tail moments in comet assays, indicative of DNA damage, between age-matched controls and RA T-cells, and found increased DNA damage in RA. The finding of increased DNA damage in the comet assay was further confirmed by detecting chemically altered DNA with probes reactive to 8-oxoguanin. Several components of the DNA repair complex had reduced expression in RA T-cells, including several members of the MRE11-RAD50-NBS1 (MRN) complex that recognize double-stranded breaks, the kinase ATM, and p53. The primary defect appeared to be the decreased expression of ATM, because overexpression of ATM in RA T-cells restored the expression of the MRN, as well as p53, and rendered RA T-cells more resistant to apoptosis.[47]

In summary, several mechanisms come together to accelerate immune aging of T-cells and possibly other hematopoietic lineages in patients with RA. Decreased capacity in the reserve of hematopoietic stem cells and shortened telomeres in

Con   RA

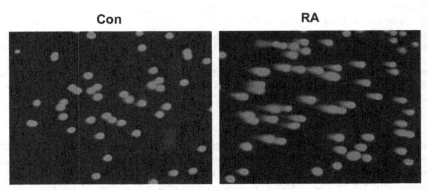

Fig. 3. DNA instability in naïve RA T-cells. Unprimed, naïve CD4 T-cells isolated from RA patients carry a high load of damaged DNA (*right panel*, RA). Broken DNA is identified by the comet assay, a single-cell gel electrophoresis assay in which DNA fragments leaking from the nucleus form a comet. DNA damage can be quantified for individual cells as a tail moment. Naive CD4 T cells from age-matched control individuals have low levels of tail moments (*left panel*, Con). (*From* Weyand CM, Fujii H, Shao L, et al. Rejuvenating the immune system in rheumatoid arthritis. Nat Rev Rheumatol 2009;5:587; with permission.)

hematopoietic stem cells appear to be at least in part genetically determined by risk factors that map to HLA-DRB*04, the same genetic region that predisposes to RA. Independent of this is a defect in RA T-cells in the maintenance of genomic integrity with age, causing excessive loss of peripheral T-cells. Molecular mechanisms include an inability to induce hTERT after stimulation and reduced expression of ATM. Whether the reduced number of TRECs is a consequence of this excessive T-cell loss or whether there is also an independent component of accelerated thymic involution remains to be determined. The net effect of these mechanisms is an excessive peripheral loss of T-cells that is compensated by homeostatic proliferation to maintain compartment size, leading to the eventual emergence of senescence biomarkers.

IMMUNE AGING AND AUTOIMMUNITY—IS THERE A PATHOGENETIC LINK?

The aging immune system is characterized by impaired immune responses to peptide antigens. At first thought, it is, therefore, paradoxic that aging of the immune system should be a risk factor for an increased response to self-antigens and autoimmunity. In one possible model, peripheral regulatory cells are lost with aging, resulting in autoreactive responses, even if the individual autoreactive T-cell has also decreased responsiveness. A population of natural regulatory cells is generated in the thymus and would, therefore, be susceptible to thymic involution; however, regulatory T-cells also are generated from existing T cell-populations in the periphery. Data on the frequency and function of regulatory T-cells with aging are conflicting, and there is no convincing evidence that regulatory function decreases with age. Also, evidence that a deficiency in the number of regulatory T-cells is involved in the pathogenesis of RA is, at this time, not convincing, suggesting that RA is not a consequence of failing regulatory T-cell function with age.

As described previously, one of the prominent defects in RA T-cells related to immune aging is the decreased survival or decreased production of T-cells, resulting into a lymphopenic state that needs to be compensated by homeostatic cytokines. Lymphopenia has been shown to be a major risk factor for autoimmunity in several animal models. Young disease-free non-obese diabetic mice that are prone to develop diabetes are mildly lymphopenic. Disease development in this strain depends on IL-21 mediated homeostatic expansion of islet-specific T cells.[61] Similarly, lymphopenia is important for the autoimmune diabetes mellitus in the biobreeding rat.[62] Also, unpublished observations from the authors' laboratory show that the SKG mouse is markedly lymphopenic (Goronzy and colleagues, unpublished observation, 2010). SKG mice have a mutation in the ZAP70 signaling molecule, causing a defect in T-cell activation and in thymic selection. These mice develop a rheumatoid arthritis-like picture at the age of 3 to 4 months that includes the production of anti-CCP antibodies and rheumatoid factors. Finally, antigen-induced arthritis in normal mouse strains can be age-dependent. Glant and colleagues[63] have shown that proteoglycan-induced arthritis is much more easily induced in middle-aged and old animals rather than in young mice. The common denominator of all these models is that lymphopenia is compensated by homeostatic proliferation, suggesting that homeostatically proliferating cells are risk factors for autoimmunity.

How can a defect in T-cell homeostasis predispose to autoimmunity and be a disease mechanism for the development of RA? At least three different models come to mind. Increased homeostatic proliferation will peripherally select the repertoire in favor of the survival of T-cells with T-cell receptors that have a higher affinity for self.[64,65] A repertoire that is biased by peripheral selection may be more difficult to control by peripheral tolerance mechanisms. This model also would explain the observation that autoantibodies in RA are preferentially specific for common self-antigens and neoantigens that may play a particular role in peripheral selection. In this model, one also would expect a contraction in the diversity of the T-cell receptor repertoire, which indeed can be found in patients with RA. A second model is that the homeostatic proliferation is sufficient to induce T-cell differentiation and lead to the generation of effector cells. Increased effector frequencies have been described in RA.[66] Although these effector populations are found frequently in the inflamed synovium, they do not appear to be specific for synovial antigens, and they also are found in peripheral blood. These effector cell populations frequently have lost the CD28 molecule, but have gained other regulatory molecules such as MHC class I recognizing receptors, the fractalkine receptor, and increased expression of LFA-1. Such changes facilitate interactions with somatic cells other than professional antigen-presenting cells and permit these T-cells to receive costimulatory signals from the environment in an inflamed tissue such as the synovium.[67–71] The authors recently found that RA patients have an altered steady-state equilibrium of the Raf-Mek-ERK signaling pathway.[72] This increased ERK responsiveness was reproduced in T-cells from normal individuals by exposure to homeostatic cytokines, but not by proinflammatory cytokines. ERK activation is central in controlling the T-cell receptor activation threshold. Active ERK serine phosphorylates Lck and prevents the recruitment of SHP-1 and early termination of T cell receptor-induced signaling. Indeed, the authors have shown that the increased ERK responses in RA patients lower the T-cell receptor threshold and confer an increased responsiveness to RA T-cells to suboptimal stimulation.[72] Obviously, these models are not mutually exclusive but can work in concert; patients with RA may have contracted T-cell repertoire biased for autoreactive specificities with an accumulation of effector cells that are responsive to suboptimal triggers. In spite of this increased responsiveness, T-cell responses to exogenous antigen that require clonal expansion are compromised because of the reduced and shortened survival of proliferating T-cells due to a defective DNA damage response.[47]

IMMUNE AGING AND RA COMORBIDITIES

RA is associated with comorbidities that significantly contribute to morbidity and mortality in this patient population. Of particular interest are cardiovascular manifestations; RA patients have an increased risk to develop accelerated coronary artery disease.[73] One possible explanation for this observation is that the chronic inflammatory process associated with RA causes vascular injury and progressive plaque formation. Indeed, plaque inflammation has been identified as a major disease mechanism in coronary artery disease in the general population, not only in patients with autoimmune conditions. The second possible explanation is that accelerated coronary artery disease is a consequence of immune aging, and that RA and coronary artery disease co-occur in a host whose immune system is prematurely aged.[74] In support of this hypothesis, evidence for accelerated immune aging also is found in patients with acute coronary symptoms who do not have an inflammatory disease. These patients frequently have an expanded population of T-effector cells that have lost the CD28 molecule.[75] They contribute to vascular damage by releasing proinflammatory cytokines[76] and also by cytotoxic activity toward vascular endothelial[77] and smooth muscle cells.[78–80] Clonally expanded effector T-cell populations are found in the inflamed coronary artery plaque.[81] These effector cell populations are not necessarily specific for one particular antigen in the vascular environment, but exert their effector function due to a lowered T-cell receptor activation threshold and, therefore, a propensity to be stimulated in low-affinity recognition processes.[82] Expansion of

CD28-negative effector cell populations, a hallmark of immune aging, therefore, is a common denominator in the pathogenesis of atherosclerotic coronary artery disease and of RA.[83]

REFERENCES

1. Kokkonen H, Soderstrom I, Rocklov J, et al. Up-regulation of cytokines and che-mokines predates the onset of rheumatoid arthritis. Arthritis Rheum 2010;62(2): 383–91.
2. Weyand CM, Goronzy JJ. Pathogenesis of rheumatoid arthritis. Med Clin North Am 1997;81(1):29–55.
3. Goronzy JJ, Weyand CM. Developments in the scientific understanding of rheumatoid arthritis. Arthritis Res Ther 2009;11(5):249.
4. Doran MF, Pond GR, Crowson CS, et al. Trends in incidence and mortality in rheu-matoid arthritis in Rochester, Minnesota, over a forty-year period. Arthritis Rheum 2002;46(3):625–31.
5. Goronzy JJ, Weyand CM. Rheumatoid arthritis. Immunol Rev 2005;204:55–73.
6. Larbi A, Fulop T, Pawelec G. Immune receptor signaling, aging and autoimmu-nity. Adv Exp Med Biol 2008;640:312–24.
7. Weyand CM, Goronzy JJ. Giant-cell arteritis and polymyalgia rheumatica. Ann Intern Med 2003;139(6):505–15.
8. Weyand CM, Goronzy JJ. Medium- and large-vessel vasculitis. N Engl J Med 2003;349(2):160–9.
9. Moulias R, Proust J, Wang A, et al. Age-related increase in autoantibodies. Lancet 1984;1(8386):1128–9.
10. Grubeck-Loebenstein B, Wick G. The aging of the immune system. Adv Immunol 2002;80:243–84.
11. Weng NP. Aging of the immune system: how much can the adaptive immune system adapt? Immunity 2006;24(5):495–9.
12. Targonski PV, Jacobson RM, Poland GA. Immunosenescence: role and measure-ment in influenza vaccine response among the elderly. Vaccine 2007;25(16): 3066–9.
13. Jefferson T, Rivetti D, Rivetti A, et al. Efficacy and effectiveness of influenza vaccines in elderly people: a systematic review. Lancet 2005;366(9492):1165–74.
14. Nichol KL, Nordin JD, Nelson DB, et al. Effectiveness of influenza vaccine in the community-dwelling elderly. N Engl J Med 2007;357(14):1373–81.
15. Donahue JG, Choo PW, Manson JE, et al. The incidence of herpes zoster. Arch Intern Med 1995;155(15):1605–9.
16. Arvin A. Aging, immunity, and the varicella-zoster virus. N Engl J Med 2005; 352(22):2266–7.
17. Thompson WW, Shay DK, Weintraub E, et al. Mortality associated with influenza and respiratory syncytial virus in the United States. JAMA 2003;289(2):179–86.
18. Looney RJ, Hasan MS, Coffin D, et al. Hepatitis B immunization of healthy elderly adults: relationship between naive CD4 + T-cells and primary immune response and evaluation of GM-CSF as an adjuvant. J Clin Immunol 2001;21(1):30–6.
19. Goronzy JJ, Weyand CM. T-cell development and receptor diversity during aging. Curr Opin Immunol 2005;17(5):468–75.
20. Naylor K, Li G, Vallejo AN, et al. The influence of age on T-cell generation and TCR diversity. J Immunol 2005;174(11):7446–52.
21. Gomez CR, Boehmer ED, Kovacs EJ. The aging innate immune system. Curr Opin Immunol 2005;17(5):457–62.

22. Niessner A, Weyand CM. Dendritic cells in atherosclerotic disease. Clin Immunol 2010;134(1):25–32.
23. Weyand CM, Younge BR, Goronzy JJ. T-cells in arteritis and atherosclerosis. Curr Opin Lipidol 2008;19(5):469–77.
24. Hakim FT, Memon SA, Cepeda R, et al. Age-dependent incidence, time course, and consequences of thymic renewal in adults. J Clin Invest 2005; 115(4):930–9.
25. Czesnikiewicz-Guzik M, Lee WW, Cui D, et al. T-cell subset-specific susceptibility to aging. Clin Immunol 2008;127(1):107–18.
26. Nikolich-Zugich J. Ageing and life-long maintenance of T-cell subsets in the face of latent persistent infections. Nat Rev Immunol 2008;8(7):512–22.
27. Hodes RJ, Hathcock KS, Weng NP. Telomeres in T- and B-cells. Nat Rev Immunol 2002;2(9):699–706.
28. Jendro MC, Ganten T, Matteson EL, et al. Emergence of oligoclonal T-cell populations following therapeutic T-cell depletion in rheumatoid arthritis. Arthritis Rheum 1995;38(9):1242–51.
29. Brett S, Baxter G, Cooper H, et al. Repopulation of blood lymphocyte sub-populations in rheumatoid arthritis patients treated with the depleting humanized monoclonal antibody, CAMPATH-1H. Immunology 1996;88(1):13–9.
30. Lorenzi AR, Clarke AM, Wooldridge T, et al. Morbidity and mortality in rheumatoid arthritis patients with prolonged therapy-induced lymphopenia: twelve-year outcomes. Arthritis Rheum 2008;58(2):370–5.
31. Jones JL, Phuah CL, Cox AL, et al. IL-21 drives secondary autoimmunity in patients with multiple sclerosis, following therapeutic lymphocyte depletion with alemtuzumab (Campath-1H). J Clin Invest 2009;119(7):2052–61.
32. Koetz K, Bryl E, Spickschen K, et al. T-cell homeostasis in patients with rheumatoid arthritis. Proc Natl Acad Sci U S A 2000;97(16):9203–8.
33. Kong FK, Chen CL, Six A, et al. T-cell receptor gene deletion circles identify recent thymic emigrants in the peripheral T-cell pool. Proc Natl Acad Sci U S A 1999;96(4):1536–40.
34. Douek DC, McFarland RD, Keiser PH, et al. Changes in thymic function with age and during the treatment of HIV infection. Nature 1998;396(6712):690–5.
35. van den Dool C, de Boer RJ. The effects of age, thymectomy, and HIV Infection on alpha and beta TCR excision circles in naive T-cells. J Immunol 2006;177(7): 4391–401.
36. Ponchel F, Morgan AW, Bingham SJ, et al. Dysregulated lymphocyte proliferation and differentiation in patients with rheumatoid arthritis. Blood 2002;100(13): 4550–6.
37. Hazenberg MD, Otto SA, Cohen Stuart JW, et al. Increased cell division but not thymic dysfunction rapidly affects the T-cell receptor excision circle content of the naive T-cell population in HIV-1 infection. Nat Med 2000;6(9): 1036–42.
38. Hazenberg MD, Borghans JA, de Boer RJ, et al. Thymic output: a bad TREC record. Nat Immunol 2003;4(2):97–9.
39. Andrews NP, Fujii H, Goronzy JJ, et al. Telomeres and immunological diseases of aging. Gerontology 2009. [Epub ahead of print].
40. Vallejo A, Nestel AR, Schirmer M, et al. Aging-related deficiency of CD28 expression in CD4+ T cells is associated with the loss of gene specific nuclear factor binding activity. J Biol Chem 1998;273:8119–29.
41. Effros RB, Dagarag M, Spaulding C, et al. The role of CD8 + T-cell replicative senescence in human aging. Immunol Rev 2005;205:147–57.

42. Schmidt D, Goronzy JJ, Weyand CM. CD4 + CD7-CD28-T cells are expanded in rheumatoid arthritis and are characterized by autoreactivity. J Clin Invest 1996; 97(9):2027–37.
43. Schmidt D, Martens PB, Weyand CM, et al. The repertoire of CD4 + CD28-T cells in rheumatoid arthritis. Mol Med 1996;2(5):608–18.
44. Wagner UG, Koetz K, Weyand CM, et al. Perturbation of the T-cell repertoire in rheumatoid arthritis. Proc Natl Acad Sci U S A 1998;95(24):14447–52.
45. Thewissen M, Somers V, Venken K, et al. Analyses of immunosenescent markers in patients with autoimmune disease. Clin Immunol 2007;123(2):209–18.
46. Schönland SO, Lopez C, Widmann T, et al. Premature telomeric loss in rheumatoid arthritis is genetically determined and involves both myeloid and lymphoid cell lineages. Proc Natl Acad Sci U S A 2003;100(23):13471–6.
47. Shao L, Fujii H, Colmegna I, et al. Deficiency of the DNA repair enzyme ATM in rheumatoid arthritis. J Exp Med 2009;206(6):1435–49.
48. Goronzy JJ, Matteson EL, Fulbright JW, et al. Prognostic markers of radiographic progression in early rheumatoid arthritis. Arthritis Rheum 2004;50(1):43–54.
49. Martens PB, Goronzy JJ, Schaid D, et al. Expansion of unusual CD4 + T-cells in severe rheumatoid arthritis. Arthritis Rheum 1997;40(6):1106–14.
50. Bryl E, Vallejo AN, Weyand CM, et al. Down-regulation of CD28 expression by TNF-alpha. J Immunol 2001;167(6):3231–8.
51. Bryl E, Vallejo AN, Matteson EL, et al. Modulation of CD28 expression with anti-tumor necrosis factor alpha therapy in rheumatoid arthritis. Arthritis Rheum 2005;52(10):2996–3003.
52. Warrington KJ, Vallejo AN, Weyand CM, et al. CD28 loss in senescent CD4 + T-cells: reversal by interleukin-12 stimulation. Blood 2003;101(9):3543–9.
53. Chapman A, Stewart SJ, Nepom GT, et al. CD11b+CD28-CD4+ human T-cells: activation requirements and association with HLA-DR alleles. J Immunol 1996; 157(11):4771–80.
54. Waase I, Kayser C, Carlson PJ, et al. Oligoclonal T-cell proliferation in patients with rheumatoid arthritis and their unaffected siblings. Arthritis Rheum 1996; 39(6):904–13.
55. van Leeuwen EM, Remmerswaal EB, Vossen MT, et al. Emergence of a CD4+CD28- granzyme B+, cytomegalovirus-specific T-cell subset after recovery of primary cytomegalovirus infection. J Immunol 2004;173(3):1834–41.
56. Palm W, de Lange T. How shelterin protects mammalian telomeres. Annu Rev Genet 2008;42:301–34.
57. Weyand CM, Fujii H, Shao L, et al. Rejuvenating the immune system in rheumatoid arthritis. Nat Rev Rheumatol 2009;5(10):583–8.
58. Fujii H, Shao L, Colmegna I, et al. Telomerase insufficiency in rheumatoid arthritis. Proc Natl Acad Sci U S A 2009;106(11):4360–5.
59. Colmegna I, Diaz-Borjon A, Fujii H, et al. Defective proliferative capacity and accelerated telomeric loss of hematopoietic progenitor cells in rheumatoid arthritis. Arthritis Rheum 2008;58(4):990–1000.
60. Lavin MF, Kozlov S, Gueven N, et al. Atm and cellular response to DNA damage. Adv Exp Med Biol 2005;570:457–76.
61. King C, Ilic A, Koelsch K, et al. Homeostatic expansion of T-cells during immune insufficiency generates autoimmunity. Cell 2004;117(2):265–77.
62. Crisa L, Mordes JP, Rossini AA. Autoimmune diabetes mellitus in the BB rat. Diabetes Metab Rev 1992;8(1):4–37.
63. Glant TT, Finnegan A, Mikecz K. Proteoglycan-induced arthritis: immune regulation, cellular mechanisms, and genetics. Crit Rev Immunol 2003;23(3):199–250.

64. Goronzy JJ, Weyand CM. Aging, autoimmunity and arthritis: T-cell senescence and contraction of T-cell repertoire diversity—catalysts of autoimmunity and chronic inflammation. Arthritis Res Ther 2003;5(5):225–34.
65. Goronzy JJ, Weyand CM. Thymic function and peripheral T-cell homeostasis in rheumatoid arthritis. Trends Immunol 2001;22(5):251–5.
66. Cope AP. T-cells in rheumatoid arthritis. Arthritis Res Ther 2008;10(Suppl 1):S1.
67. Singh K, Colmegna I, He X, et al. Synoviocyte stimulation by the LFA-1-intercellular adhesion molecule-2-Ezrin-Akt pathway in rheumatoid arthritis. J Immunol 2008;180(3):1971–8.
68. Sawai H, Park YW, Roberson J, et al. T cell costimulation by fractalkine-expressing synoviocytes in rheumatoid arthritis. Arthritis Rheum 2005;52(5):1392–401.
69. Davila E, Kang YM, Park YW, et al. Cell-based immunotherapy with suppressor CD8 + T-cells in rheumatoid arthritis. J Immunol 2005;174(11):7292–301.
70. Sawai H, Park YW, He X, et al. Fractalkine mediates T-cell dependent proliferation of synovial fibroblasts in rheumatoid arthritis. Arthritis Rheum 2007;56(10): 3215–25.
71. Goronzy JJ, Henel G, Sawai H, et al. Costimulatory pathways in rheumatoid synovitis and T-cell senescence. Ann N Y Acad Sci 2005;1062:182–94.
72. Singh K, Deshpande P, Pryshchep S, et al. ERK-dependent T-cell receptor threshold calibration in rheumatoid arthritis. J Immunol 2009;183(12):8258–67.
73. Warrington KJ, Kent PD, Frye RL, et al. Rheumatoid arthritis is an independent risk factor for multivessel coronary artery disease: a case control study. Arthritis Res Ther 2005;7(5):R984–91.
74. Crowson CS, Liang KP, Therneau TM, et al. Could accelerated aging explain the excess mortality in patients with seropositive rheumatoid arthritis? Arthritis Rheum 2010;62(2):378–82.
75. Liuzzo G, Kopecky SL, Frye RL, et al. Perturbation of the T-cell repertoire in patients with unstable angina. Circulation 1999;100(21):2135–9.
76. Liuzzo G, Vallejo AN, Kopecky SL, et al. Molecular fingerprint of interferon-gamma signaling in unstable angina. Circulation 2001;103(11):1509–14.
77. Nakajima T, Schulte S, Warrington KJ, et al. T-cell mediated lysis of endothelial cells in acute coronary syndromes. Circulation 2002;105(5):570–5.
78. Niessner A, Sato K, Chaikof EL, et al. Pathogen-sensing plasmacytoid dendritic cells stimulate cytotoxic T-cell function in the atherosclerotic plaque through interferon-alpha. Circulation 2006;114(23):2482–9.
79. Sato K, Niessner A, Kopecky SL, et al. TRAIL-expressing T-cells induce apoptosis of vascular smooth muscle cells in the atherosclerotic plaque. J Exp Med 2006; 203(1):239–50.
80. Pryshchep S, Sato K, Goronzy JJ, et al. T-cell recognition and killing of vascular smooth muscle cells in acute coronary syndrome. Circ Res 2006;98(9):1168–76.
81. Liuzzo G, Goronzy JJ, Yang H, et al. Monoclonal T-cell proliferation and plaque instability in acute coronary syndromes. Circulation 2000;101(25):2883–8.
82. Pryshchep S, Goronzy JJ, Parashar S, et al. Insufficient deactivation of the protein tyrosine kinase Lck amplifies T-cell responsiveness in acute coronary syndrome. Circ Res 2010;106:769–78.
83. Pasceri V, Yeh ET. A tale of two diseases: atherosclerosis and rheumatoid arthritis. Circulation 1999;100(21):2124–6.

Cell-cell Interactions in Rheumatoid Arthritis Synovium

David A. Fox, MD[a],*, Alison Gizinski, MD[a], Rachel Morgan, BSc[b],
Steven K. Lundy, PhD[b]

KEYWORDS

- Synovial fibroblasts • T lymphocytes • B lymphocytes
- Antigen-presenting cells • Endothelial cells • Cytokines

Although the cause of rheumatoid arthritis (RA) remains unknown, insights into the pathogenesis of RA have been achieved by careful study of inflammatory, immune, and tissue-destructive processes that take place in synovial tissue. Successful approaches have included ex vivo analysis of RA synovium, experiments in animal model systems, and use of cultured cell lines, especially fibroblast-like synoviocytes, derived from patients' synovial tissue. These insights have led to remarkable advances in the treatment of RA and other diseases, such as the use of tumor necrosis factor (TNF)-blocking biologics.

None of the molecular targets of medications currently used in the treatment of RA are expressed uniquely in synovial tissue. Instead, all of them are of great importance in host defense as well. Recent research is revealing important molecules and pathways pertinent to joint inflammation and damage that may be less central to host defense compared with currently targeted molecules. A conceptual framework for such investigations is the realization that although RA synovium can display some features of an immune organ and is justifiably regarded as a tertiary lymphoid structure, it also contains cells that are distinct from those found in primary or secondary lymphoid tissue, namely, the intrinsic structural cells of the joint such as fibroblast-like synoviocytes.

Grant support: David Fox: NIH RO-1 AR38477; Alison Gizinski: American College of Rheumatology Research and Education Foundation; Rachel Morgan: Immunology Training Grant and Rackham Pre-doctoral Merit Fellowship: Steven Lundy: Arthritis Foundation Arthritis Investigator Award and NIH K Award.
[a] Division of Rheumatology and Rheumatic Diseases Research Core Center, 3918 Taubman Center, 1500 East Medical Center Drive, The University of Michigan, Ann Arbor, MI 48109, USA
[b] Division of Rheumatology and Rheumatic Diseases Research Core Center, 109 Zina Pitcher Place, The University of Michigan, Ann Arbor, MI 48109, USA
* Corresponding author.
E-mail address: dfox@umich.edu

Rheum Dis Clin N Am 36 (2010) 311–323
doi:10.1016/j.rdc.2010.02.004
0889-857X/10/$ – see front matter © 2010 Elsevier Inc. All rights reserved.
rheumatic.theclinics.com

It is clear that no one cell type explains the pathologic behavior of RA synovial tissue. It is the interactions between these cells that define the disease. The 3 most abundant cell populations in RA synovium are the monocyte/macrophage synoviocytes (type A), the fibroblast-like synoviocytes (FLS) (type B), and T lymphocytes (which are strikingly heterogeneous). Other critically important cells of the RA synovium include B lymphocytes, plasma cells, dendritic cells, mast cells, endothelial cells, osteoclasts, and adjacent chondrocytes. These various cell types can interact in 2 general ways: first through secreted mediators, notably inflammatory cytokines such as TNF, interleukin (IL)-6, IL-17, and many others; and second through direct cell-cell contact that is mediated by cell surface receptors and ligands, including some membrane-anchored cytokines.

This article focuses on selected cell-cell interactions that may be important in the pathogenesis of RA. It is hoped that the relative molecular specificity of some of these interactions for events in the joint compared with the systemic immune response will provide more specific targets (**Table 1**) for a new generation of biologic and nonbiologic therapeutics.

HOMOTYPIC AND AUTOCRINE INTERACTIONS OF FLS
Cadherin-11

During the course of RA, the cells of the synovial lining undergo extensive hyperplasia to form the synovial pannus that invades and destroys cartilage and bone. Recent discoveries have highlighted a critical role for cadherin-11 in these events. Cadherin-11 has been identified as a strongly expressed intercellular adhesion molecule on human and mouse FLS.[1,2] Transfection of L cells with cadherin-11 led to the formation of sheet-like structures with an organization similar to that seen in synovial lining[1]; furthermore, cadherin-11 localized to cell-to-cell junctions between FLS.[2] Joints in cadherin-11 null mice had an underdeveloped synovial lining and decreased extracellular matrix.[2] These data indicate that cadherin-11 plays a vital role in the formation of the synovial lining layer by mediating FLS/FLS connections.

Cadherin-11 staining correlated strongly with cellular infiltration of macrophages and T lymphocytes in RA synovium.[3] Cadherin-11 staining also correlated with erythrocyte sedimentation rate and C-reactive protein level although not as strongly.[3] Cadherin-11 expression in synovium is not specific to RA, because cadherin-11 staining on synovial biopsies was similar in inflamed joints from RA, osteoarthritis (OA), and psoriatic arthritis (PsA).[3] There was also a positive correlation between cadherin-11 staining of lung tissue from patients with RA-associated interstitial pneumonitis (IP) and CD4$^+$ T-cell infiltration of the lung.[3] Cadherin-11 null mice showed an average of 50% reduction in clinical arthritis activity in the K/BxN serum transfer model.[2]

Table 1	
Important cell-cell interactions in RA synovium	
Cell Types	**Potential New Molecular Targets**
FLS-FLS	Cadherin-11, fractalkine
FLS-T	B7-H3, IL-15
T-APC	OX40, CCL20, IL-7
B-T	CXCL13, ICOS, OX40, BAFF
B-FLS	BAFF, osteopontin
Leucocyte-endothelial	Le^y/H

Please see text for explanation of abbreviations.

Cadherin-11 has been explored as a possible therapeutic target using the same mouse serum transfer model. Cadherin-11-Fc and an anticadherin-11 mAb ameliorated clinical arthritis when administered with arthritogenic serum.[2] More significant for potential treatment of human disease, anticadherin-11 mAb ameliorated established arthritis in a modified K/BxN serum transfer model.[2]

Fractalkine and its Receptor

Fractalkine (FKN) is a potent chemoattractant and adhesion molecule that is found in increased levels in RA synovium. RA FLS secrete FKN and express its receptor, CX_3CR1.[4] Soluble FKN induced proliferation of FLS that was blocked by addition of anti-CX_3CR1.[5] Even in the absence of sFKN, the antibody was able to decrease FLS proliferation, revealing an autocrine growth loop.[5] FKN also induced migration of RA FLS and caused significant reorganization of F-actin within FLS.[4] It is likely that FKN could act in an autocrine fashion to aid in pannus invasion of the bone and cartilage through FLS growth and migration.

FLS/T CELL INTERACTIONS

In RA, FLS and other cells produce chemokines that attract T cells to the joint. FLS and T cells then interact in the synovium through secreted factors and direct cell-to-cell interactions, resulting in activation of both cell types. FLS proliferate when cocultured with $CD4^+$ T cells, especially when RA T cells are used.[5]

Synovial T cells in RA patients include an expanded population of $CD4^+CD28^-$ cells and this subset of cells in particular greatly enhances FLS proliferation. $CD4^+CD28^-$ cells, which are sometimes considered to be senescent, aberrantly express CX_3CR1, and anti-CX_3CR1 decreases the FLS growth-promoting activity of these cells without a significant effect on $CD4^+CD28^+$ T cells.[5] Stimulation of $CD4^+CD28^-$ T cells by FKN through CX_3CR1 increases TNFα production, and TNFα can then act on FLS to increase growth, FKN secretion, and CX_3CR1 expression.[4,5] These data suggest an important relationship between TNFα and FKN/CX_3CR1 in FLS/T cell interactions in the RA joint, in which production and action of these molecules occur in linked paracrine and autocrine loops involving T cells and FLS.

IL-15

IL-15 is constitutively expressed on FLS and is a potent T-cell growth factor that can cause activation/proliferation of effector T cells (T_{eff}) and regulatory T cells (T_{reg}) in T-cell/FLS cocultures.[6] Moreover, IL-15 can decrease apoptosis of various cell types including FLS and T cells.[7,8] The IL-15 receptor is a trimer (IL-15Rα,β,γ_c) and subunits of IL-15R are expressed by various cell types, including FLS and T cells.[7] IL-15 can function as a secreted or membrane-bound cytokine, with signaling similar to other cytokines through the full trimeric IL-15R, or through dimeric IL-15Rβγ_c receptor (cis presentation).[7] IL-15 can also signal through a unique trans signaling form, in which distinct subunits of IL-15R are expressed on the surface of interacting cells. IL-15 can be recycled by the cell and presented on the cell surface by IL-15Rα, a pathway that allows for persistence of an IL-15 signal even when soluble IL-15 is no longer available.[7] In cultures containing T_{eff} and T_{reg} cocultured with RA FLS, proliferation and function of both T cell subsets were stimulated, with a net proinflammatory effect. These effects were not observed when OA FLS or dermal fibroblasts were used and were dependent on cell-to-cell contact. Neutralizing IL-15 during T-cell/FLS cocultures significantly attenuated the proliferation of T_{eff} and T_{reg}, T_{eff} production of TNFα and IFNγ, and T_{reg} inhibition of T_{eff}.[6] The overall proinflammatory effect of

IL-15 makes it a potential target for RA therapy. A proof-of-concept study has been conducted using a human immunoglobulin (Ig)G1 anti-IL-15 monoclonal antibody in RA. This antibody suppressed effects of IL-15 in vitro, and showed meaningful efficacy in phase I and II trials.[8]

FLS as Antigen-presenting Cells

FLS can also act as antigen-presenting cells (APCs) in the initiation of T-lymphocyte responses. For example, FLS induced secretion of IL-2 by class II MHC-restricted CD4$^+$ T-cell hybridomas specific for arthritogenic autoantigens, specifically human cartilage gp-39 (HC gp-39) and human type II collagen (CII).[9] The T-cell hybridomas in these experiments were developed from HLA-DR4 transgenic mice, and therefore respond to peptide antigens that are loaded onto and presented by HLA-DR4. Activation of the hybridomas required reexpression of class II on the FLS, which occurs in vivo in RA and is reinduced in vitro by IFNγ. The T-cell response to peptide antigen presented by FLS was exquisitely MHC-restricted, identical to experiments in which professional APCs were used,[9] and blocking antibodies to human class II MHC or murine CD4 prevented IL-2 production. Because T-cell hybridomas do not require a second signal to respond to peptide antigen, this system was not useful for defining potential costimulatory ligands on FLS. FLS do not express the classic APC costimulatory molecules CD80 or CD86 (B7-1, B7-2) at functionally relevant levels.[10]

B7-H3

Of the molecules that belong to the B7 family, B7-H3 is expressed strongly and constitutively on FLS in vitro.[10] Moreover, immunostaining of RA synovium showed broad B7-H3 expression nearly identical in distribution to the FLS marker cadherin-11. Dual-color immunohistochemical analysis showed CD3$^+$ T cells in close proximity to FLS expressing B7-H3.[10] Furthermore, in coculture experiments, B7-H3 localized to the contact point between FLS and cytokine-activated T cells (Tck) or during FLS presentation of superantigen to T cells.[10] Previous studies had indicated that B7-H3 can have either stimulatory or inhibitory effects on T cells, and results with FLS/T-cell cocultures were consistent with a dual role for B7-H3. RNAi knockdown of B7-H3 in FLS decreased production of TNFα, IFNγ, and IL-2 by cocultured Tck but increased production of these cytokines by resting T cells.[10] The T-cell ligand or ligands for B7-H3 have not yet been defined. B7-H3, in contrast to B7-1 and B7-2, is expressed on human solid tumors,[11] in part controlled by the microRNA miR-29.[12] In early-phase human clinical trials, the B7-H3–specific mAb 8H9 was reported to prolong survival in patients with solid tumors and central nervous system metastasis.[12] Further trials of anti-B7-H3 in cancer could yield safety information pertinent to consideration of therapeutic trials of this antibody in RA.

T CELLS AND APCS IN THE RA SYNOVIUM

The following sections highlight examples of selected cytokine-mediated and cognate cell-cell contact-driven interactions between T cells and synovial APCs that are current or potential therapeutic targets for the treatment of RA. Interruption of T-cell costimulation between T cells and APCs in the synovium is a worthwhile approach given the clinical success of blocking T-cell costimulation with CTLA-4Ig in RA. Resting T cells require at least 2 signals to differentiate into effector T cells: the first signal through engagement of the T-cell antigen receptor by the antigen-MHC complex on the APC, and the second signal by engagement of costimulatory molecules such as CD28, on T cells by ligands such as CD80/86 on APCs. Effector

T-cell differentiation leads to the expression of additional surface molecules. These inducible structures may have stimulatory (ICOS, OX40) or inhibitory (CTLA-4) potential.

CTLA-4 and Indoleamine Dioxygenase

CD28 is the prototypic T-cell receptor (TCR) for costimulatory signals. The ligation of CD28 by CD80/86 (B7-1 and B7-2) sends activating signals into the T cell and the APC. CTLA-4 (CD152) is up-regulated on activated T cells and binds to the CD28 ligands CD80/86. The ligation of CD80/86 by CTLA-4 sends inhibitory signals directly into the T cell. The ligation of CD80/86 by CTLA-4 can also deliver regulatory signals to the APC. The interaction of CD80/86 with CTLA-4 leads to the induction of indoleamine dioxygenase (IDO) in APCs.[13] IDO is believed to be critical in inducing anergy in T cells, because IDO depletes tryptophan that is necessary for T-cell activation. Blocking the activity of IDO in a mouse model of arthritis led to increased severity of arthritis and accumulation of Th1 and Th17 cells in the inflamed joints.[14,15] Conversely, administration of L-kynurenine, a metabolite of L-tryptophan, resulted in amelioration of arthritis. These findings suggest manipulation of tryptophan degradation as a therapeutic target in RA.[15]

OX40/OX40L

OX40 (CD134) is predominantly expressed on activated CD4 and CD8 T cells following stimulation via TCR and CD28. Proinflammatory cytokines, IL-1, IL-2, and TNFα can further augment the expression of OX40. The ligand of OX40 and OX40L (CD252) is expressed on APCs including dendritic cells, B cells, and macrophages.[16] OX40L is induced on APCs after stimulation via CD40.[17] There is bidirectional activation of T cells and APCs via the OX40/OX40L pathway. Stimulation of OX40 on T cells induces proliferation and cytokine secretion, and signaling via OX40L into APCs induces the secretion of proinflammatory cytokines by APCs.[17]

In RA, there is increased expression of OX40 on peripheral blood CD4 T cells with a trend toward a positive correlation with serum C-reactive protein levels.[18] OX40 is expressed on CD4- and CD8-positive synovial T cells, more so on CD4-positive T cells, and levels of expression correlate with disease activity.[19–21] OX40 and OX40L expressing cells are also present in the RA synovium.[19] Although there is increased expression of OX40 and OX40L in the RA synovium, the role of OX40/OX40L in mediating immune events in RA is unclear. However, preclinical studies in animal models blocking the interaction of OX40/OX40L have shown promise.[19]

CCL20

Chemokines mediate inflammatory responses by stimulating the recruitment of leucocytes. The chemokine CCL20 (MIP-3α) and its receptor CCR6 play a role in the migration of different cell types to the RA synovium. CCL20 is a CC-chemokine expressed on macrophages, dendritic cells, and lymphocytes. CCR6, the receptor for CCL20, is expressed on Th17 cells, immature dendritic cells, and B cells. CCL20 is chemotactic for Th17 cells and dendritic cells, which express CCR6. Th17 cells secrete CCL20 and recruit other CCR6-expressing Th17 cells to the site of Th17 cell-mediated damage.[22] Increased levels of CCL20 have been observed in the synovial fluid of RA patients compared with OA patients, and protein concentrations of CCL20 are increased in the peripheral blood of patients with RA.[23,24] Expression of CCL20 is induced in FLS by the synergistic interaction of proinflammatory cytokines, including TNFα, IL-1β and IL-17, and cytokine-stimulated FLS can recruit mononuclear cells in a CCL20/CC6–dependent manner.[25,26] The results suggest that CCL20 produced by FLS recruits monocytes and Th17 T cells to the synovium and is an important chemokine in the pathogenesis of RA. Moreover, blockade of CCL20 binding to CCR6 with a neutralizing antibody was effective in treating arthritis in a T-cell transfer model in mice.[22] Further supporting the role of CCL20 as an important chemokine in RA, a recent study demonstrated that treatment with infliximab, etanercept, or tocilizumab reduced serum levels of CCL20 in patients with RA.[27]

IL-7

IL-7 is a member of the IL-2 family. IL-7 is associated with endothelial cells, FLS, and macrophages in the RA synovium and colocalizes with deposits of extracellular matrix collagen IV.[28] IL-7R is composed of IL-7Rα and IL-2Rγ and is expressed on CD4$^+$ and CD8$^+$ T cells, NK T cells, and monocytes. IL-7 levels are increased in RA compared with OA synovial fluid. Serum IL-7 levels correlate with disease activity in RA.[29] In RA patients who are poor responders to anti-TNF therapy, persistently increased serum levels of IL-7 are seen.[29] Moreover, reduced levels of serum IL-7 were observed in patients with early RA treated with methotrexate, and the reduction correlated with disease suppression.[29]

Within RA synovial biopsies, samples with lymphoid follicles demonstrated consistent IL-7 staining, and gene expression analysis of RA synovial samples revealed increased expression of genes involved in IL-7 signal transduction.[28] IL-7 may be responsible for generation of tertiary lymphoid follicles observed in RA synovium, because IL7 is known to be crucial for the development of lymphoid tissue. Enhanced expression of IL-7Rα and IL-7 in patients with RA may contribute to joint inflammation by activating T cells, B cells, and macrophages because treatment with soluble human IL-7Rα inhibited IL-7R–mediated immune activation in vitro.[30] These research findings suggest that IL-7 and its receptor are potential targets for immune modulation in RA therapy.

B-CELL INTERACTIONS WITH SYNOVIAL T CELLS

Recent successes of therapeutic interventions using B-cell–depleting reagents have highlighted the importance of B cells in the pathogenesis of RA.[31] These current therapies, which target CD20-positive B cells, and several others that are in the pipeline that target other B-cell markers, are designed to eliminate or disrupt the activation of a large percentage of the entire population of B cells. Although effective as treatment for RA in the short-term, each of these reagents has the potential to have long-term deleterious effects on the immune response to common infectious microorganisms. Therefore, it is desirable to continue pursuing B-cell–directed treatments that are more specific to the pathogenic subset of B cells that mediate joint inflammation. The following is a summary of some recently recognized cell-cell interactions involving synovial B cells that point to emerging potential targets of interest.

Germinal Centers in RA Synovium

It has been established that structures resembling lymph node germinal centers can be found in the inflamed synovium of a subset of RA patients. The recently described expression of activation-induced cytidine deaminase (AID) within these ectopic germinal centers supports the hypothesis that maturation of the antibody response through somatic hypermutation and class-switch recombination could occur within the RA synovium.[32] This study went on to show that germinal centers remained functionally active following implantation of RA synovial tissue in SCID mice.[32] Analysis of a panel of cytokines and chemokines that are believed to contribute to germinal center formation showed correlations between the presence of germinal centers and TNFα, lymphotoxin-β, APRIL, and B-lymphocyte chemoattractant (BLC, CXCL13). Another study by the same researchers demonstrated that mononuclear cells from RA synovium had 400-fold higher expression of CXCL13 than cells isolated from the peripheral blood of the same patients.[33] Most synovial CXCL13 was produced by CD45RO[+]/CD4[+]/CD3[+] T lymphocytes, suggesting that this T-cell subset was of an activated phenotype. Further analysis of surface markers on these T cells suggested a phenotype that was distinct from T follicular helper cells found in other lymphoid structures. Although systemic blockade of CXCL13 or its receptor CXCR5 may be expected to interrupt T cell–B cell interactions that are important to host defenses, the findings concerning CXCL13 expression within the RA synovium open the possibility of intra-articular immune therapy directed at CXCL13/CXCR5 or other contributors to germinal center formation. Localized neutralization of other cytokines or cytokine receptors involved in germinal center formation including lymphotoxin, IL-21, APRIL, and B-cell–activating factor (BAFF) may also provide therapeutic benefit in some patients.

ICOS and Its Ligand

As described earlier, B cells constitute an important APC population for T-lymphocyte activation. Therapies directed at OX40/OX40L, CD80, and CD86 are expected to act on B-cell antigen presentation as well as dendritic cells and macrophages. Another notable interaction between CD4[+] T helper cells and B cells that has gained interest recently is that of T-cell–expressed inducible costimulator (ICOS, CD278) with its ligand on B cells, B7RP-1 (ICOS-L, CD275). These molecules are also involved in the formation of germinal centers and are critical to the initiation and further development of antigen-specific antibody responses. Disruption of interactions between ICOS and its ligand has been shown to diminish arthritis incidence and severity in 2 independent studies.[34,35] In the latter study, treatment with a blocking antibody decreased the number of T follicular helper cells and germinal center B cells in the draining lymph nodes and spleens of mice in the collagen-induced arthritis model. This led to an overall reduction in T-cell cytokine production and titers of anticollagen antibodies in the serum. ICOS/ICOS-L blockade was also effective in the NZB/NZW F_1 model of lupus nephritis. As described earlier for CXCL13, systemic blockade of ICOS/ICOS-L interactions may not prove to be desirable because of adverse side effects, but local inhibition of ICOS/ICOS-L in the synovium may be a viable treatment option.

Regulatory B Cells and NK T Cells

Not all interactions between B cells and T cells result in increased disease pathogenesis in arthritis. Regulatory B cells that express IL-10 have been studied for many years, but have recently gained prominence through the demonstration that they have unique surface markers (CD1d[hi]CD5[+]) and may represent a subset of B cells distinct from those that are pathogenic in autoimmune diseases.[36] The high expression of CD1d by these regulatory B cells suggests that they may present antigens to invariant NK T cells. The role of NK T cells in arthritis has been controversial with almost an equal number of articles suggesting a pathogenic or suppressive phenotype.[37] The conflicting roles of NK T cells in arthritis might be explained by differences in the B-cell populations that are presenting antigen to them. A recent study has demonstrated the increased presence of invariant NK T cells with regulatory phenotype following depletion of B cells with anti-CD20 therapy.[38] This study suggests a novel mechanism contributing to the success of B-cell depletion therapy, and demonstrates the potential efficacy of targeting the interaction of B cells with iNK T cells.

B-CELL INTERACTIONS WITH OTHER SYNOVIAL CELL POPULATIONS

Although B-cell interactions with T cells in the RA synovium may present important and obvious targets for future therapy, it is critical to understand that signaling between B cells and other synovial cell populations may also contribute to joint pathology.

BAFF

A recent study has shown that BAFF is expressed on the cell surface of RA FLS but not on OA FLS.[39] This RA FLS-associated BAFF acted as a first signal for the transcription of recombinase-activating genes (RAG) in B cells that are involved in maturation of the antibody response. RAG expression in B cells cocultured with RA FLS was blocked by interference with BAFF gene translation or by neutralization of IL-6. Forced expression of membrane-associated BAFF in OA FLS did not result in RAG gene transcription unless IL-6 was also present in the coculture. These results highlight that RA FLS can have a direct effect on B-cell activation through the combined expression of cell surface BAFF and IL-6. Evidence for the importance of local synovial BAFF expression to the pathogenesis of arthritis comes from a study in which intra-articular injection of a lentiviral vector containing a BAFF-silencing reagent provided long-term protection from joint inflammation in the collagen-induced arthritis model.[40] This protective effect of BAFF gene silencing within the joint was accompanied by decreases in production of anticollagen antibodies and IL-17 by cells of the joint and draining lymph node, but not in the spleen of treated mice. This study demonstrates another potential approach to localized treatment of arthritic inflammation.

Osteopontin

Another notable interaction between RA FLS and B cells that may contribute to joint inflammation was found to be associated with the expression of an RA-associated isoform of osteopontin (OPN).[41] This larger form of OPN was preferentially detected in RA FLS on Western blot analysis, and was found to form a unique macrocomplex with fibrinogen on the cell surface of RA FLS. Cocultures of purified B cells with OPN-fibrinogen complex–positive FLS led to increased expression of IL-6, an effect that was blocked by specific inhibition of OPN production. Immunohistochemistry of RA synovial tissue demonstrated the colocalization of OPN, IL-6, and B cells to highly inflamed areas of the joint.

RANK-L on B Cells

Provocative new data suggest that B cells can express the receptor activator of nuclear factor-κB ligand (RANK-L).[42] The expression of RANK-L in the synovium drives differentiation of osteoclasts that mediate the erosion of bone in RA. The study by Han and colleagues[42] demonstrated that RANK-L expression was stimulated on rat splenic B cells by culture with the inactivated bacterium, *Aggregatibacter actinomycetemcomitans*, a pathogenic microbe associated with human periodontal disease. Purified splenic B cells from rats infected with *A actinomycetemcomitans* stimulated a reporter cell line to differentiate toward osteoclasts.[42] Thus, oral infection has systemic effects on RANK-L expression by B cells and may be a partial explanation of the association between RA and periodontal disease. Although the expression of RANK-L by synovial B cells has not yet been reported, it will be interesting to determine whether B cells contribute to RA tissue damage through this mechanism, and what local or systemic signals might be involved in B cell expression of RANK-L.

LEUCOCYTE-ENDOTHELIAL INTERACTIONS IN RA SYNOVIUM

Cell migration into inflammatory lesions is a tightly regulated and complex process that involves adhesion receptors on leucocytes and vascular endothelial cells, multiple chemokines, and retention signals within target tissues. Space does not permit a comprehensive description of the extensive knowledge concerning these processes in RA synovium; they have been recently reviewed elsewhere.[43] Relevant adhesion molecules include selectins, integrins, and members of the immunoglobulin gene superfamily.[43] These molecules are also used in various combinations in leucocyte efflux into nonsynovial tissues, but it seems likely that in some respects, the synovial vasculature and the cell homing mechanisms to synovium are unique.

Neutrophil Recruitment

Intravital microscopy has emerged as an elegant technique for assessing leucocyte ingress into synovium, at least in animal model systems.[44] Such studies have revealed an unexpected prominence of neutrophil versus lymphocyte recruitment that, in RA, could be reflected by the cell composition of synovial fluid more than synovial tissue. In the mouse model of proteoglycan-induced arthritis, neutrophil expression of CD44 and CD62L (L-selectin) is crucial for entry into the joint.[45] In human RA, in vitro studies suggest that FLS control neutrophil recruitment indirectly through their influence on endothelial cells.[46] Coculture of endothelial cells with RA FLS but not RA dermal fibroblasts markedly augmented adherence of neutrophils to the endothelial cells, a process that depended on IL-6 production by the FLS. A role for FLS IL-6 was also identified in a similar coculture system that measured lymphocyte recruitment by endothelial cells.[47] In these experiments, OA FLS and RA FLS behaved similarly, but FLS from injured but otherwise normal joints or dermal fibroblasts inhibited lymphocyte-endothelial adhesion. Although limited by the use of umbilical vein rather than synovial microvascular endothelial cells, these interesting studies provide striking evidence for a role of FLS in the control of endothelial cell function.

Permeability of the Synovial Vasculature

Ingress of leucocytes into synovium may also be facilitated by unique permeability properties of the synovial microvasculature that have been revealed by experiments in a murine immune-complex model of acute joint inflammation that is induced by serum transfer (as described earlier). Intravital microscopy was used to show that joints destined to become inflamed developed a unique degree of vascular leakage on systemic administration of arthritogenic sera or even nonarthritogenic immune complexes, through a process dependent on mast cells and vasoactive amines.[48] Such studies may point to hitherto unappreciated physiologic functions of normal synovium, and explain the high propensity for systemic inflammatory processes to target the joints. The relationship of this model system to chronic arthritis, particularly RA, is still difficult to define.

Blood Vessel Growth in RA Synovium

Vasculogenesis and angiogenesis are distinct but related events that occur in RA synovium.[43] Vasculogenesis, the de novo formation of blood vessels from circulating endothelial cell precursors (EPCs), is believed to occur in RA synovium and in corresponding animal models.[43,49] Coculture studies have implicated cell-cell contact between RA EPCs and RA FLS, mediated by binding of vascular cell adhesion molecule 1 (VCAM-1) to the integrin VLA-4, as critical to such interactions, which could retain EPCs in synovial tissue long enough to allow vasculogenesis to occur.[49] New blood vessel formation in RA synovium also depends on TNF and can be reversed by TNF blockade.[50] TNF and other proinflammatory cytokines can induce molecules that are involved in angiogenesis, leucocyte-endothelial adhesion, or both. One example is the group of molecules termed Le^y/H (identified by a carbohydrate-binding antibody termed 4A11) or its analog H-2 g.[51] These molecules not only promote angiogenesis and expression of adhesion ligands by endothelial cells, but also stimulate monocyte migration. This latter effect was observed in vitro and in vivo in assays of monocyte recruitment to human RA synovial tissues implanted into SCID mice.[51]

Lymphocyte Egress

Little is known about the control of lymphocyte egress versus retention in RA synovium. It is possible that some current treatment approaches, such as TNF blockade, do stimulate cell egress, although this is difficult to prove. Some data exist to suggest that expression of chemokine receptors on T lymphocytes is altered on entry into RA synovium, and that chemokine gradients in synovial lymphatics, endothelium, and stromal cells are distorted to discourage lymphocyte egress.[52] Readjustment of these gradients to deplete synovial tissue of inflammatory cells is a particularly compelling approach to resolving joint inflammation.

SUMMARY

Analysis of cell-cell interactions in RA synovium is providing a vivid and detailed understanding of RA pathogenesis. Current biologic and nonbiologic therapies are likely to be already targeting some of these interactions in ways that are still poorly understood. Several new possibilities for more targeted therapies have been identified based on interactions that are unique, or uniquely important, in the inflamed joint.

REFERENCES

1. Valencia X, Higgins JM, Kiener HP, et al. Cadherin-11 provides specific cellular adhesion between fibroblast-like synoviocytes. J Exp Med 2004;200:1673.
2. Lee DM, Kiener HP, Agarwal SK, et al. Cadherin-11 in synovial lining formation and pathology in arthritis. Science 2007;315:1006.
3. Vandooren B, Cantaert T, ter Borg M, et al. Tumor necrosis factor alpha drives cadherin 11 expression in rheumatoid inflammation. Arthritis Rheum 2008;58: 3051.
4. Volin MV, Huynh N, Klosowska K, et al. Fractalkine is a novel chemoattractant for rheumatoid arthritis fibroblast-like synoviocyte signaling through MAP kinases and Akt. Arthritis Rheum 2007;56:2512.
5. Sawai H, Park YW, He X, et al. Fractalkine mediates T cell-dependent proliferation of synovial fibroblasts in rheumatoid arthritis. Arthritis Rheum 2007;56:3215.
6. Benito-Miguel M, Garcia-Carmona Y, Balsa A, et al. A dual action of rheumatoid arthritis synovial fibroblast IL-15 expression on the equilibrium between CD4+CD25+ regulatory T cells and CD4+CD25− responder T cells. J Immunol 2009;183:8268.
7. Dubois S, Mariner J, Waldmann TA, et al. IL-15Ralpha recycles and presents IL-15 in trans to neighboring cells. Immunity 2002;17:537.
8. Baslund B, Tvede N, Danneskiold-Samsoe B, et al. Targeting interleukin-15 in patients with rheumatoid arthritis: a proof-of-concept study. Arthritis Rheum 2005;52:2686.

9. Tran CN, Davis MJ, Tesmer LA, et al. Presentation of arthritogenic peptide to antigen-specific T cells by fibroblast-like synoviocytes. Arthritis Rheum 2007;56: 1497.

10. Tran CN, Thacker SG, Louie DM, et al. Interactions of T cells with fibroblast-like synoviocytes: role of the B7 family costimulatory ligand B7-H3. J Immunol 2008;180:2989.

11. Modak S, Kramer K, Gultekin SH, et al. Monoclonal antibody 8H9 targets a novel cell surface antigen expressed by a wide spectrum of human solid tumors. Cancer Res 2001;61:4048.

12. Xu H, Cheung IY, Guo HF, et al. MicroRNA miR-29 modulates expression of immunoinhibitory molecule B7-H3: potential implications for immune based therapy of human solid tumors. Cancer Res 2009;69:6275.

13. Munn DH, Sharma MD, Mellor AL. Ligation of B7-1/B7-2 by human CD4 + T cells triggers indoleamine 2,3-dioxygenase activity in dendritic cells. J Immunol 2004; 172:4100.

14. Szanto S, Koreny T, Mikecz K, et al. Inhibition of indoleamine 2,3-dioxygenase-mediated tryptophan catabolism accelerates collagen-induced arthritis in mice. Arthritis Res Ther 2007;9:R50.

15. Criado G, Simelyte E, Inglis JJ, et al. Indoleamine 2,3 dioxygenase-mediated tryptophan catabolism regulates accumulation of Th1/Th17 cells in the joint in collagen-induced arthritis. Arthritis Rheum 2009;60:1342.

16. Zola H, editor. Leucocyte and stromal cell molecules: the CD markers. Hoboken (NJ): Wiley-Liss; 2007. p. 412.

17. Ohshima Y, Tanaka Y, Tozawa H, et al. Expression and function of OX40 ligand on human dendritic cells. J Immunol 1997;159:3838.

18. Brugnoni D, Bettinardi A, Malacarne F, et al. CD134/OX40 expression by synovial fluid CD4+ T lymphocytes in chronic synovitis. Br J Rheumatol 1998;37:584.

19. Yoshioka T, Nakajima A, Akiba H, et al. Contribution of OX40/OX40 ligand interaction to the pathogenesis of rheumatoid arthritis. Eur J Immunol 2000; 30:2815.

20. Giacomelli R, Passacantando A, Perricone R, et al. T lymphocytes in the synovial fluid of patients with active rheumatoid arthritis display CD134-OX40 surface antigen. Clin Exp Rheumatol 2001;19:317.

21. Passacantando A, Parzanese I, Rascente M, et al. Synovial fluid OX40T lymphocytes of patients with rheumatoid arthritis display a Th2/Th0 polarization. Int J Immunopathol Pharmacol 2006;19:499.

22. Hirota K, Yoshitomi H, Hashimoto M, et al. Preferential recruitment of CCR6-expressing Th17 cells to inflamed joints via CCL20 in rheumatoid arthritis and its animal model. J Exp Med 2007;204:2803.

23. Ruth JH, Shahrara S, Park CC, et al. Role of macrophage inflammatory protein-3alpha and its ligand CCR6 in rheumatoid arthritis. Lab Invest 2003;83:579.

24. Kageyama Y, Ichikawa T, Nagafusa T, et al. Etanercept reduces the serum levels of interleukin-23 and macrophage inflammatory protein-3 alpha in patients with rheumatoid arthritis. Rheumatol Int 2007;28:137.

25. Chabaud M, Page G, Miossec P. Enhancing effect of IL-1, IL-17, and TNF-alpha on macrophage inflammatory protein-3alpha production in rheumatoid arthritis: regulation by soluble receptors and Th2 cytokines. J Immunol 2001; 167:6015.

26. Tanida S, Yoshitomi H, Nishitani K, et al. CCL20 produced in the cytokine network of rheumatoid arthritis recruits CCR6+ mononuclear cells and enhances the production of IL-6. Cytokine 2009;47:112.

27. Kawashiri SY, Kawakami A, Iwamoto N, et al. Proinflammatory cytokines synergistically enhance the production of chemokine ligand 20 (CCL20) from rheumatoid fibroblast-like synovial cells in vitro and serum CCL20 is reduced in vivo by biologic disease-modifying antirheumatic drugs. J Rheumatol 2009; 36:2397.

28. Timmer TC, Baltus B, Vondenhoff M, et al. Inflammation and ectopic lymphoid structures in rheumatoid arthritis synovial tissues dissected by genomics technology: identification of the interleukin-7 signaling pathway in tissues with lymphoid neogenesis. Arthritis Rheum 2007;56:2492.

29. van Roon JA, Jacobs K, Verstappen S, et al. Reduction of serum interleukin 7 levels upon methotrexate therapy in early rheumatoid arthritis correlates with disease suppression. Ann Rheum Dis 2008;67:1054.

30. Hartgring SA, van Roon JA, Wenting-van Wijk M, et al. Elevated expression of interleukin-7 receptor in inflamed joints mediates interleukin-7-induced immune activation in rheumatoid arthritis. Arthritis Rheum 2009;60:2595.

31. Levesque MC. Translational mini-review series on B cell-directed therapies: recent advances in B cell-directed biological therapies for autoimmune disorders. Clin Exp Immunol 2009;157:198.

32. Humby F, Bombardieri M, Manzo A, et al. Ectopic lymphoid structures support ongoing production of class-switched autoantibodies in rheumatoid synovium. PLoS Med 2009;6:e1.

33. Manzo A, Vitolo B, Humby F, et al. Mature antigen-experienced T helper cells synthesize and secrete the B cell chemoattractant CXCL13 in the inflammatory environment of the rheumatoid joint. Arthritis Rheum 2008;58:3377.

34. Iwai H, Kozono Y, Hirose S, et al. Amelioration of collagen-induced arthritis by blockade of inducible costimulator-B7 homologous protein costimulation. J Immunol 2002;169:4332.

35. Hu YL, Metz DP, Chung J, et al. B7RP-1 blockade ameliorates autoimmunity through regulation of follicular helper T cells. J Immunol 2009;182:1421.

36. Matsushita T, Yanaba K, Bouaziz JD, et al. Regulatory B cells inhibit EAE initiation in mice while other B cells promote disease progression. J Clin Invest 2008;118: 3420.

37. Coppieters K, Dewint P, Van Beneden K, et al. NKT cells: manipulable managers of joint inflammation. Rheumatology (Oxford) 2007;46:565.

38. Parietti V, Chifflot H, Sibilia J, et al. Rituximab treatment overcomes reduction of regulatory iNKT cells in patients with rheumatoid arthritis. Clin Immunol 2009;134:331–9.

39. Rochas C, Hillion S, Saraux A, et al. Transmembrane BAFF from rheumatoid synoviocytes requires interleukin-6 to induce the expression of recombination-activating gene in B lymphocytes. Arthritis Rheum 2009;60:1261.

40. Lai Kwan Lam Q, King Hung Ko O, Zheng BJ, et al. Local BAFF gene silencing suppresses Th17-cell generation and ameliorates autoimmune arthritis. Proc Natl Acad Sci U S A 2008;105:14993.

41. Take Y, Nakata K, Hashimoto J, et al. Specifically modified osteopontin in rheumatoid arthritis fibroblast-like synoviocytes supports interaction with B cells and enhances production of interleukin-6. Arthritis Rheum 2009;60:3591.

42. Han X, Lin X, Seliger AR, et al. Expression of receptor activator of nuclear factor-kappaB ligand by B cells in response to oral bacteria. Oral Microbiol Immunol 2009;24:190.

43. Szekanecz Z, Koch AE. Vascular involvement in rheumatic diseases: 'vascular rheumatology'. Arthritis Res Ther 2008;10:224.

44. Gal I, Bajnok E, Szanto S, et al. Visualization and in situ analysis of leukocyte trafficking into the ankle joint in a systemic murine model of rheumatoid arthritis. Arthritis Rheum 2005;52:3269.
45. Sarraj B, Ludanyi K, Glant TT, et al. Expression of CD44 and L-selectin in the innate immune system is required for severe joint inflammation in the proteoglycan-induced murine model of rheumatoid arthritis. J Immunol 1932;177:2006.
46. Lally F, Smith E, Filer A, et al. A novel mechanism of neutrophil recruitment in a coculture model of the rheumatoid synovium. Arthritis Rheum 2005;52:3460.
47. McGettrick HM, Smith E, Filer A, et al. Fibroblasts from different sites may promote or inhibit recruitment of flowing lymphocytes by endothelial cells. Eur J Immunol 2009;39:113.
48. Binstadt BA, Patel PR, Alencar H, et al. Particularities of the vasculature can promote the organ specificity of autoimmune attack. Nat Immunol 2006;7:284.
49. Silverman MD, Haas CS, Rad AM, et al. The role of vascular cell adhesion molecule 1/very late activation antigen 4 in endothelial progenitor cell recruitment to rheumatoid arthritis synovium. Arthritis Rheum 2007;56:1817.
50. Izquierdo E, Canete JD, Celis R, et al. Immature blood vessels in rheumatoid synovium are selectively depleted in response to anti-TNF therapy. PLoS One 2009;4:e8131.
51. Amin MA, Ruth JH, Haas CS, et al. H-2g, a glucose analog of blood group H antigen, mediates mononuclear cell recruitment via Src and phosphatidylinositol 3-kinase pathways. Arthritis Rheum 2008;58:689.
52. Burman A, Haworth O, Hardie DL, et al. A chemokine-dependent stromal induction mechanism for aberrant lymphocyte accumulation and compromised lymphatic return in rheumatoid arthritis. J Immunol 2005;174:1693.

B Cell Therapies for Rheumatoid Arthritis: Beyond B cell Depletion

Ismael Calero, MD[a], Jose Antonio Nieto, MD[a], Iñaki Sanz, MD[b,c],*

KEYWORDS

- B cell • Rheumatoid Arthritis • Biologic • Plasma cell

Although widely accepted that rheumatoid arthritis (RA) is mediated by inflammatory cytokines produced by macrophages and synovial fibroblasts in a T-dependent fashion, the success of B cell depletion (BCD) has prompted a re-evaluation of the place occupied by B cells in the pathogenesis and treatment of this disease.[1,2] Indeed, a first glimpse of B cell abnormalities in RA was provided by the description more than 50 years ago of the presence in most patients of increased levels of autoantibodies directed against immunoglobulin G (IgG) (rheumatoid factor, RF),[3] and more recently by the recognition of autoantibodies against neo-antigens created by the citrullination of cyclic peptides (CCP).[4] It is still uncertain, however, whether these autoantibodies play a direct pathogenic role or are simply produced as a by-product of inflammation as illustrated by the production of RF in situations characterized by polyclonal B cell activation (including nonautoimmune bacterial endocarditis and hepatitis C infection). Nonetheless, multiple lines of evidence strongly indicate that the production of RF in RA is mediated by antigen-driven processes that are locally amplified in the synovium. Thus, early human work demonstrated that synovial antibody production was enriched for RF and did not reflect systemic immune responses induced by

This work was supported by NIH grants U19 AI56390 (Rochester Autoimmunity Center of Excellence-IS); R01 AI049660 (IS); and N01-AI50029 (IS) Rochester Center for Biodefense of Immunocompromised Populations.

Dr Sanz has served as a paid consultant for Genentech (B Cell Summit participation) and Biogen (<$10,000 each).

[a] Internal Medicine Department, Hospital Virgen de la Luz, Calle de la Hermandad de Donantes de Sangre, Cuenca 16002, Spain
[b] Department of Microbiology and Immunology, University of Rochester Medical Center, 601 Elmwood Avenue, Rochester, NY 14642, USA
[c] Division of Allergy, Immunology and Rheumatology, University of Rochester Medical Center, 601 Elmwood Avenue, Rochester, NY 14642, USA
* Corresponding author.
E-mail address: Ignacio_Sanz@URMC.rochester.edu

Rheum Dis Clin N Am 36 (2010) 325–343
doi:10.1016/j.rdc.2010.02.003
0889-857X/10/$ – see front matter © 2010 Elsevier Inc. All rights reserved.

rheumatic.theclinics.com

immunization, thereby suggesting enhanced migration or expansion of autoreactive B cells within the target organ.[5,6] Subsequently, work in autoimmune prone MRL-lpr mice demonstrated that the production of RF was the result of strong antigen-driven selection of oligoclonal B cells.[7] Finally, in keeping with the mouse data, clonal expansions of RF-producing synovial B cells also can be found in the human rheumatoid synovium.[8] Collectively, the evidence indicates that antigen selection plays a critical role in the local expansion of synovial RF B cells and provides at least strong circumstantial evidence for a pathogenic role of autoantibodies or the B cells producing them.

Indeed, the rationale initially posited by Jonathan Edwards to pursue his pioneering studies of BCD in RA was based on the implications that the RF might have for disease pathogenesis. He astutely postulated that in addition to conventional immune complex-mediated inflammatory mechanisms, B cells expressing surface antibodies with RF properties could serve as universal antigen-presenting cells capable of amplifying autoimmune responses through RF-mediated capture and internalization of circulating immune complexes containing any type of autoantigens.[9] This hypothesis had strong experimental underpinnings provided by the experiments of Roosnek and Lanzavecchia.[10] More recent studies have unraveled other mechanisms whereby immune complexes could contribute to disease pathogenesis either through the costimulation of Toll-like receptors (TLR) and Fcγ receptors in dendritic cells and B cells and costimulation of synovial macrophages through Fcγ and C5a receptors.[1,11,12]

The potential contributions of B cells have been significantly extended by numerous studies demonstrating that B cells also play many antibody-independent proinflammatory that are likely to the pathogenesis of RA. These functions include activation of CD4 and CD8 T cells, maintenance of CD8 T cell memory, induction of Th1 and Th17 effector cells, recruitment of dendritic cells (DC), suppression of T regulatory cells (Tregs), lymphangiogenesis and production of proinflammatory cytokines including tumor necrosis factor (TNF) and interleukin (IL)-6[13,14] and polyclonal B cell activators such as IL-6 and osteopontin.[15] Of particular relevance to RA, synovial B cells are essential to sustain CD4 T cell activation in explanted RA synovium, an effect reversed by anti-CD20 mediated B cell depletion.[16]

B cells are also critical for the organization of the lymphoid architecture through membrane-bound LTα1β2 induction of LTβR signaling.[17–19] The latter function may be highly relevant to the pathogenesis of RA, since lymphoid infiltrates organized as B/T cell areas and in some cases with germinal center-like structure and function can be found in the RA synovium and have been postulated to play a pathogenic role through local amplification of autoimmune B cells and plasma cell generation.[20,21] The actual significance of synovial GCs remains controversial due to the relatively small fraction of cases in which this configuration is detected (5% to 25%, possibly on the basis of sampling variability and patchy disease) and the lack of correlation in some studies between these findings and local autoimmunity.[22] These studies stand in contrast to the recent demonstration that in 25% of RA patients analyzed, ectopic synovial lymphoid structures containing follicular dendritic cells express molecular markers of in situ somatic hypermutation and class switch recombination and are highly enriched for plasma cells locally producing antibodies against citrullinated fibrinogen.[23] This study conclusively demonstrates the ability of synovial lymphoid structures to locally support the generation and diversification of RA-specific B cell autoreactivity. This is in keeping with earlier indication that synovial memory B cells could be generated locally, a concept later disputed by the finding of clonally related B cells in separate joints and in the systemic circulation,[8,24,25] which suggests that, alternatively, pathogenic B cells may arise systemically and then migrate to the inflamed synovium where they could be diversified further in ectopic GC-like structures. Although the limited available data cannot establish whether pathogenic B cells could originate initially in the joint and then metastasize to other joints, the notion that a constant supply of recirculating B cells is important for maintaining the B cell microenvironment of inflamed joints bears significant connotations for the understanding of the mechanisms of action of B cell-targeted therapies in RA.

CURRENT B CELL THERAPIES—LIMITATIONS AND CHALLENGES OF UNIVERSAL B CELL DEPLETION

Rituximab-induced BCD is US Food and Drug Administration (FDA)-approved, in combination with methotrexate, for the treatment of RA patients who fail or are unable to tolerate anti-TNF drugs.[26,27] Although significant favorable responses are attained in this difficult to treat group, only 50% to 65% of patients maintain ACR20 or moderate-to-good European League Against Rheumatism responses 6 months after treatment, and disease relapses frequently ensue after B cell repopulation, which typically occurs 6 to 9 months after treatment. As a result, systematic retreatment with Rituximab every 6 to 9 months is becoming a frequent practice.[26] Repeated retreatment tends to be beneficial in patients who respond to the first treatment and has proven largely safe in patients receiving six to eight cycles of therapy.[28,29] However, serum IgM levels below normal values and a downward trend in IgG levels are seen with repeated treatment and vaccine responses are likely to be compromised in chronically depleted patients.[30,31] Moreover, the effect of chronic B cell depletion on protective T cell immunity also remains to be properly studied. Therefore, the need for indefinite retreatment should create significant concern that is further compounded by the report of progressive multifocal leukoencephalopathy (PML) in three RA patients treated with Rituximab (out of approximately 100,000 patients treated), including one recent case who had not received previous treatment with anti-TNF agents.[32,33]

Typically, Rituximab achieves almost universal peripheral blood B cell depletion defined as less than 5 CD19+ cell/μL but less consistent profound depletion of less than 0.01 cells/μL, a level that seems to correlate with greater and more sustained clinical response.[34] As it is also the case with systemic lupus erythematosus (SLE), B cell reconstitution in patients with good clinical responses is initiated by enhanced bone marrow generation of transitional B cells, whereas relapsing patients are characterized by relative expansion of memory cells that presumably Rituximab failed to deplete in the first place.[35–37] In tissue, some studies have shown a correlation between clinical response to Rituximab, relatively early declines in numbers of synovial B cells, and decreased frequencies of plasma cells and immunoglobulin synthesis activity, whereas other studies have found no correlation between early synovial B cell decline and clinical response.[1,38–40] All these studies have used limited numbers of patients, and their interpretation is confounded by the intrinsic variability and limitations of tissue sampling and disease heterogeneity. Nonetheless, the collective information available has been used by Silverman and Boyle to formulate the roadblock hypothesis, which postulates that the benefit of Rituximab could be mediated by interruption of the supply to the synovium of circulating B cells, leading to the progressive attrition of synovial B cells, plasma cells, and other inflammatory cells, particularly macrophages.[1]

Therefore, the current goal of BCD is to achieve complete and sustained B cell depletion in blood and synovium of pathogenic B cells whose elimination might account for initial disease improvement even in the absence of significant autoantibody changes. This goal could be accomplished with either more intensive Rituximab regimens, more efficient anti-CD20 agents, or with combination therapy with other agents (including BAFF blockade to be discussed further). More extensive B cell depletion also could be achieved with antibodies that target surface antigens expressed more widely than CD20 whose expression begins in pre-B cells and is extinguished in most immature plasma cells (a pattern accounting for the limited efficacy of Rituximab to target plasma cells). In contrast, CD19 expression is initiated in pro-B cells and persists even in a fraction of mature CD138 + PC (F-EH Lee and I Sanz, unpublished data, 2010). Accordingly, anti-CD19 antibodies represent a promising alternative, and trials with humanized anti-CD19 antibodies are under development.[41,42]

Potentially, more effective targeting of B cells and preplasma cells could be achieved by antibodies against CD79α/β, which in addition to a direct killing effect, also inhibit B cell receptor (BCR) activation, display clinical efficacy in lupus-prone MRL/lpr mice,[43] and induce profound GC depletion in cynomolgus monkeys.[44]

However, indiscriminate B cell depletion also may have a dark side, as this intervention also would compromise regulatory B cells capable of delaying progression in untreated patients or sustain the initial remission induced by the depletion of pathogenic B cells. Of note, B cell measurements used in published studies lacked the ability to differentiate between pathogenic and protective B cells. Protective B cell effects can be mediated by several direct mechanisms, including induction of T cell anergy, induction of Tregs or production of anti-inflammatory cytokines including IL-10 or TGFβ.[13,45] The latter possibility is illustrated by the recent description of IL-10 producing B regulatory cells (Bregs) with a transitional phenotype capable of suppressing arthritis in animal models and by a growing body of knowledge regarding Breg functions in multiple other autoimmune diseases.[46] It therefore could be envisioned that strategies to selectively deplete pathogenic B cells, expand in vivo Bregs, or infuse Breg cells previously expanded in vitro might represent future avenues for B cell therapies in RA.[47,48]

Undoubtedly, there is a formidable challenge to understanding the different roles of B cells in RA (which could change at different times in the natural history of the disease or differ among disease subsets) and the relative balance between pathogenic and protective B cells at different times after B cell depletion. Collectively, these considerations suggest a model (**Fig. 1**), in which the best risk/benefit ratio would be provided by induction therapies aimed at profound B cell depletion (or selective depletion of pathogenic B cells) followed by maintenance regimens that promote an environment dominated by protective B cells). The following sections provide a discussion of alternative strategies for B cell targeting (summarized in **Table 1** and illustrated by **Fig. 2**).

TARGETING B CELL ACTIVATION AND COSTIMULATION

In addition to anti-CD79 antibodies, multiple strategies could be pursued to inhibit B cell activation either through the BCR or costimulatory molecules central to the necessary cross-talk between B cells and T cells or dendritic cells. Potential targets include BCR signaling pathways, inducible T-cell co-stimulator (ICOS), and TLR signaling. The therapeutic potential of BCR inhibition has been suggested by an early clinical trial of the spleen tyrosine kinase (Syk) inhibitor R406 in RA patients. An Src family of nonreceptor kinase, Syk is required for proximal BCR signaling and mediates positive selection of immature B cells, a critical checkpoint for the censoring of autoreactive B cells.[49] In this phase 1 placebo-controlled trial, clinical benefit was obtained as early as 1 week after treatment and was maintained through the 12 weeks duration of the study.[50] Unfortunately, no B cell data were provided by this study, and therefore the

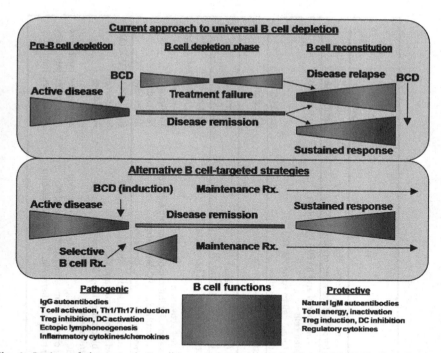

Fig. 1. Design of therapeutic B cell targeting in rheumatoid arthritis (RA). The proposed therapeutic strategies are based on the duality of B cells, which can play both protective and pathogenic functions (selected functions are presented at the bottom). Throughout the figure, pathogenic and protective functions are color coded (red to blue shading, respectively). Current approaches use indiscriminate B cell deletion with initial response based on elimination of pathogenic functions. In this model, treatment failure is caused by insufficient depletion or preferential re-expansion of pathogenic cells. Such imbalance also would underlie the relapse commonly seen with B cell reconstitution and creates the need for additional cycles of B cell depletion. B cell reconstitution dominated by protective B cells might account for sustained responses in a small fraction of RA patients who would not need frequent retreatment. Alternative approaches include the integration of induction and maintenance strategies aimed at creating a favorable functional B cell balance. Thus, remission induction could be attained with profound B cell depletion (plus or minus plasma cell [PC] depletion); by selective depletion of pathogenic B cells (or blockade of pathogenic B cell cytokines); or by preferential expansion of regulatory B cells. The latter two approaches also could be used for maintenance therapy. In addition, maintenance could be accomplished by targeting pathways that promote survival, expansion or migration of pathogenic B cells and PC (BAFF, cytokines, chemokines).

actual mechanism of Syk inhibition remains to be clarified since Syk inhibition also interferes with T cell receptor and Fcγ and Fcε receptor signaling, thereby impacting other cells of relevance for the pathogenesis of RA including T cells, mast cells, neutrophils, and osteoclast activation.[51] These studies should provide the impetus to pursue the use of other BCR signaling inhibitors acting downstream of Syk such as PI3 K inhibitors and in particular specific PI3 Kδ inhibitors given the critical and nonredundant role played by this isoform in B cell development.[52]

Upon interaction with activated T cells, B cells are themselves activated through several surface molecules including CD40, CD27, and the inducible costimulatory

Table 1
Mechanistic overview of current and potential B cell targeted therapies

Mechanism	Target	Effect	Agents
B cell killing	CD20	Depletion (pre-B cell to some PB)	Rituximab, others
	CD19	Depletion (pro-B cell to some mature PC)	Antibodies
B cell killing + inhibition	CD22	Depletion (transitional and B cells) Inhibition of activated cells	Antibodies
	CD79a/b	Depletion (pre-B cell to some PB, GC) Inhibition of activated cells	Antibodies
B cell signaling	Syk	B cell inactivation and secondary death	Inhibitors
	PI3 K		
B cell survival	BAFF	Depletion (transitional, naïve)	Belimumab
	BAFF+APRIL	Depletion (transitional, naïve, SLPC)	Atacicept
B cell costimulation and differentiation; inhibition of B cell effector functions	TLR	B cell inactivation, ↓ M cell homeostasis	Inhibitors
	TNF	↓ M cells, ↓ PC survival	ETN, HMR, IFM, GLM
	ICOS	↓ GC, ↓ M cell activation	Antibodies
	IL-6	↓ PC generation, inhibit proinflammatory Beff cells	Tocilizumab
	IL-17	↓ GC, ↓ autoantibody, ↓ PC generation	Antibodies
	IL-21	↓ M cells maintenance, ↓ PC generation	Antibodies
B cell homing and organization	TNF, LT	Inhibit formation—disrupts systemic and ectopic lymphoid architecture and GC	ETN, ADM, IFM, GLM
	LTβR		Baminercept
	CXCL13/CXCR5	As above; blocks B cell–F$_{TH}$ cell cross-talk, GC organization	Antibodies
	CXCL12/CXCR4	Disrupts GC organization, ↓ LLPC homing survival	Antibodies, inhibitors
	CCL10/CXCR3	↑ Homing of proinflammatory Beff cells and PC	Antibodies, inhibitors
	CCL20/CCR6	↓ Homing of CCR6 + Beff cells, ↓ IL-17 stimulation of B cells	Antibodies, inhibitors

Breg expansion	B cell depletion	Promote dominance of Breg upon reconstitution	B cell depleting agents
	CD40 agonists	Induce in vivo expansion of Breg cells	Antibodies
	GM-CSF/IL-15	Induce in vivo expansion of Breg cells	GM-CSF/IL15 Fusokine
Plasma cell killing	Proteasome	Depletion of PC, activated B cells, ↓ proinflammatory cytokine secretion by Beff cells[120]	Proteasome inhibitors
	CD38, CD27, others	Depletion of PC	ATG
	BCMA	Depletion of LLPC	Antibodies
	FcγR2b	Depletion of PC, inhibit antibody production	IVIG, antibodies
Plasma cell inhibition	CCL2/CCR2	Suppress antibody production by PC	Antibodies, inhibitors

This table summarizes different mechanisms of action whereby different agents could interfere with pathogenic B cell functions or promote protective B cell functions for the treatment of rheumatoid arthritis. For the sake of brevity, only the more prominent and immediate B cell effects of the corresponding interventions are included. To avoid redundancy, with the exception of B cell-depleting and antitumor necrosis factor (TNF) drugs, agents that could work through different mechanisms are mentioned only once. In most cases, the proposed effect of the mechanism in question is derived from mouse or human studies. In a few cases, highlighted in italics, the proposed mechanism is based on the speculative integration by the authors of known biologic effects. Finally, drugs currently used in clinical practice or in advanced stages of development for human autoimmune diseases are mentioned by name. Otherwise, they are generically identified as antibodies or inhibitors (the latter to indicate class agents such as specific enzymatic inhibitors or small molecules).

Abbreviations: ADM, adalimumab; ATG, antithymocyte globulin; Beff, cytokine-producing effector B cells; ETN, etanercept; F_TH, follicular T helper cells; GC, germinal center; GLM, golimumab; IFM, infliximab; IL, interleukin; LLPC, long-lived plasma cells; M, memory; PB, plasmablasts; PC, plasma cells; SLPC, short-lived PC.

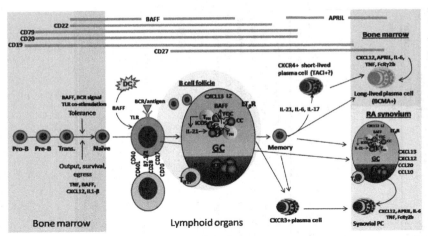

Fig. 2. The biologic basis for targeting pathogenic B cells in RA. Schematic representation of different molecular and cellular B cell targets. The recruitment of B cells into the pathogenic process could be interrupted at multiple levels including early bone marrow generation, survival, release, and censoring of autoreactive B cells. In the mature, postantigenic compartments, the pathogenic process could be blocked by inhibition of the B cell receptor (BCR) signaling complex or costimulation (the B cell-T_H cell cross-talk is illustrated here for naïve B cells and for GC cells; memory cells may share similar pathways, but response to BCR/TLR/BAFF/APRIL and other stimulatory cytokines may differ significantly). GC reactions and their progeny of pathogenic memory and plasma cells can be attenuated either by disrupting microarchitecture (LTβR/CXCL13), migration/organization/duration (CXC13/CXCL12/ interleukin [IL]-17/BAFF), or co-stimulation (IL-21). Blockade of different cytokines (IL-21, IL-6, IL-17) would decrease memory survival or differentiation into PC. Synovial generation of GC, memory, and plasma cells could be attenuated by similar interventions, and recruitment of systemic B cells into the inflamed synovium could be blocked by inhibition of chemo attraction by several chemokines including (but not limited to) CXCL12, CXCL13, CCL20, and CCL10. Finally, long-lived PC could be targeted either by depleting agents or by blocking survival factors as indicated in the figure and **Table 1**. Pathogenic B cell functions also could be interrupted by depleting antibodies directed against surface antigens. The expression of the most relevant markers is indicated at the top. Also shown is the breadth of B cell populations whose survival depends on either BAFF or APRIL stimulation.

molecule ligand (ICOS-L or B7RP1).[53] These molecules therefore represent attractive candidates for the inhibition of B cells, although a trial of anti-CD40L antibodies had to be discontinued in SLE because of thromboembolism. Targeting the ICOS pathway is of particular interest given the role played by ICOS+ T follicular helper cells (T_FH) in autoimmune B cell germinal center reactions,[54] the expression of ICOS by rheumatoid synovial T cell and CD14+ monocytes,[55] its ability to regulate IL-17 production, and the essential role it plays in collagen-induced arthritis.[56] Anti-ICOS antibodies (AMG557) are under development for autoimmune indications.

Recent data showing that B7-1/2 (CD80/86) also can transmit activation signals to B cells suggest that other members of the B7 family could represent additional targets for inhibitory antibodies.[57] These results also beg the question as to whether the interruption of CD28 signaling by CTLA4-Ig (abatacept, an effective, FDA-approved treatment), also could result in B cell inactivation and disruption of their antigen-presenting cell function. Finally, blocking of CD70-induced CD27 stimulation has been shown to improve mouse collagen-induced arthritis (CIA) disease and provides another example of the therapeutic potential of blocking costimulatory TNF superfamily members that participate in B cell–T cell costimulation.[58,59]

TLRs represent important pharmacologic targets for the treatment of RA as evidenced by the benefit imparted in this disease by hydroxychloroquine, whose activity is mediated at least in part by relatively weak TLR9 inhibition.[60] In addition to inducing receptor activator for nuclear factor κ B ligand in synovial fibroblasts (TLR2, 3 and 4),[61] TLRs also provide critical costimulation to autoreactive B cells and at least in SLE, TLR3, 7, and 9 regulate the generation of RF as well as anti-DNA and anti-RBP (RNA-binding proteins such as Ro, LA, Sm/RNP).[62,63] Other potentially important contributions of TLR9 activation of B cells in RA include the production of cytokines such as IL-6 and RANTES/CCL5.[64] Powerful and specific TLR inhibitors, including a combined TLR9/7 inhibitor (DV1079) and TLR7/8/9 antagonists, are under development for RA and SLE.[65,66] Potential drawbacks of this approach are illustrated by the exacerbation of murine lupus observed in the absence of TLR9[62] and by the dampening effect of TLR activation of B cells in autoimmune T cell responses.[67,68]

TARGETING B CELL SURVIVAL AND DIFFERENTIATION BY CYTOKINE BLOCKADE

In this category, BAFF (B lymphocyte activation factor/BLyS) and APRIL (a proliferation-inducing ligand) are of particular interest because of their central role in B cell homeostasis and the availability of inhibitory agents tested in large numbers of patients with SLE.[69] Human BAFF signals through three different receptors (BAFF-R, TACI, and BCMA), whereas APRIL only signals through TACI and BCMA. Accordingly, anti-BAFF antibodies (Belimumab) or BAFF-R-Ig provide selective BAFF blockade, whereas agents that bind TACI (TACI-Ig; Atacicept) interrupt both BAFF and APRIL-mediated signaling. BAFF is essential for the survival of late transitional, naïve, and marginal zone B cells but does not influence the survival of memory cells. In contrast, APRIL is important for the survival of short-lived and long-lived plasma cells through TACI and BCMA, and the viability of these antibody-producing cells is severely compromised by combined blockade of BAFF and APRIL but not BAFF alone.[69] BAFF levels also regulate the stringency of censoring of early autoreactive B cells, and the subversion of such censoring by excess BAFF is likely to play a major role in the generation of B cell autoimmunity in both RA and SLE.[70]

A role for BAFF/APRIL in RA is suggested by multiple lines of evidence including elevated BAFF levels in human RA and in mouse models as well as production of BAFF in the rheumatoid synovium by fibroblasts (under stimulation by TNF and interferon [IFN]γ)[71] and macrophages, production of APRIL by DCs, and production of both cytokines by synovial B cells.[69] Elegant studies of BAFF/APRIL blockade using TACI-Ig in human RA synovium explanted into SCID mice demonstrated dramatic improvement of the inflammatory process and collapse of GC-like structures in the samples with this type of B cell infiltrate. Of great interest however, TACI-Ig increased the degree of inflammation (including IFNγ production) present in explanted tissues without GC structures, thereby suggesting that BAFF/APRIL also could mediate protective functions possibly through T cells.[72] The possibility that protective BAFF/APRIL functions could have been delivered through Bregs was not addressed by this study, however.

Despite these potentially deleterious consequences, clinical blockade of BAFF/APRIL has shown clinical promise and safety in a phase 2 study of Belimumab and a phase 1b study of Atacicept.[73,74] Consistent with mouse and human SLE studies, BAFF blockade resulted in decreased numbers of transitional and naïve B cells without a major impact on memory cells or plasma cells. Also consistent with mouse studies and suggesting a preferential effect on the survival of short-lived plasma cells, Atacicept induced significant declines in IgM but not IgG levels and did not impact serum levels of antimicrobial antibodies. A preferential decline in these studies of RF versus CCP antibodies also suggests that the latter type may be largely generated by long-lived plasma cells.

As discussed in other sections of this article and in **Table 1**, multiple other cytokines may impact the survival of B cells or their differentiation into plasma cells; therefore cytokine blockade provides many opportunities for the therapeutic B cell targeting. This concept is illustrated by the powerful B cell effects of several cytokines whose inhibition is of proven clinical benefit in RA: TNF, IL-6, and IL-17.[75–77] Thus, IL-6 contributes significantly to plasma cell differentiation,[78] and B cell-produced IL-6 is critical to induce systemic autoimmunity in Lyn-deficient mice[79]; IL-17 enhances GC reactions and autoantibody production and synergizes with BAFF to enhance plasma cell differentiation.[80,81] A similar synergistic effect has been shown for IL-21, which also appears to be important for maintenance of memory B cells.[82,83] Clearly, the actual role of B cell-mediated mechanisms in the clinical benefit of these drugs merits additional investigation. IL-21 blockade is beneficial in animal models of arthritis and also represents a future avenue of significant interest.[84]

Finally, the benefit of agents capable of blocking lymphotoxin (LT) and TNF functions in RA is worth discussing in the context of B cell therapies.[85] Indeed, naïve B cells expressing surface LTα1β2 provide critical signaling through the LTβR to induce expression of CXCL13 by stromal cells leading to the expansion of follicular dendritic cells (FDCs) and organization of B cell and T cell areas and polarized GCs in systemic lymphoid tissue.[17–19] This pathway also is considered central to the formation of ectopic lymphoid structures in the target organs of multiple autoimmune diseases including RA.[54] TNF deficiency additionally has been shown to decrease CXC13 expression and disrupt lymphoid architecture. Therefore, both LT blockade and TNF blockade have direct and indirect effects on B cell function, and recent work has in fact shown that etanercept, capable of binding both these cytokines, may disrupt GC architecture and decrease memory B cells.[86] Proof of principle for the clinical efficacy of blocking this pathway initially was provided by the ability of a LTβR-Ig fusion protein to improve disease in established CIA.[87] Enthusiasm for this approach, however, has been damped somewhat by the disappointing results reported for 114 RA patients enrolled in a phase 2B study of Baminercept despite strong signals of biologic activity including increased numbers of circulating lymphocytes and a 50% reduction in serum levels of CXCL13.[88] Whether the lack of clinical benefit was caused by insufficient blockade of the LTβR pathway or the existence of redundant pathways remains to be determined. It is also likely that, as shown for LTβR-Ig protein in passive antibody transfer models, effector pathways mediated by preformed autoantibodies would not be impacted by this intervention.[87] If so, this approach still could provide significant benefit either in combination with antibody-depleting drugs or as maintenance therapy. Alternatively, as proposed by other studies, these results could indicate that ectopic lymphoid neogenesis is more a by-product of inflammation rather than a causative agent of synovial B cell-mediated autoimmunity.[22]

TARGETING B CELLS THROUGH CHEMOKINE INHIBITION

Multiple chemokines may participate in RA through B cells by

Facilitating the bone marrow egress of immature cells (CXCL12) promoted by TNF,[89] which in combination with excess BAFF could lead to defective early B cell tolerance checkpoints[90]

Organizing systemic and ectopic GC reactions (CXCL12 and CXCL13)[91,92]

Directing the homing of pathogenic CXCR4+ bone marrow plasma cells (CXCL12) and synovial CXCR3+ plasma cells (CXCL9/10/11)[93]

Contributing to the survival of long-lived plasma cells in either locale (CXCL12) mediating the invasion of subcortical bone marrow spaces by B cells and plasma cells (CXCL13 and CCL-21).[94]

Accordingly, chemokine inhibition represents an important avenue for B cell targeting. CXCL13 and CXCL12 in particular represent prime targets given their increased expression in the rheumatoid synovium.[92,95] As previously indicated, CXCL13 works downstream of LTβR signaling in stromal cells to attract B cells and promote productive engagement in the light zones of GCs with CXCR5 + T_{FH} cells, which are critical for the induction of autoimmunity,[96] and neutralization of CXCL13 ameliorates substantially established CIA in DBA/1 mice.[97] Moreover, CXCL13 inhibition also induces remarkably clinical, histologic, and radiological improvement of arthritis in TNF transgenic mice by inhibiting translocation of follicular CXCR5 + B cells and re-establishing proper compartmentalization into B cell and T cell zones.[98] Of note, increased levels of synovial CXCL13 correlate with local inflammation in human RA and predict favorable response to Rituximab.[99] As shown by these studies, development of CXCL13 antagonists is in preclinical stages.

CXCL12 also is expressed abundantly by fibroblast-like synoviocytes and plays a major pathogenic role through the promotion of angiogenesis, recruitment of proinflammatory cells, and enhancing survival of CXCR4+ plasma cells.[93,100,101] Of significant importance, the rheumatoid synovial milieu also can induce local upregulation of CXCR4, thereby contributing to lymphocyte retention and compromised lymphatic drainage due to high expression of CXCL12 in the vascular and lymphatic endothelium.[102] The importance of this chemokine in RA is illustrated further by the association reported between genetic polymorphisms of CXCL12 and progression of joint destruction in RA.[103] Accordingly, significant interest exists in the potential of CXCL12 inhibitors for the treatment of RA.[104] Recent studies indicate that in addition to CXCR4, CXCL12 inhibition also could block signaling through a second receptor, CXCR7,[105] which also is expressed abundantly in the RA synovium.[106]

Promising results in RA also have been reported using inhibitors of other chemokines with important B cell effects including a phase 2 placebo-controlled study of CXCL10, an IFNγ-induced chemokine that attracts CXCR3 + B cells and plasma cells to Th1-infiltrated inflammatory tissues.[107]

Finally, another important chemokine axis of significant importance in RA pathogenesis merits discussion here. Thus, recruitment of CCR6 + Th17 cells to the rheumatoid synovium is powerfully mediated by CCL20, and anti-CCR6 antibodies can inhibit arthritis in animal models.[108] Given that CCR6 also is expressed by activated human B cells[109] and the B cell effects of IL-17 stimulation previously discussed, it will be important to understand the B cell impact of CCR6 inhibition and its benefit in RA.

TARGETING PLASMA CELLS IN RHEUMATOID ARTHRITIS

PC contributes to RA pathogenesis through the production of autoantibodies both systemically (from lymphoid and bone marrow plasma cells) and locally within the RA synovium. The pathogenic role of PC is illustrated further by their prominence within the RA joint and by the correlation found in at least some Rituximab studies between decline in local PC and disease amelioration.[39,110] These observations clearly identify PC elimination as an important therapeutic goal, which, as previously discussed, could be indirectly achieved by the blockade of multiple cytokines and chemokines.

A more direct approach to depleting PC is provided by agents capable of directly killing these cells including antithymocyte globulin, a compound used in transplantation and autoimmunity for its anti-T cell effects but which has also powerful anti-B cell and PC activity.[111] In addition, a new class of anti-PC drugs is represented by proteasome inhibitors (PIs) such as bortezomib, approved for the treatment of multiple myeloma. A selective inhibitor of the 26S ubiquitin–proteasome, bortezomib activates the terminal unfolded protein response (UPR), which eventually leads to cell cycle arrest and apoptosis. Because of their extremely high immunoglobulin synthesis, which primes an initial UPR, plasma cells are particularly sensitive to PI.[112] In addition, PIs block NFκB and can inhibit activated B cells, GC cells, dendritic cells, and the release of NFκB-induced proinflammatory cytokines (including TNF, IL-1, and IL-6) from RA activated T cells.[113,114] PIs have shown efficacy in the treatment of murine models of RA and SLE.[113] In particular, an immunoproteasome-specific inhibitor (PR-957) can attenuate disease progression in experimental arthritis by a combination of cytokine inhibition, decreased cellular infiltrates, and decreased autoantibody production.[115] Of interest, PR-957 is related to carfilzomib, an irreversible inhibitor of the chymotrypsin-like activity of the 20S proteasome, currently under development for multiple myeloma and solid tumor treatment.[116] Recently presented results indicating that the newer PI inhibitors have a much lower incidence of painful peripheral neuropathy than bortezomib should buttress the development of these powerful drugs for RA.[117]

Finally, the pathogenic role of PC in RA could be diminished by interventions aimed at inhibiting their secretory function. This paradigm is illustrated by the ability of inhibitory CCL2 variants produced by mesenchymal stem cells (MSC) to suppress PC antibody production.[118] These studies provide rationale for the therapeutic B cell potential of inhibitory anti-CCR2 antibodies.

SUMMARY AND FUTURE DIRECTIONS

The therapeutic benefit of targeting B cells, either by killing, attrition, or inhibition has been made apparent by the experience with Rituximab. Moreover, other effective RA treatments are likely to have substantial B cell effects that could be elucidated by a more probing B cell analysis of clinical trials and patients treated in clinical practice. The observations discussed in this article, however, also paint a nuanced picture and indicate that universal B cell depletion may not be the best goal because of

  Difficulty in eliminating (mostly in the synovium, lymphoid tissue, and bone marrow)[119] pathogenic B cells
  Elimination of Breg cells or preferential repopulation with pathogenic B cells thereby contributing to an undesirable under-representation of protective B cells
  The need for inducing chronic B cell depletion with repeated courses of treatment.

Hence, while these caveats will apply in some measure to other B cell manipulations, more specific B cell interventions aimed at the elimination of pathogenic B cells or expansion or preservation of regulatory B cells will be of the essence. Accomplishing these goals will require a more precise understanding of the phenotypic diversity of human B cells and the functional division of labor among different subsets. This basic knowledge should contribute to the recognition of disease heterogeneity in RA and ultimately will allow investigators and clinicians alike to devise rational interventions capable of targeting specific components of the autoimmune and regulatory B cell response tailored to the pathogenic underpinnings of different disease subsets. Improved understanding of these critical issues also should facilitate the development of biomarkers of disease susceptibility and response to B cell therapies.

REFERENCES

1. Silverman GJ, Boyle DL. Understanding the mechanistic basis in rheumatoid arthritis for clinical response to anti-CD20 therapy: the B cell roadblock hypothesis. Immunol Rev 2008;223(1):175–85.
2. Edwards JCW, Szczepanski L, Szechinski J, et al. Efficacy of B-Cell-targeted therapy with rituximab in patients with rheumatoid arthritis. N Engl J Med 2004;350(25):2572–81.
3. Morris Z, Patricia B, Joseph L, et al. Agglutination and inhibition by serum globulin in the sensitized sheep cell agglutination reaction in rheumatoid arthritis. Am J Med 1956;20(4):500–9.
4. Schellekens GA, de Jong BA, van den Hoogen FHJ, et al. Citrulline is an essential constituent of antigenic determinants recognized by rheumatoid arthritis-specific autoantibodies. J Clin Invest 1998;101(1):273–81.
5. Mellors RC, Nowoslawski A, Korngold L, et al. Rheumatoid factor and the pathogenesis of rheumatoid arthritis. J Exp Med 1961;113(2):475–84.
6. Herman JH, Bradley J, Ziff M, et al. Response of the rheumatoid synovial membrane to exogenous immunization. J Clin Invest 1971;50(2):266–73.
7. Shlomchik MJ, Marshak-Rothstein A, Wolfowicz CB, et al. The role of clonal selection and somatic mutation in autoimmunity. Nature 1987;328(6133):805–11.
8. Schroder AE, Greiner A, Seyfert C, et al. Differentiation of B cells in the nonlymphoid tissue of the synovial membrane of patients with rheumatoid arthritis. Proc Natl Acad Sci U S A 1996;93(1):221–5.
9. Edwards JC, Cambridge G, Abrahams V. Do self-perpetuating B lymphocytes drive human autoimmune disease? Immunology 1999;97(2):188–96.
10. Roosnek E, Lanzavecchia A. Efficient and selective presentation of antigen–antibody complexes by rheumatoid factor B cells. J Exp Med 1991;173(2):487–9.
11. Huang QQ, Pope RM. The role of toll-like receptors in rheumatoid arthritis. Curr Rheumatol Rep 2009;11(5):357–64.
12. Lau CM, Broughton C, Tabor AS, et al. RNA-associated autoantigens activate B cells by combined B cell antigen receptor/toll-like receptor 7 engagement. J Exp Med 2005;202(9):1171–7.
13. Manjarrez-Orduno N, Quach TD, Sanz I. B cells and immunological tolerance. J Invest Dermatol 2009;129(2):278–88.
14. Sanz I, Anolik JH, Looney RJ. B cell depletion therapy in autoimmune diseases. Front Biosci 2007;12:2546–67.
15. Rothstein TL, Guo B. Receptor crosstalk: reprogramming B cell receptor signaling to an alternate pathway results in expression and secretion of the auto-immunity-associated cytokine, osteopontin. J Intern Med 2009;265(6):632–43.
16. Takemura S, Klimiuk PA, Braun A, et al. T Cell activation in rheumatoid synovium is B cell dependent. J Immunol 2001;167(8):4710–8.
17. Gonzalez M, Mackay F, Browning JL, et al. The sequential role of lymphotoxin and B cells in the development of splenic follicles. J Exp Med 1998;187(7):997–1007.

18. Endres R, Alimzhanov MB, Plitz T, et al. Mature follicular dendritic cell networks depend on expression of lymphotoxin {beta} receptor by radioresistant stromal cells and of lymphotoxin {beta} and tumor necrosis factor by B cells. J Exp Med 1999;189(1):159–68.

19. Ngo VN, Korner H, Gunn MD, et al. Lymphotoxin {alpha}/{beta} and tumor necrosis factor are required for stromal cell expression of homing chemokines in B and T cell areas of the spleen. J Exp Med 1999;189(2):403–12.

20. Takemura S, Braun A, Crowson C, et al. Lymphoid neogenesis in rheumatoid synovitis. J Immunol 2001;167(2):1072–80.

21. Weyand C, Seyler T, Goronzy J. B cells in rheumatoid synovitis. Arthritis Res Ther 2005;7(Suppl 3):S9–12.

22. Cantaert T, Kolln J, Timmer T, et al. B lymphocyte autoimmunity in rheumatoid synovitis is independent of ectopic lymphoid neogenesis. J Immunol 2008; 181(1):785–94.

23. Humby F, Bombardieri M, Manzo A, et al. Ectopic lymphoid structures support ongoing production of class-switched autoantibodies in rheumatoid synovium. PLoS Med 2009;6(1):e1.

24. Voswinkel J, Weisgerber K, Pfreundschuh M, et al. The B lymphocyte in rheumatoid arthritis: recirculation of B lymphocytes between different joints and blood. Autoimmunity 1999;31(1):25–34.

25. Souto-Carneiro MM, Krenn V, Hermann R, et al. IgVH genes from different anatomical regions, with different histopathological patterns, of a rheumatoid arthritis patient suggest cyclic re-entry of mature synovial B-cells in the hypermutation process. Arthritis Res 2000;2(4):303–14.

26. Smolen JS, Keystone EC, Emery P, et al. Consensus statement on the use of rituximab in patients with rheumatoid arthritis. Ann Rheum Dis 2007;66(2):143–50.

27. Cohen SB, Emery P, Greenwald MW, et al. Rituximab for rheumatoid arthritis refractory to anti-tumor necrosis factor therapy: results of a multicenter, randomized, double-blind, placebo-controlled, phase III trial evaluating primary efficacy and safety at twenty-four weeks. Arthritis Rheum 2006;54(9):2793–806.

28. Thurlings RM, Vos K, Gerlag DM, et al. Disease activity-guided rituximab therapy in rheumatoid arthritis: the effects of re-treatment in initial nonresponders versus initial responders. Arthritis Rheum 2008;58(12):3657–64.

29. Keystone E, Fleischmann R, Emery P, et al. Safety and efficacy of additional courses of rituximab in patients with active rheumatoid arthritis: an open-label extension analysis. Arthritis Rheum 2007;56(12):3896–908.

30. Bingham CO III, Looney RJ, Deodhar A, et al. Immunization responses in rheumatoid arthritis patients treated with rituximab: Results from a controlled clinical trial. Arthritis Rheum 2010;62(1):64–74.

31. van Assen S, Holvast A, Benne CA, et al. Humoral responses after influenza vaccination are severely reduced in patients with rheumatoid arthritis treated with rituximab. Arthritis Rheum 2010;62(1):75–81.

32. Genentech. Important drug warning regarding Rituxan® (Rituximab). Available at: http://www.gene.com/gene/products/information/pdf/rituxan_dhcp_letter_1009.pdf 2009. Accessed January 19, 2010.

33. Molloy ES, Calabrese LH. Progressive multifocal leukoencephalopathy: a national estimate of frequency in systemic lupus erythematosus and other rheumatic diseases. Arthritis Rheum 2009;60(12):3761–5.

34. Dass S, Rawstron AC, Vital EM, et al. Highly sensitive B cell analysis predicts response to rituximab therapy in rheumatoid arthritis. Arthritis Rheum 2008; 58(10):2993–9.

35. Leandro MJ, Cooper N, Cambridge G, et al. Bone marrow B-lineage cells in patients with rheumatoid arthritis following rituximab therapy. Rheumatology 2007;46(1):29–36.
36. Roll P, Dörner T, Tony H- P. Anti-CD20 therapy in patients with rheumatoid arthritis: predictors of response and B cell subset regeneration after repeated treatment. Arthritis Rheum 2008;58(6):1566–75.
37. Nakou M, Katsikas G, Sidiropoulos P, et al. Rituximab therapy reduces activated B cells in both the peripheral blood and bone marrow of patients with rheumatoid arthritis: depletion of memory B cells correlates with clinical response. Arthritis Res Ther 2009;11:R131.
38. Kavanaugh A, Rosengren S, Lee SJ, et al. Assessment of rituximab's immunomodulatory synovial effects (ARISE trial). 1: clinical and synovial biomarker results. Ann Rheum Dis 2008;67(3):402–8.
39. Thurlings RM, Vos K, Wijbrandts CA, et al. Synovial tissue response to rituximab: mechanism of action and identification of biomarkers of response. Ann Rheum Dis 2008;67(7):917–25.
40. Teng YKO, Levarht EWN, Hashemi M, et al. Immunohistochemical analysis as a means to predict responsiveness to rituximab treatment. Arthritis Rheum 2007;56(12):3909–18.
41. Tedder TF. CD19: a promising B cell target for rheumatoid arthritis. Nat Rev Rheumatol 2009;5(10):572–7.
42. Cardarelli PM, Blanset D, Rao-Naik C, et al. A nonfucosylated human antibody to CD19 with potent B-cell depletive activity for treatment of autoimmune diseases presentation. Presented at the Annual Meeting of the American College of Rheumatology. Philadelphia (PA), October 17–21, 2009.
43. Li Y, Chen F, Putt M, et al. B Cell depletion with anti-CD79 mAbs ameliorates autoimmune disease in MRL/lpr mice. J Immunol 2008;181(5):2961–72.
44. Zheng B, Fuji RN, Elkins K, et al. In vivo effects of targeting CD79b with antibodies and antibody-drug conjugates. Mol Cancer Ther 2009;8(10):2937–46.
45. Fillatreau S, Gray D, Anderton SM. Not always the bad guys: B cells as regulators of autoimmune pathology. Nat Rev Immunol 2008;8:391–7.
46. Evans JG, Chavez-Rueda KA, Eddaoudi A, et al. Novel suppressive function of transitional 2 B cells in experimental arthritis. J Immunol 2007;178(12):7868–78.
47. Blair PA, Chavez-Rueda KA, Evans JG, et al. Selective targeting of B cells with agonistic anti-CD40 is an efficacious strategy for the generation of induced regulatory T2-like B cells and for the suppression of lupus in MRL/lpr mice. J Immunol 2009;182(6):3492–502.
48. Rafei M, Hsieh J, Zehntner S, et al. A granulocyte–macrophage colony-stimulating factor and interleukin-15 fusokine induces a regulatory B cell population with immune suppressive properties. Nat Med 2009;15(9):1038–45.
49. Wardemann H, Yurasov S, Schaefer A, et al. Predominant autoantibody production by early human B Cell precursors. Science 2003;301(5638):1374–7.
50. Weinblatt M, Kavanaugh A, Burgos-Vargas R, et al. Treatment of rheumatoid arthritis with a syk kinase inhibitor: a twelve-week, randomized, placebo-controlled trial. Arthritis Rheum 2008;58(11):3309–18.
51. Ghosh D, Tsokos GC. Spleen tyrosine kinase: an Src family of non-receptor kinase has multiple functions and represents a valuable therapeutic target in the treatment of autoimmune and inflammatory diseases. Autoimmunity 2010;43(1):48–55.

52. Rommel C, Camps M, Ji H. PI3K[delta] and PI3K[gamma]: partners in crime in inflammation in rheumatoid arthritis and beyond? Nat Rev Immunol 2007;7(3): 191–201.

53. Liossis SN, Sfikakis PP. Costimulation blockade in the treatment of rheumatic diseases. BioDrugs 2004;18(2):95–102.

54. Vinuesa CG, Sanz I, Cook MC. Dysregulation of germinal centres in autoimmune disease. Nat Rev Immunol 2009;9(12):845–57.

55. Ruth JH, Rottman JB, Kingsbury GA, et al. ICOS and B7 costimulatory molecule expression identifies activated cellular subsets in rheumatoid arthritis. Cytometry A 2007;71(5):317–26.

56. Nurieva RI, Treuting P, Duong J, et al. Inducible costimulator is essential for collagen-induced arthritis. J Clin Invest 2003;111(5):701–6.

57. Rau FC, Dieter J, Luo Z, et al. B7-1/2 (CD80/CD86) direct signaling to B cells enhances IgG secretion. J Immunol 2009;183(12):7661–71.

58. Oflazoglu E, Boursalian TE, Zeng W, et al. Blocking of CD27-CD70 pathway by anti-CD70 antibody ameliorates joint disease in murine collagen-induced arthritis. J Immunol 2009;183(6):3770–7.

59. Croft M. The role of TNF superfamily members in T-cell function and diseases. Nat Rev Immunol 2009;9(4):271–85.

60. Lafyatis R, York M, Marshak-Rothstein A. Antimalarial agents: closing the gate on toll-like receptors? Arthritis Rheum 2006;54(10):3068–70.

61. Brentano F, Kyburz D, Gay S. Toll-like receptors and rheumatoid arthritis. Methods in Molecular Biology 2009;517:1–15.

62. Christensen SR, Shupe J, Nickerson K, et al. Toll-like receptor 7 and TLR9 dictate autoantibody specificity and have opposing inflammatory and regulatory roles in a murine model of lupus. Immunity 2006;25(3):417–28.

63. Kono DH, Haraldsson MK, Lawson BR, et al. Endosomal TLR signaling is required for anti-nucleic acid and rheumatoid factor autoantibodies in lupus. Proc Natl Acad Sci U S A 2009;106(29):12061–6.

64. Avalos AM, Latz E, Mousseau B, et al. Differential cytokine production and bystander activation of autoreactive B cells in response to CpG-A and CpG-B oligonucleotides. J Immunol 2009;183(10):6262–8.

65. Barrat FJ, Coffman RL. Development of TLR inhibitors for the treatment of autoimmune diseases. Immunol Rev 2008;223(1):271–83.

66. Lipford G, Forsbach A, Zepp C, et al. Selective toll-like receptor 7/8/9 antagonists for the oral treatment of autoimmune diseases. Presented at the Annual Meeting of the American College of Rheumatology. Boston (MA), November 7–11, 2007.

67. Lenert P, Brummel R, Field EH, et al. TLR-9 activation of marginal zone B cells in lupus mice regulates immunity through increased IL-10 production. J Clin Immunol 2005;25(1):29–40.

68. Lampropoulou V, Hoehlig K, Roch T, et al. TLR-activated B cells suppress T cell-mediated autoimmunity. J Immunol 2008;180(7):4763–73.

69. Moisini I, Davidson A. BAFF: a local and systemic target in autoimmune diseases. Clin Exp Immunol 2009;158(2):155–63.

70. Cancro MP. The BLyS/BAFF family of ligands and receptors: key targets in the therapy and understanding of autoimmunity. Ann Rheum Dis 2006; 65(Suppl 3):iii34–6.

71. Ohata J, Zvaifler NJ, Nishio M, et al. Fibroblast-like synoviocytes of mesenchymal origin express functional B cell-activating factor of the TNF family in response to proinflammatory cytokines. J Immunol 2005;174(2):864–70.

72. Seyler TM, Park YW, Takemura S, et al. BLyS and APRIL in rheumatoid arthritis. J Clin Invest 2005;115(11):3083–92.
73. Tak PP, Thurlings RM, Rossier C, et al. Atacicept in patients with rheumatoid arthritis: results of a multicenter, phase ib, double-blind, placebo-controlled, dose-escalating, single- and repeated-dose study. Arthritis Rheum 2008; 58(1):61–72.
74. Huizinga TW. Genetic and environmental risk factors, disease outcome and responses to anti B-cell therapy belimumab indicate anti-CCP positive RA is a distinct disease entity. Presented at the Annual Meeting of the American College of Rheumatology. Washington, DC, November 11–15, 2006.
75. Kievit W, Fransen J, Oerlemans AJM, et al. The efficacy of anti-TNF in rheumatoid arthritis, a comparison between randomised controlled trials and clinical practice. Ann Rheum Dis 2007;66(11):1473–8.
76. Nishimoto N, Yoshizaki K, Miyasaka N, et al. Treatment of rheumatoid arthritis with humanized anti-interleukin-6 receptor antibody: a multicenter, double-blind, placebo-controlled trial. Arthritis Rheum 2004;50(6):1761–9.
77. van den Berg WB, Miossec P. IL-17 as a future therapeutic target for rheumatoid arthritis. Nat Rev Rheumatol 2009;5(10):549–53.
78. Jego G, Palucka AK, Blanck JP, et al. Plasmacytoid dendritic cells induce plasma cell differentiation through type I interferon and interleukin 6. Immunity 2003;19(2):225–34.
79. Tsantikos E, Oracki SA, Quilici C, et al. Autoimmune disease in lyn-deficient mice is dependent on an inflammatory environment established by IL-6. J Immunol 2010;184(3):1348–60.
80. Hsu H-C, Yang P, Wang J, et al. Interleukin 17-producing T helper cells and interleukin 17 orchestrate autoreactive germinal center development in autoimmune BXD2 mice. Nat Immunol 2008;9(2):166–75.
81. Doreau A, Belot A, Bastid J, et al. Interleukin 17 acts in synergy with B cell-activating factor to influence B cell biology and the pathophysiology of systemic lupus erythematosus. Nat Immunol 2009;10(7):778–85.
82. Ettinger R, Sims GP, Robbins R, et al. IL-21 and BAFF/BLyS synergize in stimulating plasma cell differentiation from a unique population of human splenic memory B cells. J Immunol 2007;178(5):2872–82.
83. Avery DT, Deenick EK, Ma CS, et al. B cell-intrinsic signaling through IL-21 receptor and STAT3 is required for establishing long-lived antibody responses in humans. J Exp Med 2010;207(1):155–71.
84. Young DA, Hegen M, Ma HLM, et al. Blockade of the interleukin-21/interleukin-21 receptor pathway ameliorates disease in animal models of rheumatoid arthritis. Arthritis Rheum 2007;56(4):1152–63.
85. Browning JL. Inhibition of the lymphotoxin pathway as a therapy for autoimmune disease. Immunol Rev 2008;223(1):202–20.
86. Anolik JH, Ravikumar R, Barnard J, et al. Cutting edge: antitumor necrosis factor therapy in rheumatoid arthritis inhibits memory B lymphocytes via effects on lymphoid germinal centers and follicular dendritic cell networks. J Immunol 2008;180(2):688–92.
87. Fava RA, Notidis E, Hunt J, et al. A role for the lymphotoxin/LIGHT axis in the pathogenesis of murine collagen-induced arthritis. J Immunol 2003;171(1):115–26.
88. Genovese MC, Greenwald MW, Alloway JA, et al. Efficacy and safety of Baminercept in the treatment of rheumatoid arthritis (RA)—results of the phase 2B study in the TNF-IR population. Presented at the Annual Meeting of the American College of Rheumatology. Philadelphia (PA), October 17–21, 2009.

89. Ueda Y, Yang K, Foster SJ, et al. Inflammation controls B lymphopoiesis by regulating chemokine CXCL12 expression. J Exp Med 2004;199(1):47–58.

90. Samuels J, Ng Y-S, Coupillaud C, et al. Impaired early B cell tolerance in patients with rheumatoid arthritis. J Exp Med 2005;201(10):1659–67.

91. Ansel KM, Ngo VN, Hyman PL, et al. A chemokine-driven positive feedback loop organizes lymphoid follicles. Nature 2000;406(6793):309–14.

92. Shi K, Hayashida K, Kaneko M, et al. Lymphoid chemokine B cell-attracting chemokine-1 (CXCL13) is expressed in germinal center of ectopic lymphoid follicles within the synovium of chronic arthritis patients. J Immunol 2001;166(1):650–5.

93. Radbruch A, Muehlinghaus G, Luger EO, et al. Competence and competition: the challenge of becoming a long-lived plasma cell. Nat Rev Immunol 2006; 6(10):741–50.

94. Jimenez-Boj E, Redlich K, Turk B, et al. Interaction between synovial inflammatory tissue and bone marrow in rheumatoid arthritis. J Immunol 2005;175(4): 2579–88.

95. Manzo A, Paoletti S, Carulli M, et al. Systematic microanatomical analysis of CXCL13 and CCL21 in situ production and progressive lymphoid organization in rheumatoid synovitis. Eur J Immunol 2005;35(5):1347–59.

96. Linterman MA, Rigby RJ, Wong RK, et al. Follicular helper T cells are required for systemic autoimmunity. J Exp Med 2009;206(3):561–76.

97. Zheng B, Ozen Z, Zhang X, et al. CXCL13 neutralization reduces the severity of collagen-induced arthritis. Arthritis Rheum 2005;52(2):620–6.

98. Li J, Turner A, Kuzin I, et al. CXCL13-mediated translocation of B cells in the draining lymph node of inflamed joints: a potential mechanism for arthritic flare. Presented at the Annual Meeting of the American College of Rheumatology. San Francisco (CA), October 25–29, 2008.

99. Boyle DL, Rosengren S, Lee S, et al. Synovial CXCL13 expression is associated with localized inflammation and predicts synovial response to rituximab in rheumatoid arthritis. Presented at the Annual Meeting of the American College of Rheumatology. San Francisco (CA), October 25–29, 2008.

100. Murdoch C. CXCR4: chemokine receptor extraordinaire. Immunol Rev 2000; 177(1):175–84.

101. Nanki T, Takada K, Komano Y, et al. Chemokine receptor expression and functional effects of chemokines on B cells: implication in the pathogenesis of rheumatoid arthritis. Arthritis Res Ther 2009;11(5):R149.

102. Burman A, Haworth O, Hardie DL, et al. A chemokine-dependent stromal induction mechanism for aberrant lymphocyte accumulation and compromised lymphatic return in rheumatoid arthritis. J Immunol 2005;174(3):1693–700.

103. Joven B, González N, Aguilar F, et al. Association between stromal cell-derived factor 1 chemokine gene variant and radiographic progression of rheumatoid arthritis. Arthritis Rheum 2005;52(1):354–6.

104. Tamamura H, Tsutsumi H, Masuno H, et al. Development of low molecular weight CXCR4 antagonists by exploratory structural tuning of cyclic tetra- and pentapeptide-scaffolds towards the treatment of HIV infection, cancer metastasis and rheumatoid arthritis. Curr Med Chem 2007;14(1):93–102.

105. Burns JM, Summers BC, Wang Y, et al. A novel chemokine receptor for SDF-1 and I-TAC involved in cell survival, cell adhesion, and tumor development. J Exp Med 2006;203(9):2201–13.

106. Watanabe K, Nanki T, Penfold ME, et al. Pathogenic role of CXCR7 in rheumatoid arthritis. Presented at the Annual Meeting of the American College of Rheumatology. San Francisco (CA), October 25–29, 2008.

107. Yellin M, Paliienko I, Balanescu A, et al. A phase II, randomized, double-blind, placebo-controlled study to evaluate the efficacy and safety of MDX-1100, a fully human anti-CXCL10 monoclonal antibody, in combination with methotrexate (MTX) in patients with rheumatoid arthritis (RA). Presented at the Annual Meeting of the American College of Rheumatology. Philadelphia (PA), October 17–21, 2009.

108. Hirota K, Yoshitomi H, Hashimoto M, et al. Preferential recruitment of CCR6-expressing Th17 cells to inflamed joints via CCL20 in rheumatoid arthritis and its animal model. J Exp Med 2007;204(12):2803–12.

109. Liao F, Shirakawa A-K, Foley JF, et al. Human B cells become highly responsive to macrophage-inflammatory protein-3{alpha}/CC chemokine ligand-20 after cellular activation without changes in CCR6 expression or ligand binding. J Immunol 2002;168(10):4871–80.

110. Dechanet J, Merville P, Durand I, et al. The ability of synoviocytes to support terminal differentiation of activated B cells may explain plasma cell accumulation in rheumatoid synovium. J Clin Invest 1995;95(2):456–63.

111. Zand MS, Vo T, Huggins J, et al. Polyclonal rabbit antithymocyte globulin triggers B cell and plasma cell apoptosis by multiple pathways. Transplantation 2005;79(11):1507–15.

112. Obeng EA, Carlson LM, Gutman DM, et al. Proteasome inhibitors induce a terminal unfolded protein response in multiple myeloma cells. Blood 2006; 107(12):4907–16.

113. Neubert K, Meister S, Moser K, et al. The proteasome inhibitor bortezomib depletes plasma cells and protects mice with lupus-like disease from nephritis. Nat Med 2008;14(7):748–55.

114. van der Heijden JW, Oerlemans R, Lems WF, et al. The proteasome inhibitor bortezomib inhibits the release of NFkappaB-inducible cytokines and induces apoptosis of activated T cells from rheumatoid arthritis patients. Clin Exp Rheumatol 2009;27(1):92–8.

115. Muchamuel T, Basler M, Aujay MA, et al. A selective inhibitor of the immunoproteasome subunit LMP7 blocks cytokine production and attenuates progression of experimental arthritis. Nat Med 2009;15(7):781–7.

116. Demo SD, Kirk CJ, Aujay MA, et al. Antitumor activity of PR-171, a novel irreversible inhibitor of the proteasome. Cancer Res 2007;67(13):6383–91.

117. Siegel D, Wang L, Orlowski RZ, et al. PX-171–004, an ongoing open-label, phase II study of single-agent carfilzomib (CFZ) in patients with relapsed or refractory myeloma (MM); updated results from the bortezomib-treated cohort. Presented at the 51st Annual Meeting of the American Society for Hematology, 2009.

118. Rafei M, Hsieh J, Fortier S, et al. Mesenchymal stromal cell-derived CCL2 suppresses plasma cell immunoglobulin production via STAT3 inactivation and PAX5 induction. Blood 2008;112(13):4991–8.

119. Boumans M, Tak P. Rituximab treatment in rheumatoid arthritis: how does it work? Arthritis Res Ther 2009;11(6):134.

120. Lund FE. Cytokine-producing B lymphocytes – key regulators of immunity. Curr Opin Immunol 2008;20(3):332–8.

Targeting IL-17 and Th17 Cells in Rheumatoid Arthritis

Sujata Sarkar, MD[a],*, David A. Fox, MD[b]

KEYWORDS

- Cytokines • T-cell differentiation • Biologic therapeutics
- Interleukin-6 • Interleukin-23 • Interleukin-17

CD4+ T cells differentiate into distinct subsets with unique functions and patterns of cytokine secretion, such as the subsets termed Th1 and Th2.[1] Th1 cells produce interferon (IFN)-γ and induce cell-mediated immunity against intracellular pathogens, while Th2 cells produce interleukin (IL)-4 and stimulate humoral immunity against parasitic helminths. This model was revised in 2005 to include a third Th subset, known as Th17.[2,3] Th17 cells produce IL-17, and are important in host defense against microbes against which Th1 or Th2 immunity are not fully effective, such as extracellular bacteria and some fungi. Human IL-17 was cloned in 1995, and early reports demonstrated multiple inflammatory and hematopoietic effects.[4–6] Th17 cells have received considerable attention in recent years because they appear to be principal mediators of pathogenesis in several autoimmune and inflammatory disorders, including rheumatoid arthritis (RA) and its animal models.[7]

Both T-helper cell differentiation, and the cytokine networks that control it, are remarkably complex and tightly regulated. Although many principles of mouse Th17 biology are widely accepted, important questions regarding human Th17 cells are still under dispute. Given the wide array of human diseases associated with aberrant Th17 responses, a thorough understanding of Th17 biology in humans is essential for designing the safest and most effective approaches to regulating these cells in disease.

TH17 DIFFERENTIATION

Naïve T cells stimulated in the presence of IL-12 become Th1 cells and express the transcription factor T-bet while Th2 cells express the transcription factor GATA-3.[8]

---

[a] Section of Rheumatology, Department of Medicine, The University of Arizona, 1501 North Campbell Avenue, Tucson, AZ 85724, USA
[b] Division of Rheumatology, Department of Medicine, The University of Michigan, 1500 East Medical Center Drive, Ann Arbor, MI 48109, USA
* Corresponding author.
E-mail address: ssarkar@email.arizona.edu

Rheum Dis Clin N Am 36 (2010) 345–366
doi:10.1016/j.rdc.2010.02.006
0889-857X/10/$ – see front matter
rheumatic.theclinics.com

Initial studies in mice suggested that IL-23, a heterodimeric cytokine that shares a subunit with IL-12, induced IL-17 expression.[2,3,9,10] However, subsequent studies demonstrated that the IL-23 receptor is only expressed on T cells after activation, and therefore IL-23 can up-regulate IL-17 in memory T cells but cannot act on naïve T cells to induce Th17 differentiation.[10] Instead, the key to Th17 differentiation in the mouse is the combination of transforming growth factor (TGF)-β and IL-6.[11–13] Tumor necrosis factor (TNF)-α and IL-1β can further enhance mouse Th17 differentiation, but only in the presence of TGF-β and IL-6.[13–15]

Whereas Th1 and Th2 cells follow similar rules in humans as in mice, Th17 differentiation may not be as conserved, and IL-1β, IL-6, and IL-23 all appear to be important.[16,17] Several studies suggest that TGF-β, a crucial cytokine for mouse Th17 differentiation, actually inhibits human Th17 development.[16–18] Notwithstanding these claims, TGF-β likely is an inducer of human Th17 cells, but the effects of TGF-β are extremely concentration dependent; low doses induce Th17 differentiation, while high doses inhibit Th17 development and induce Tregs.[19] T cells from cord blood, which represent a more naïve state than those in adult peripheral blood, do in fact require TGF-β to differentiate into Th17 cells.[20] Additional recent studies also support a role for TGF-β in human Th17 differentiation.[21,22]

IL-12, IFN-γ, and IL-4 can inhibit Th17 differentiation in both mouse and human.[2,3,16,17,23–25] IL-17, on the other hand, does not appear to inhibit Th1 or Th2 differentiation, or does so very weakly, and so Th1 and Th2 cells typically dominate over Th17.[15] This domination explains one of the ways in which TGF-β can promote Th17 differentiation—by suppressing production of the inhibitory cytokines IFN-γ and IL-4—but TGF-β also has direct roles in Th17 differentiation because it is required even in the absence of IFN-γ and IL-4.[11–13] TGF-β synergizes with IL-6 to induce expression of the transcription factor RORγt, a key regulator of Th17 differentiation. In mice RORγt is both necessary and sufficient for IL-17 expression in vitro and in vivo,[26] although its induction and action may be facilitated by a distinct transcription factor, Runx1.[27] In humans RORC (the human orthologue of RORγt) is induced by IL-1β, IL-6 and IL-23, the same cytokines that induce IL-17.[16,17] In addition, RORC expression is restricted to IL-17–producing clones.[23]

In addition to RORγt, Th17 development in mice depends on the transcription factor STAT3, which is activated by IL-6 and IL-23. STAT3 has multiple roles in Th17 development: in activated Th17 cells stimulated with IL-23 it binds directly to the IL-17 promoter and induces IL-17 expression, and in naïve T cells stimulated with TGF-β and IL-6 it is required for induction of RORγt expression. IL-23 also activates STAT4, which is the primary mediator of IL-12 signaling and is required for Th1 differentiation, yet is still important for IL-23–induced IL-17 production.[28] Thus STAT4 may inhibit Th17 development downstream of IL-12, while also supporting IL-17 expression downstream of IL-23.

CYTOKINES EXPRESSED BY TH17 CELLS

Mouse Th17 cells specifically express IL-21 soon after activation, and autocrine IL-21 plays an important role in RORγt and IL-17 expression. IL-21 can also partially replace IL-6 during Th17 differentiation, giving established Th17 cells the ability to promote further Th17 development in neighboring cells. IL-23 in combination with TGF-β can also induce RORγt and IL-17 expression, but only after IL-6 or IL-21 induce IL-23 receptor expression.[29–33] Thus IL-6, IL-21, and IL-23 act sequentially: first IL-6 up-regulates IL-21, then both IL-6 and IL-21 up-regulate IL-23 receptor, and finally IL-23 appears to up-regulate effector function and pathogenicity in Th17 cells. Recent evidence points to a role for IL-21 in human Th17 differentiation,[22] and human IL-21 can also counteract suppression by Tregs.[34,35]

IL-17, or IL-17A, is one member of a family of 6 cytokines known as IL-17A through F. Th17 cells specifically express IL-17F in addition to IL-17A. IL-17A and IL-17F are closely related, with 55% amino acid identity as well as a common receptor.[36] IL-17A and IL-17F are both homodimeric cytokines, but human and mouse T cells also produce an IL-17A/F heterodimer that has potent inflammatory effects.[37,38] It may be important to measure, as well as to target, both IL-17A and IL-17F in disease. Other proinflammatory cytokines produced by both mouse and human Th17 cells include TNF-α and IL-22.[16,17,39–43] IL-22 induces antimicrobial proteins, defensins, acute-phase proteins, inflammatory cytokines, chemokines, and hyperplasia.[44–46] However, IL-22 protects hepatocytes during acute liver inflammation[47]; thus IL-22 may either enhance inflammation or limit tissue damage induced by IL-17, depending on the type of tissue.

Unexpectedly, a subset of Th17 cells coexpresses IFN-γ, particularly in humans, where as many as half of all the IL-17 positive cells also express IFN-γ.[16,17,39,41] These double positive cells complicate the idea that Th17 cells are a unique subset distinct from Th1 cells, and are particularly hard to explain given that IFN-γ has been shown to inhibit IL-17 expression. It is not clear yet whether these cells represent a stable phenotype, or a transitional phase from Th17 to Th1 or vice versa. Although there are no data on the specific role of these double positive cells, both IFN-γ and IL-17 are important mediators of inflammation, and cells that produce both cytokines are likely to contribute to pathogenesis in certain environments. Also unexpected is that Th17 cells coexpress IL-10, an anti-inflammatory cytokine. T-cell sources of IL-10 include Th2 cells and various types of Tregs, but Th1 cells also secrete IL-10 in certain conditions.[48,49] In mice the combination of TGF-β and IL-6, which synergize to induce IL-17 production, also synergize to induce IL-10, such that half of the IL-17 positive cells coexpress IL-10.[50,51] IL-10 produced by mouse Th17 cells may serve an important protective function by limiting inflammation and tissue damage normally caused by IL-17, through antagonistic effects on target tissues.[50] It is not yet known whether human Th17 cells ever coexpress IL-10.

TRAFFICKING OF TH17 CELLS

Human and mouse Th17 cells express the chemokine receptor CCR6, including memory cells from healthy peripheral blood and inflamed tissue, as well as in vitro primed naïve T cells.[16,23,41,52,53] Although not all CCR6-positive cells are Th17, within the CCR6-positive population, those that coexpress CXCR3 are either Th1 or IFNγ-IL-17 double positive, whereas those that coexpress CCR4 secrete only IL-17. The majority of RORC expression is restricted to the CCR6+CCR4+ population, with a small amount in the CCR6+CXCR3+ population.[41] CCR6 mediates homing to skin and mucosal tissues and is important in recruitment of pathogenic T cells in many inflammatory diseases now associated with IL-17, including psoriasis, inflammatory bowel disease, allergic asthma, and RA.[52,54–57] Of note, the CCR6 ligand CCL-20 is expressed by Th17 cells and is up-regulated in stromal cells by IL-17, allowing Th17 cells in inflamed tissues to attract additional Th17 and Th1 cells.[17,52,58,59] Another group found human memory Th17 cells within the CCR2+CCR5− population and Th1 cells within the CCR2+CCR5+ population.[60] It is not yet clear whether the CCR6+CCR4+ population overlaps with the CCR2+CCR5−, but the combination of all 4 markers may be useful for isolating human Th17 cells from blood and sites of inflammation.

ROLE OF TH SUBSETS IN COLLAGEN-INDUCED ARTHRITIS AND OTHER RA MODELS

RA is traditionally classified as a Th1-mediated disease,[61–64] but mice treated with neutralizing antibodies to IFN-γ and IFN-γ receptor deficient mice develop more severe arthritis,[65,66] and IFN-γ deficiency renders resistant strains of mice susceptible to collagen-induced arthritis (CIA).[67–69] Further insight arises from the discovery that the IL-12 p40 subunit is shared by IL-23. IL-23 p19 deficient mice do not develop CIA, while IL-12 p35 deficient mice actually develop more severe disease.[70] Both IL-12 and IFN-γ are potent suppressors of Th17 differentiation in vitro, suggesting a mechanism for the protective function of these cytokines. In vivo, arthritic mice deficient in IFN-γ or treated with neutralizing antibody to IFN-γ have elevated IL-17 in serum and in cultures of collagen restimulated spleens and lymph nodes.[7,68,71]

The importance of IL-17 in the pathogenesis of arthritis has been shown in a variety of animal models, both genetic and adaptive. IL-17 knockout mice develop significantly less arthritis, and treatment with neutralizing antibodies to IL-17 or soluble IL-17 receptor alleviates joint inflammation.[72–74] IL-17 receptor signaling in radiation-resistant cells of the joint is required for the induction of chronic destructive synovitis, cartilage damage, bone erosion, and inflammatory cytokine expression in acute streptococcal cell wall arthritis.[75,76] In rat adjuvant-induced arthritis, IL-17 is important for both inflammation and joint destruction.[77] In TNF-deficient mice, IL-17 can drive cartilage and bone destruction.[78] IL-17 is also required for the development of spontaneous arthritis in other mouse models of RA, such as IL-1Ra deficient mice and SKG mice.[79,80] IFN-γ plays a protective role in CIA by inhibiting Th17 cell development, but it may still have pathogenic effects in some instances. For example, the effect of neutralizing IFN-γ in CIA varies depending on the timing of administration, demonstrating that IFN-γ may be pathogenic in the early phases of CIA but protective in the later stages.[81] In addition, the mouse model proteoglycan-induced arthritis is dependent on IFN-γ.[82] Similarly, there may be subsets of RA patients with Th1- or Th17-dominant disease.

THE ROLE OF IL-17 IN RA

IL-17 is increased in RA sera and synovial fluid, and is present in the T-cell rich areas of the synovium.[83–86] RA serum and synovial fluid contains much more IL-17 than osteoarthritis serum or synovial fluid.[85,87] T cells cultured from normal donors or RA patients produce IL-17 in vitro following activation.[83,88,89] A specific response of RA T cells to citrullinated but not uncitrullinated aggrecan is accompanied by robust secretion of IL-17.[90] Increased levels of IL-17 and TNF-α mRNA expression in early RA synovium are predictive of more severe joint damage progression, whereas high levels of IFN-γ mRNA are predictive of protection from damage progression.[91]

Further support for the role of Th17 cells in RA comes from in vitro studies showing the robust and widespread inflammatory effects of IL-17 on cells of the joint,[92–100] IL-17 induces the production of inflammatory cytokines such as IL-1β, TNF-α, IL-6, and IL-23 by synovial fibroblasts, monocytes, and macrophages, all of which promote inflammation and Th17 development.[92] IL-17 also induces an array of chemokines, including CXCL-1, CXCL-2, CXCL-5, CXCL-8, CCL-2, and CCL-20, leading to recruitment of T cells, B cells, monocytes, and neutrophils. Moreover, IL-17 directly stimulates monocyte migration.[93] Leukocyte recruitment is further enhanced by up-regulation of granulocyte-colony stimulating factor and granulocyte macrophage-colony stimulating factor, as well as vascular endothelial growth factor (VEGF), an inducer of angiogenesis, and other angiogenic factors.[94,97] IL-17 has been reported to induce production of proangiogenic factors from synovial fibroblasts, and to synergize with TNF-α in this effect.[95] IL-17 can also orchestrate bone and carti-lage damage. matrix metalloproteinases, nitric oxide, and RANK/RANKL, as well as inflammatory cytokines and chemokines, are up-regulated in chondrocytes and oste-oblasts by IL-17. Th17 cells can also induce osteoclastogenesis directly by expressing RANKL (receptor activator of nuclear factor κB ligand) on their cell surface.[96–98] SDF-1, which is abundant in RA synovium and promotes recruitment of CD4+ memory T cells, monocytes, and B cells, is induced by IL-17, although IL-1β and TNF-α are not efficient in inducing this factor.[99]

TNF blockade does lower serum IL-17 levels,[101] but IL-17 can induce inflammation and enhance cartilage and bone erosion in mice even under TNF and IL-1 neutralizing conditions.[100,102,103] Combined TNF, IL-1β, and IL-17 blockade, was more effective at controlling IL-6 production and collagen degradation than was blocking TNF-α alone, in cultures of RA synovium.[104] Similarly, combination blockade of TNF-α and IL-17 sup-pressed ongoing CIA and was more effective than neutralization of TNF-α alone.[102] These results suggest that treatments designed to block IL-17 could be beneficial in RA.

Th17 cells produce IL-21, which acts to further enhance Th17 development and plays a role in CIA and RA. IL-21 is increased in RA serum and synovial fluid. Its receptor is highly expressed on peripheral blood and synovial fluid lymphocytes, as well as on synovial fibroblasts and macrophages from patients with RA.[105,106] Admin-istration of IL-21R fusion protein significantly reduced disease in CIA and rat antigen-induced arthritis.[107]

IL-23, which enhances IL-17 production and Th17 effector function in humans and mice, is also implicated in arthritis. Mice deficient in the IL-23 p19 subunit develop less severe CIA.[70] In RA patients IL-23 is elevated in sera and synovial fluid, with increased expression of IL-23 p19 subunit in synovial fibroblasts.[108,109] Recently STAT4 has been identified as a susceptibility gene for RA.[110,111] STAT4 is important in the signaling pathway through IL-12/IL-23 receptors, and is critical to the generation and maintenance of Th17 cells.[28] STAT4 knockout mice are resistant to arthritis, and antisense STAT4 suppresses ongoing CIA.[112]

There is increased expression of IL-22 and IL-22R in the synovium in RA,[113] but the effects of this cytokine on cells of the joint are still unknown. Another cytokine that may play a role in Th17 biology is IL-15. IL-15 is overexpressed in RA synovial fluid and peripheral blood T cells, and can induce the secretion of IL-17 from PBMCs.[85] RA synovial fibroblasts produce IL-15, which up-regulates IL-17 and TNF-α production by T cells. IL-17 and TNF-α then, in turn, stimulate production of IL-15 and IL-6 by the synovial fibroblasts (FLS), creating a positive feedback loop.[114] In mice, insertion of an IL-15 transgene on an arthritis resistant strain increases severity of arthritis asso-ciated with increased IL-17 and IL-23 receptor expression,[115] while an IL-15 receptor antagonist ameliorates CIA and down-regulates TNF-α, IL-1β, IL-6, and IL-17.[116]

IL-17 can synergize with resting T cells to stimulate RA FLS to secrete IL-6, IL-8, and prostaglandin E$_2$.[117] Cytokine-activated T cells can adhere avidly to RA FLS and induce IL-6 and IL-8 production from the FLS, which is further enhanced by exoge-nous IL-17. Neutralization of TNF-α, a cytokine that is both upstream and downstream of IL-17, inhibits the production of these proinflammatory cytokines, which are impor-tant in mediating joint inflammation in RA and CIA.[118] T cells can also induce IL-6 production by osteoblasts, an effect that is augmented by IL-17.[119] Such findings provide clues to pathways for in situ stimulation of T cells that could foster chronic inflammation in RA synovium.

Understanding the regulation of Th17 cells will be important in designing therapeutic options targeting IL-17. IL-4 is a potent suppressor of IL-17, both in vitro and in vivo. Dendritic cells genetically modified to express IL-4 have been shown to inhibit collagen-specific IL-17 production and reduce the incidence and severity of CIA.[120,121] The suppression mediated by IL-4 dendritic cells is robust and not reversed by exogenous IL-23. Similarly, injection of an adenoviral vector expressing IL-4 has been shown to ameliorate CIA by down-regulating joint IL-17 levels and reducing bone and cartilage damage.[122]

OVERVIEW OF APPROACHES TO TH17 INHIBITION IN RA

It is possible that current biologic and even nonbiologic disease-modifying antirheumatic drugs (DMARDs) used in RA work in part through effects (largely indirect) on Th17 cells, but much more evidence is needed to support this notion. For example, masking of CD28 ligands by CTLA-4Ig could deprive Th17 cells of a critical second activation signal early in their differentiation. Depletion of B cells by anti-CD20 could deprive Th17 cells of an important source of IL-6 while also diminishing the pools of antigen-presenting cells. Inhibition of IL-1 and possibly even TNF would tend to diminish Th17 differentiation. The subsequent paragraphs do not consider all of these approaches in the context of Th17 cells, but instead focus on the more recent strategies that neutralize IL-23/IL-12, block the IL-6 receptor, or inhibit IL-17 directly.

ANTI–IL-12/IL-23

Ustekinumab is a human monoclonal antibody targeting the shared subunit p40 of IL-12 and IL-23. This antibody is being extensively tested in psoriasis, and clinical studies are also being undertaken in other diseases that may involve IL-12 and IL-23, such as psoriatic arthritis, Crohn disease, and multiple sclerosis. Inhibition of IL-23 is of great interest in diseases that involve pathogenic Th17 cells, while inhibition of IL-12 is logical in diseases that are mediated by Th1 cells, or both Th1 and Th17 cells, but could be counterproductive in a disease in which Th1 cells play a regulatory role vis-à-vis Th17 cells.

Safety and initial clinical efficacy was shown in phase 1 and 2 trials with ustekinumab in psoriasis.[123–125] Two phase 3 studies have been done with ustekinumab in psoriasis: PHOENIX 1 and PHOENIX 2.[126,127] Both PHOENIX 1 and PHOENIX 2 used similar doses of ustekinumab and similar trial design for the initial part of the study, but there were differences in the study design for the latter part of each study. In the initial phase of both studies patients received ustekinumab at 45 mg or 90 mg every 12 weeks, or placebo. Patients who were started on placebo were switched to the active drug at 12 weeks. In PHOENIX 1, patients were assessed for withdrawal of ustekinumab during the latter half of the study. In PHOENIX 2, effects of dose escalation of ustekinumab were assessed in partial responders from the initial part of this study. A significantly greater number of patients on ustekinumab achieved 75% improvement in the psoriasis area and severity index scores (PASI 75) compared with patients receiving placebo. In addition, patients who were started on placebo and subsequently switched to ustekinumab achieved a degree of clinical improvement similar to patients started on the active drug from the beginning of the study. Moreover, PHOENIX 1 showed that withdrawal of ustekinumab was associated with relapses that were responsive to retreatment with ustekinumab. PHOENIX 2 showed that in nonresponders to ustekinumab reducing the interval of drug administration from every 12 weeks to 8 weeks was beneficial for those who were on the 90-mg dosage from the start of the study. Patients who were on 45 mg of ustekinumab every 12 weeks did not have any further improvement in their PASI 75 responses on reducing the interval of dosing to every 8 weeks.

In a recently reported trial, ustekinumab was compared with etanercept in patients with plaque psoriasis.[128] In this 12-week study patients were randomized to receive either etanercept (50 mg twice weekly) or ustekinumab 45 mg or 90 mg at weeks 0 and 4. The patients in the etanercept group who did not have significant improvement at week 12, received ustekinumab (2 doses, 4 weeks apart). In addition, patients who had received at least 1 cycle of ustekinumab and were experiencing relapses also received repeat doses of ustekinumab. The patients receiving ustekinumab had better therapeutic responses than those receiving etanercept. PASI 75 scores were seen in 67.5% of patients on 45 mg of ustekinumab, and in 73.8% of patients on 90 mg of ustekinumab versus 56.8% of patients on etanercept. Among the patients who did not have clinical improvement on etanercept and were switched to ustekinumab, 48.9% had improvement in their PASI 75 scores.

Ustekinumab has also shown promise in a trial involving patients with psoriatic arthritis.[129] In this study 146 patients were randomized to either a ustekinumab group or a placebo group. Patients in the ustekinumab group received 63 to 90 mg of the drug weekly for the first 4 weeks followed by placebo on weeks 12 and 16. Patients assigned to the placebo group received placebo weekly for the first 4 weeks and then 63 to 90 mg of ustekinumab on weeks 12 and 16. All patients were followed for 36 weeks. During the first 12 weeks of the study, 52% of patients in the ustekinumab group achieved a PASI 75 response in comparison to 5% in the placebo group. Forty-two percent of patients in the ustekinumab group had achieved ACR20 (American College of Rheumatology 20% improvement measure) responses versus 14% in the placebo group in the first 12 weeks. At 12 weeks, the ACR50 and ACR70 responses were significantly better in the ustekinumab group than in the placebo group. ACR50 responses were 25% versus 7% in the ustekinumab and placebo groups, respectively. Similarly, the ACR70 responses were 11% and 0% in the ustekinumab and placebo groups, respectively. Patients who received placebo in the first 4 weeks then received 2 doses of ustekinumab at weeks 16 and 20 showed improvement in their ACR20 responses. The ACR20 responses in this group at 24 weeks was 51%, at 28 weeks 45%, and at 36 weeks 42%, which were very similar to those who had received the active drug from the start of the study. As stated previously, patients in the ustekinumab group received active drug for the first 4 weeks but were followed for 36 weeks. In these patients ACR20, ACR50, and ACR70 responses peaked at 16 to 20 weeks, and mostly stayed steady or had a very slow decline up to 36 weeks. The adverse events, including headaches, diarrhea, back pain, and nausea, were similar in the 2 groups. The rates of infections were similar overall, 36% in the ustekinumab group and 30% in the placebo group, and upper respiratory tract infection was 13% in the ustekinumab group versus 9% in the placebo group. At present there is a phase 3 study underway in patients with psoriatic arthritis (NCT01009086).

In a clinical trial involving patients with Crohn disease, administration of ustekinumab was associated with significantly better therapeutic improvement than placebo.[130] Of note, in another clinical trial involving patients with relapsing-remitting multiple sclerosis, administration of ustekinumab was not associated with clinical improvement.[131]

The immunologic mechanism underlying a therapeutic response to ustekinumab remains to be evaluated. Ustekinumab inhibited the production of IFN-γ and IL-17A by normal human peripheral blood mononuclear cells stimulated by IL-12 and IL-23. Further, there was inhibition of the up-regulation of cutaneous lymphocyte antigen, IL-2 receptor, IL-12 receptor, and CD40 ligand, and reduced secretion of TNF-α, IL-2, and IL-10.[132] In the phase 1 study in psoriasis, a single dose of anti-p40 antibody led to down-regulation of both p40 and IL-23 p19 expression in skin lesions.[133]

Data regarding efficacy of ustekinumab in RA are not yet available. It is possible that the approach of inhibiting both IL-12 and IL-23 action will be inferior in RA, compared with inhibition of IL-23 alone, if RA turns out to be primarily a Th17 disease rather than a mixed Th1/Th17 disease. It is also possible that the primary pathogenic Th subset in RA may differ between patients, or over time during the evolution of RA in an individual patient.

ANTI–IL-6 RECEPTOR

The role of IL-6 in mediating inflammation in arthritis has been confirmed in several preclinical studies. Administration of anti–IL-6 receptor antibody (tocilizumab) reduced severity of inflammatory arthritis in mice as well as in monkeys.[134] Mice with a point mutation in the regulatory pathway that controls signaling through the IL-6 receptor develop spontaneous arthritis due to prolonged unrestrained stimulation of this receptor.[135] IL-6 is elevated in the synovial fluid and sera of patients with RA, and its level correlates with disease activity.[62,136–139] IL-6 has effects on various cell types including neutrophils, T cells, B cells, monocytes, and osteoclasts. The IL-6 receptor is also expressed on hepatocytes and IL-6 can directly induce C-reactive protein (CRP) production from hepatocytes, thus elevating serum levels of CRP during inflammatory arthritis.[140] The key role of IL-6 in Th17 cell development potentially places it as an upstream target in immune/inflammatory cascade in RA, along with its obvious role as a downstream target that is prominent in the effector phases of joint inflammation and damage.

A phase 1 study of tocilizumab in RA was not associated with significant adverse events.[141] In a phase 2 study,[142] 164 patients with refractory RA were randomized to receive MRA (the anti–IL-6R antibody now named tocilizumab), at 8 mg/kg, 4 mg/kg, or placebo every 4 weeks for 24 weeks. At 24 weeks patients receiving MRA had significantly improved clinical responses. The ACR20/50/70 responses were 78%/40%/16% in the MRA 8 mg/kg group, 57%/26%/20% in the MRA 4 mg/kg group, and 11%/1.9%/0% in the placebo group. DAS28 (disease activity score for 28 joints) scores also reflected similar improvements in the patients receiving MRA. Patients in the MRA (tocilizumab) arm of this trial were followed in an open-label extension for 5 years in the STREAM study. At the end of 5 years the ACR20/50/70 responses were 84%/69%/43.6%. The clinical efficacy peaked in the first year and remained at that level for the entire 5 years.[143]

In contrast to the above trial, which compared tocilizumab with placebo, the CHARISMA trial was performed to compare the clinical efficacy of tocilizumab with that of methotrexate. Three hundred and fifty-nine patients were randomized to receive tocilizumab (at 2 mg/kg, 4 mg/kg, or 8 mg/kg every 4 weeks) alone or in combination with methotrexate for 16 weeks. The control group received methotrexate only. There was significant clinical improvement with tocilizumab alone or in combination with methotrexate. Among the groups that received tocilizumab alone, those patients who received 4 mg/kg or 8 mg/kg of tocilizumab had higher ACR20/50/70 responses when compared with the 2 mg/kg tocilizumab group or methotrexate alone group. The ACR20 responses were 63%, 61%, 31%, and 41% in the tocilizumab 8 mg/kg, 4 mg/kg, 2 mg/kg, and the methotrexate group, respectively. The ACR50 responses were higher in the tocilizumab 8 mg/kg group than in the 4 mg/kg group, 41% versus 28%. Similarly, the ACR70 responses were higher in the 8 mg/kg group; 16% versus 6% in the tocilizumab 4 mg/kg group. When tocilizumab was administered along with methotrexate, the ACR20/50/70 responses were significantly improved in all groups including the group receiving 2 mg/kg of tocilizumab. The ACR20/50/70 responses were 74%/53%/37% in the tocilizumab 8 mg/kg + methotrexate group; 63%/37%/ 12% in the tocilizumab 4 mg/kg + methotrexate group; 64%/32%/14% in the tocilizumab 2 mg/kg + methotrexate group in comparison with methotrexate alone, which was 41%/29%/16%. Similar improvements were seen when DAS28 scores were used to measure responses. The clinical improvement was apparent by 1 month after starting infusion and continued to increase during the 16-week study.[144]

The phase 3 OPTION trial was similar to the CHARISMA trial except that this study was continued for 24 weeks.[145] In this study, 623 patients were randomized into 3 groups: (i) 205 patients receiving tocilizumab at 8 mg/kg every 4 weeks + methotrexate, (ii) 214 patients receiving tocilizumab at 4 mg/kg every 4 weeks + methotrexate, and (iii) 204 patients on placebo + methotrexate. Patients were followed for 24 weeks. At the conclusion of this period patients on tocilizumab had significantly better responses than those on methotrexate alone: 59% of patients in the 8 mg/kg group, 48% of patients in the 4 mg/kg group, and 26% in the placebo group achieved ACR20 responses at 24 weeks. A similar trend was seen with the ACR50 and ACR70 responses, with 44% in the 8 mg/kg, 31% in the 4 mg/kg, and 11% in the placebo group achieving ACR50 responses. Twenty-two percent in the 8 mg/kg, 12% in the 4 mg/kg, and 2% in the placebo groups achieved ACR70 responses. In addition, 27% of patients in the 8 mg/kg and 13% in the 4 mg/kg groups compared with 0.8% in the placebo group achieved DAS28 responses of less than 2.6, consistent with remission. Therapeutic efficacy was seen after the first dose and continued to improve up to 24 weeks. There were improvements in the HAQ-DI (Health Assessment Questionnaire Disability Index) and fatigue scores as well.

In the phase 3 TOWARD trial the therapeutic efficacy of tocilizumab in combination with other DMARDs was assessed.[146] In this trial, 1220 patients on stable DMARD doses were randomized to receive either tocilizumab 8 mg/kg every 4 weeks or placebo for 24 weeks. The patients receiving tocilizumab in combination with DMARDs had superior clinical efficacy compared with the DMARDs + placebo group. ACR20 responses were 61% in the tocilizumab + DMARD group versus 25% in the placebo + DMARD group. The ACR50/70 responses were 38%/21% in the tocilizumab group and 9%/3% in the placebo group. Thirty percent of patients in the tocilizumab group achieved DAS28 scores less than 2.6 versus 3% in the DMARD only group. The clinical responses were seen across all DMARDs, including methotrexate, leflunomide, sulfasalazine, hydroxychloroquine, and azathioprine. The rate of clinical improvement was similar whether patients were on 1, 2, or 3 DMARDs.[146]

Furthermore, tocilizumab + methotrexate was shown to be effective in patients who had failed anti-TNF agents in the RADIATE trial.[147] In this 24-week trial 499 patients who were refractory to anti-TNF therapy were randomized to receive tocilizumab 8 mg/kg + methotrexate, or tocilizumab 4 mg/kg + methotrexate, or placebo + methotrexate. The ACR20 responses were 50%/30.4%/10% in the 8 mg/kg, 4 mg/kg, and placebo groups, respectively. The clinical efficacy of tocilizumab was independent of the specific anti-TNF agent that was used previously. Similarly, the ACR50 responses were 28.8%, 16.8%, and 3.8% in the tocilizumab 8 mg/kg, 4 mg/kg, and placebo groups. The ACR70 responses were 12.4%, 5%, and 1.3% in the tocilizumab 8 mg/ kg, 4 mg/kg, and placebo groups. The DAS28 remission (<2.6) was achieved in 30%, 7.6%, and 1.6% among the 8 mg/kg, 4 mg/kg, and the placebo groups, respectively.

In the AMBITION study, tocilizumab monotherapy was compared with methotrexate monotherapy in patients who had not failed methotrexate or anti-TNF agents in the past. In this 24-week study, 673 patients were randomized to receive tocilizumab 8 mg/kg every 4 weeks, methotrexate starting at 7.5 mg weekly, increasing to 20 mg in 8 weeks, or placebo for 8 weeks followed by tocilizumab 8 mg/kg weekly. The ACR20 responses were 70% in the tocilizumab group versus 52.5% in the methotrexate group. 33.6% of patients in the tocilizumab group achieved DAS28 scores of less than 2.6 versus 12.1% in the methotrexate group.[148]

Tocilizumab has also been shown to slow radiographic bone damage in the SAMURAI trial. In this study, 306 patients were randomized to receive 8 mg/kg of tocilizumab weekly or conventional DMARDs for 52 weeks. At 52 weeks the mean total van der Heijde scores were lower in the tocilizumab group than in the DMARD group.[149] In this study 306 patients with RA of less than 5 years' duration were randomized to receive tocilizumab 8 mg/kg every 4 weeks or DMARDs for 52 weeks. The modified total Sharp score (TSS) at entry was 29.4. At the conclusion of the study, patients in the tocilizumab group had lower increments in their TSS than those in the DMARDs group (2.3 vs 6.1). Clinical improvement was similar to previous trials.

Finally, efficacy of tocilizumab was shown in methotrexate nonresponders in the SATORI trial. In this trial 127 patients were randomized to receive tocilizumab 8 mg/kg or weekly methotrexate (8 mg/wk—the most commonly used dosage in Japan) for 24 weeks. 80.3% of patients in the tocilizumab group achieved ACR20 responses compared with 25% in the control group. The ACR50 and ACR70 responses were 49.2% and 29.5%, respectively in the tocilizumab group compared with 10.9% and 6.3% in the control group. These differences in ACR responses were corroborated by improvements in the DAS28 responses. The clinical effects were evident at 4 weeks and continued up to 24 weeks.[150]

In this trial, serum VEGF levels dropped by 346.9 pg/mL in the tocilizumab group compared with the control group, in which VEGF levels dropped by 74.0 pg/mL.[150] VEGF is an angiogenic factor that can induce growth of new blood vessels required to sustain synovial hypertrophy and inflammation in RA. VEGF is produced by macrophages, vascular smooth muscle cells, synovial lining cells, neutrophils from synovial fluid, and peripheral blood mononuclear cells. VEGF can also facilitate migration of cells from blood into the synovium and thus maintain synovial inflammation. VEGF is increased in the sera of patients with RA.[151–153]

A 2-year trial is currently underway to determine the safety and efficacy of tocilizumab + methotrexate in methotrexate nonresponders, the LITHE trial.[154] In this trial, 1200 patients were randomized to receive tocilizumab 4 mg/kg + methotrexate, tocilizumab 8 mg/kg + methotrexate, or methotrexate + placebo. The dose of methotrexate is 10 to 25 mg weekly, which is higher than the previous SATORI trial where it was used at 8 mg weekly. Patients in the placebo arm were given the option of switching to blinded rescue therapy from week 16. At the initial 52-week analysis of this study, the ACR20 responses were 56%, 47%, and 25% in the tocilizumab 8 mg/kg, tocilizumab 4 mg/kg, and placebo groups, respectively. Similarly, the ACR50 and ACR70 responses were higher in the tocilizumab group, with the 8 mg/kg group showing higher responses than the 4 mg/kg group. The mean change in the Genant modified TSS from baseline was 0.29, 0.34, and 1.13 in the tocilizumab 8 mg/kg, tocilizumab 4 mg/kg, and placebo groups, respectively.

Safety of Tocilizumab

All clinical trials with tocilizumab have shown that the infusion is well tolerated without significant infusion reactions. However, most studies concur that administration of tocilizumab is associated with increased adverse events compared with placebo. The percentage of patients experiencing adverse events in the various trials ranged from 59% to 92% in the tocilizumab groups in comparison to 51% to 82% in the placebo groups. The most common adverse event was nasopharyngitis, and other adverse events included rash, headaches, and gastrointestinal disturbances. Serious adverse events were typically similar in the tocilizumab and control groups, but in one trial serious adverse events were higher in the tocilizumab group, 18% versus 13% in the DMARD only group.[149] The serious adverse events in this trial included pneumonia and cellulitis.

Administration of tocilizumab is also associated with several laboratory abnormalities including neutropenia, elevations in transaminases, total bilirubin, total cholesterol, low-density lipoprotein (LDL), and high-density lipoprotein (HDL). The proportion of patients developing laboratory abnormalities ranged between 56% and 76% in the tocilizumab groups versus 23% to 41% in the control groups. Serum total cholesterol was elevated in 38% to 44% of patients on tocilizumab, LDL in 26%, and HDL in 24%. No adverse cardiovascular events were reported from the clinical trials to date.

Alanine aminotransferase (ALT) was frequently elevated at 2 to 3 times normal. The elevation of ALT was associated with each infusion and came down to baseline levels before the next infusion.[144] Some patients also developed elevations in total bilirubin without overt hepatic failure.

Of note, neutropenia is seen in a significant number of patients receiving tocilizumab, and could contribute to its therapeutic efficacy in RA. Neutropenia is temporally related to the drug and improves on discontinuation of tocilizumab. There were no reported increases in infection associated with tocilizumab-induced neutropenia. The tendency of tocilizumab to induce neutropenia, in comparison to anti-TNF agents, was assessed in a recent study. In this study patients received tocilizumab 8 mg/kg, infliximab 3 mg/kg, etanercept 25 mg subcutaneously, or adalimumab 40 mg subcutaneously. There was a 70% incidence of decrease in neutrophil counts with tocilizumab versus 45% in the infliximab group, 20% in the etanercept group, and 28% in the adalimumab group. Neutropenia with tocilizumab occurred 2 days after the infusion and recovered before the next infusion.[155] Further studies are needed to carefully assess the long-term risks of tocilizumab-induced neutropenia, particularly because in clinical practice patients have other comorbid conditions and may be on moderate doses of steroids.

Early in 2010 tocilizumab was approved in the United States for the treatment of RA.

IL-17 NEUTRALIZING THERAPIES

Two different clones of anti–IL-17 antibody are currently undergoing clinical trials in patients with RA. LY2439821, developed by Eli Lilly, has recently completed a phase 1 trial and a phase 2 trial is currently underway. The phase 1 study had 2 parts. During part A of the study a single dose was administered to 20 patients with dose escalation to evaluate safety. Patients were followed for 8 weeks. In part B, 77 patients were divided among 4 treatment groups and received 0.2, 0.6, or 2.0 mg/kg of LY2439821, or placebo every 2 weeks for a total of 8 weeks, and were followed for an additional 8 weeks. The most frequent adverse event reported in the single dose group was headache and diarrhea. Patients receiving multiple doses of LY2439821 had increased incidences of leukopenia, neutropenia, rhinitis, and vertigo. These adverse events were not dose dependent. Leukopenia (<3000 white blood cells/μl) was reported in 3 patients and neutropenia (<1500 neutrophils/μl) was reported in 5 patients receiving the active drug. Only one patient required withdrawal of the drug for leukopenia. There was no reported increased incidence of infections in patients with leucopenia or neutropenia. At 10 weeks, patients receiving LY2439821 at all doses (0.2 mg/kg, 0.6 mg/kg, or 2 mg/kg) had significant improvement of their

DAS28 scores and ACR20 responses. DAS28 scores decreased by −2.3, −2.2, and −2.4 with LY2439821 0.2 mg/kg, 0.6 mg/kg, and 2 mg/kg, respectively, and by 0.5 in the placebo group. Seventy-four percent, 70%, and 90% of patients achieved ACR20 responses in LY2439821 0.2, 0.6, and 2 mg/kg groups. ACR50 responses were in the range of 35% to 42% among the various treatment groups. ACR70 responses were 20% to 25% among the different treatment groups receiving LY2439821. ACR20/50/70 responses were 55.6%, 16.7%, and 5.6% among patients in the placebo group.[156]

A phase 2 trial with this antibody (LY2439821) in 372 patients is currently underway (NCT00966875). This study has 2 parts. In part A, patients will be randomized to receive varying doses of active drug for 16 weeks followed by part B, in which patients will be followed in an open-label extension for a total of 60 weeks. In this study, 2 patient populations will be evaluated: (i) DMARD and biologic naïve and, (ii) inadequate responders to TNF-targeted therapy. During part A of this study biologic and DMARD naïve patients will receive 3, 10, 30, 80, or 180 mg of active drug or placebo. TNF nonresponders will receive 80 or 180 mg of active drug or placebo at weeks 0, 1, 2, 4, 6, 8, and 10. During part B patients will receive 160 mg of active drug at 16, 18, and 20 weeks and then every 4 weeks up to week 60. The primary end points are DAS28 and ACR20 responses.

AIN457 is an anti-IL-17A monoclonal antibody developed by Novartis. A phase 1 trial was recently completed. In this study 52 patients with RA were randomized to receive 2 doses of 10 mg/kg of AIN457, administered intravenously 3 weeks apart, or placebo. Forty-six percent of patients in the active drug group achieved ACR20 responses at 6 weeks in comparison to 27% in the placebo group. ACR50 responses were 27% in the AIN457 group versus 15% in the placebo group. ACR70 responses at 6 weeks were 8% in both groups. There was a slightly higher frequency of adverse events in the AIN457 group, at 81% versus 65% in the placebo group. Overall the types of adverse events were similar between the 2 groups.[157]

At present, a phase 2 study evaluating efficacy and safety of AIN457 in patients with active RA on methotrexate is ongoing (NCT00928512). In this 16-week study, followed by an extension phase up to a total of 60 weeks, patients will be randomized into 4 active drug groups receiving different doses of AIN457 + methotrexate or placebo + methotrexate. Clinical trials are underway with AIN457 in several other autoimmune diseases in which Th17 or IL-17 plays a pathogenic role, such as psoriasis, psoriatic arthritis, ankylosing spondylitis, Crohn disease, uveitis, and multiple sclerosis.

CURRENT STATUS OF IL-17 AND TH17 CELLS AS VALID TARGETS IN THE TREATMENT OF RA

Direct approaches to blocking IL-17 action include neutralization of IL-17 or the IL-17 receptor. Although animal data and in vitro studies suggest that this would be effective in RA, the clinical results available are only preliminary and are clouded by high response rates in placebo groups. At least 2 isoforms of IL-17 that are proinflammatory, IL-17A and IL-17F, appear to play a role in RA. Each of these can exist as a homodimer, and IL-17A and IL-17F can also form heterodimers. It is possible that effective blockade of IL-17 will need to neutralize all of these molecules. Although worrisome toxicities have not yet been reported, the role in IL-17 in host defenses against gram-negative bacteria and fungi is a reason for caution. The IL-17 receptor is also complex, employs several subunits, and may exist in more than one type of molecular assembly; the optimal subunit to target in therapeutic blockade by an antibody is currently uncertain.

Table 1
IL-17 and the treatment of RA: potential approaches

Target	Agent	Mechanism: Known or Postulated
IL-17 (A, F, or A/F)	Anti–IL-17	Neutralization of IL-17
IL-17 receptor	Anti–IL-17R	Receptor blockade
IL-6 receptor	Tocilizumab	Inhibition of Th17 differentiation
IL-23	Ustekinumab	Inhibition of Th17 differentiation
IL-1	Anakinra Anti–IL-1	Inhibition of Th17 differentiation
CD28 ligands	Abatacept	Blockade of costimulation required for Th17 cell activation
B lymphocytes	Rituximab	Depletion of B cells that can assist in Th17 cell differentiation by presenting antigen, engaging costimulatory receptors and secreting IL-6
Th17 cells	Vitamin D	Inhibition of Th17 cell differentiation
Th17 cells	Sulforophane	Inhibition of IL-17 secretion by Th17 cells

Indirect approaches to lowering IL-17 levels involve inhibition of the differentiation or activation of Th17 cells. In view of the role of cytokines at several steps in these processes, a variety of targets are available, such as IL-6, IL-23, IL-21, IL-1, and others. Each of these cytokines has multiple effects other than stimulating Th17 differentiation that could also be relevant to their roles in RA. Thus therapeutic success from targeting these molecules would not necessarily be primarily due to effects on the Th17 axis. Unfortunately, clinical trials in patients with RA have generally not included measurement of IL-17 in serum or cell culture supernatants, or enumeration of Th17 cells. Mechanistic studies of this type in the context of clinical trials are sorely needed.

Other possible approaches could be the development of inhibitors of key transcription factors in Th17 cells (especially RORC), or inhibitors of signal transduction through either the IL-17 receptor itself or through receptors for cytokines that are important in the development of Th17 cells. Nutritional approaches may also be relevant. For example, suppressive effects of vitamin D on human Th17 differentiation have been documented.[158] A vegetable-derived isothiocyanate termed sulforaphane inhibits IL-17 production by RA T cells and suppresses CIA.[159] Further complicating the situation is the ability of Th17 cells to produce a variety of other proinflammatory (and occasionally anti-inflammatory) cytokines. Moreover, IL-17 production is not the sole property of Th17 lymphocytes, but can also occur in subsets of CD8+ cells and even leukocytes other than T cells.

In view of the complexity of the Th17 axis and the many areas of uncertainty, careful testing of a variety of approaches is logical. It is likely that clinical trials of various anti–IL-17 strategies have the potential to fortify basic understanding of the regulation of IL-17 production and action in humans, as well as the roles of IL-17 and Th17 cells in RA and other immune-mediated diseases (**Table 1**).

REFERENCES

1. Mosmann TR, Cherwinski H, Bond MW, et al. Two types of murine helper T cell clone. I. Definition according to profiles of lymphokine activities and secreted proteins. 1986. J Immunol 2005;175:5.

2. Harrington LE, Hatton RD, Mangan PR, et al. Interleukin 17-producing CD4+ effector T cells develop via a lineage distinct from the T helper type 1 and 2 lineages. Nat Immunol 2005;6:1123.

3. Park H, Li Z, Yang XO, et al. A distinct lineage of CD4 T cells regulates tissue inflammation by producing interleukin 17. Nat Immunol 2005;6:1133.

4. Yao Z, Painter SL, Fanslow WC, et al. Human IL-17: a novel cytokine derived from T cells. J Immunol 1995;155:5483.

5. Yao Z, Fanslow WC, Seldin MF, et al. Herpesvirus Saimiri encodes a new cytokine, IL-17, which binds to a novel cytokine receptor. Immunity 1995;3:811.

6. Fossiez F, Djossou O, Chomarat P, et al. T cell interleukin-17 induces stromal cells to produce proinflammatory and hematopoietic cytokines. J Exp Med 1996;183:2593.

7. Sarkar S, Cooney LA, White P, et al. Regulation of pathogenic IL-17 responses in collagen-induced arthritis: roles of endogenous interferon-gamma and IL-4. Arthritis Res Ther 2009;11:R158.

8. Murphy KM, Reiner SL. The lineage decisions of helper T cells. Nat Rev Immunol 2002;2:933.

9. Langrish CL, Chen Y, Blumenschein WM, et al. IL-23 drives a pathogenic T cell population that induces autoimmune inflammation. J Exp Med 2005;201:233.

10. Aggarwal S, Ghilardi N, Xie MH, et al. Interleukin-23 promotes a distinct CD4 T cell activation state characterized by the production of interleukin-17. J Biol Chem 2003;278:1910.

11. Bettelli E, Carrier Y, Gao W, et al. Reciprocal developmental pathways for the generation of pathogenic effector TH17 and regulatory T cells. Nature 2006; 441:235.

12. Mangan PR, Harrington LE, O'Quinn DB, et al. Transforming growth factor-beta induces development of the T(H)17 lineage. Nature 2006;441:231.

13. Veldhoen M, Hocking RJ, Atkins CJ, et al. TGFbeta in the context of an inflammatory cytokine milieu supports de novo differentiation of IL-17-producing T cells. Immunity 2006;24:179.

14. Sutton C, Brereton C, Keogh B, et al. A crucial role for interleukin (IL)-1 in the induction of IL-17-producing T cells that mediate autoimmune encephalomyelitis. J Exp Med 2006;203:1685.

15. Nakae S, Iwakura Y, Suto H, et al. Phenotypic differences between Th1 and Th17 cells and negative regulation of Th1 cell differentiation by IL-17. J Leukoc Biol 2007;81:1258.

16. Acosta-Rodriguez EV, Napolitani G, Lanzavecchia A, et al. Interleukins 1beta and 6 but not transforming growth factor-beta are essential for the differentiation of interleukin 17-producing human T helper cells. Nat Immunol 2007;8:942.

17. Wilson NJ, Boniface K, Chan JR, et al. Development, cytokine profile and function of human interleukin 17-producing helper T cells. Nat Immunol 2007;8:950.

18. Evans HG, Suddason T, Jackson I, et al. Optimal induction of T helper 17 cells in humans requires T cell receptor ligation in the context of Toll-like receptor-activated monocytes. Proc Natl Acad Sci U S A 2007;104:17034.

19. Zhou L, Lopes JE, Chong MM, et al. TGF-beta-induced Foxp3 inhibits T(H)17 cell differentiation by antagonizing RORgammat function. Nature 2008;453: 236.

20. Manel N, Unutmaz D, Littman DR. The differentiation of human T(H)-17 cells requires transforming growth factor-beta and induction of the nuclear receptor RORgammat. Nat Immunol 2008;9:641.

21. Volpe E, Servant N, Zollinger R, et al. A critical function for transforming growth factor-beta, interleukin 23 and proinflammatory cytokines in driving and modulating human T(H)-17 responses. Nat Immunol 2008;9:650.
22. Yang L, Anderson DE, Baecher-Allan C, et al. IL-21 and TGF-beta are required for differentiation of human T(H)17 cells. Nature 2008;454:350.
23. Annunziato F, Cosmi L, Santarlasci V, et al. Phenotypic and functional features of human Th17 cells. J Exp Med 2007;204:1849.
24. Amadi-Obi A, Yu CR, Liu X, et al. TH17 cells contribute to uveitis and scleritis and are expanded by IL-2 and inhibited by IL-27/STAT1. Nat Med 2007;13:711.
25. Hoeve MA, Savage ND, de Boer T, et al. Divergent effects of IL-12 and IL-23 on the production of IL-17 by human T cells. Eur J Immunol 2006;36:661.
26. Ivanov II, McKenzie BS, Zhou L, et al. The orphan nuclear receptor RORgammat directs the differentiation program of proinflammatory IL-17+ T helper cells. Cell 2006;126:1121.
27. Zhang F, Meng G, Strober W. Interactions among the transcription factors Runx1, RORgammat and Foxp3 regulate the differentiation of interleukin 17-producing T cells. Nat Immunol 2008;9:1297.
28. Mathur AN, Chang HC, Zisoulis DG, et al. Stat3 and Stat4 direct development of IL-17-secreting Th cells. J Immunol 2007;178:4901.
29. Wei L, Laurence A, Elias KM, et al. IL-21 is produced by Th17 cells and drives IL-17 production in a STAT3-dependent manner. J Biol Chem 2007;282:34605.
30. Fantini MC, Rizzo A, Fina D, et al. IL-21 regulates experimental colitis by modulating the balance between Treg and Th17 cells. Eur J Immunol 2007;37:3155.
31. Zhou L, Ivanov II, Spolski R, et al. IL-6 programs T(H)-17 cell differentiation by promoting sequential engagement of the IL-21 and IL-23 pathways. Nat Immunol 2007;8:967.
32. Korn T, Bettelli E, Gao W, et al. IL-21 initiates an alternative pathway to induce proinflammatory T(H)17 cells. Nature 2007;448:484.
33. Nurieva R, Yang XO, Martinez G, et al. Essential autocrine regulation by IL-21 in the generation of inflammatory T cells. Nature 2007;448:480.
34. Peluso I, Fantini MC, Fina D, et al. IL-21 counteracts the regulatory T cell-mediated suppression of human CD4+ T lymphocytes. J Immunol 2007;178:732.
35. Onoda T, Rahman M, Nara H, et al. Human CD4+ central and effector memory T cells produce IL-21: effect on cytokine-driven proliferation of CD4+ T cell subsets. Int Immunol 2007;19:1191.
36. Kuestner RE, Taft DW, Haran A, et al. Identification of the IL-17 receptor related molecule IL-17RC as the receptor for IL-17F. J Immunol 2007;179:5462.
37. Wright JF, Guo Y, Quazi A, et al. Identification of an interleukin 17F/17A heterodimer in activated human CD4+ T cells. J Biol Chem 2007;282:13447.
38. Liang SC, Long AJ, Bennett F, et al. An IL-17F/A heterodimer protein is produced by mouse Th17 cells and induces airway neutrophil recruitment. J Immunol 2007;179:7791.
39. Chen Z, Tato CM, Muul L, et al. Distinct regulation of interleukin-17 in human T helper lymphocytes. Arthritis Rheum 2007;56:2936.
40. Zheng Y, Danilenko DM, Valdez P, et al. Interleukin-22, a T(H)17 cytokine, mediates IL-23-induced dermal inflammation and acanthosis. Nature 2007;445:648.
41. Acosta-Rodriguez EV, Rivino L, Geginat J, et al. Surface phenotype and antigenic specificity of human interleukin 17-producing T helper memory cells. Nat Immunol 2007;8:639.

42. Liang SC, Tan XY, Luxenberg DP, et al. Interleukin (IL)-22 and IL-17 are coexpressed by Th17 cells and cooperatively enhance expression of antimicrobial peptides. J Exp Med 2006;203:2271.

43. Chung Y, Yang X, Chang SH, et al. Expression and regulation of IL-22 in the IL-17-producing CD4+ T lymphocytes. Cell Res 2006;16:902.

44. Boniface K, Bernard FX, Garcia M, et al. IL-22 inhibits epidermal differentiation and induces proinflammatory gene expression and migration of human keratinocytes. J Immunol 2005;174:3695.

45. Wolk K, Witte E, Wallace E, et al. IL-22 regulates the expression of genes responsible for antimicrobial defense, cellular differentiation, and mobility in keratinocytes: a potential role in psoriasis. Eur J Immunol 2006;36:1309.

46. Andoh A, Zhang Z, Inatomi O, et al. Interleukin-22, a member of the IL-10 subfamily, induces inflammatory responses in colonic subepithelial myofibroblasts. Gastroenterology 2005;129:969.

47. Zenewicz LA, Yancopoulos GD, Valenzuela DM, et al. Interleukin-22 but not interleukin-17 provides protection to hepatocytes during acute liver inflammation. Immunity 2007;27:647.

48. Anderson CF, Oukka M, Kuchroo VJ, et al. CD4(+)CD25(−)Foxp3(−) Th1 cells are the source of IL-10-mediated immune suppression in chronic cutaneous leishmaniasis. J Exp Med 2007;204:285.

49. Jankovic D, Kullberg MC, Feng CG, et al. Conventional T-bet(+)Foxp3(−) Th1 cells are the major source of host-protective regulatory IL-10 during intracellular protozoan infection. J Exp Med 2007;204:273.

50. McGeachy MJ, Bak-Jensen KS, Chen Y, et al. TGF-beta and IL-6 drive the production of IL-17 and IL-10 by T cells and restrain T(H)-17 cell-mediated pathology. Nat Immunol 2007;8:1390.

51. Stumhofer JS, Silver JS, Laurence A, et al. Interleukins 27 and 6 induce STAT3-mediated T cell production of interleukin 10. Nat Immunol 2007;8:1363.

52. Hirota K, Yoshitomi H, Hashimoto M, et al. Preferential recruitment of CCR6-expressing Th17 cells to inflamed joints via CCL20 in rheumatoid arthritis and its animal model. J Exp Med 2007;204:2803.

53. Singh SP, Zhang HH, Foley JF, et al. Human T cells that are able to produce IL-17 express the chemokine receptor CCR6. J Immunol 2008;180:214.

54. Lundy SK, Lira SA, Smit JJ, et al. Attenuation of allergen-induced responses in CCR6−/− mice is dependent upon altered pulmonary T lymphocyte activation. J Immunol 2005;174:2054.

55. Teraki Y, Miyake A, Takebayashi R, et al. Homing receptor and chemokine receptor on intraepidermal T cells in psoriasis vulgaris. Clin Exp Dermatol 2004;29:658.

56. Varona R, Cadenas V, Flores J, et al. CCR6 has a non-redundant role in the development of inflammatory bowel disease. Eur J Immunol 2003;33:2937.

57. Ruth JH, Shahrara S, Park CC, et al. Role of macrophage inflammatory protein-3alpha and its ligand CCR6 in rheumatoid arthritis. Lab Invest 2003;83:579.

58. Kao CY, Huang F, Chen Y, et al. Up-regulation of CC chemokine ligand 20 expression in human airway epithelium by IL-17 through a JAK-independent but MEK/NF-kappaB-dependent signaling pathway. J Immunol 2005;175:6676.

59. Chabaud M, Page G, Miossec P. Enhancing effect of IL-1, IL-17, and TNF-alpha on macrophage inflammatory protein-3alpha production in rheumatoid arthritis: regulation by soluble receptors and Th2 cytokines. J Immunol 2001;167:6015.

60. Sato W, Aranami T, Yamamura T. Cutting edge: Human Th17 cells are identified as bearing CCR2+CCR5− phenotype. J Immunol 2007;178:7525.

61. van der Graaff WL, Prins AP, Niers TM, et al. Quantitation of interferon gamma- and interleukin-4-producing T cells in synovial fluid and peripheral blood of arthritis patients. Rheumatology (Oxford) 1999;38:214.
62. Steiner G, Tohidast-Akrad M, Witzmann G, et al. Cytokine production by synovial T cells in rheumatoid arthritis. Rheumatology (Oxford) 1999;38:202.
63. Isomaki P, Luukkainen R, Lassila O, et al. Synovial fluid T cells from patients with rheumatoid arthritis are refractory to the T helper type 2 differentiation-inducing effects of interleukin-4. Immunology 1999;96:358.
64. Berner B, Akca D, Jung T, et al. Analysis of Th1 and Th2 cytokines expressing CD4+ and CD8+ T cells in rheumatoid arthritis by flow cytometry. J Rheumatol 2000;27:1128.
65. Manoury-Schwartz B, Chiocchia G, Bessis N, et al. High susceptibility to collagen-induced arthritis in mice lacking IFN-gamma receptors. J Immunol 1997;158:5501.
66. Vermeire K, Heremans H, Vandeputte M, et al. Accelerated collagen-induced arthritis in IFN-gamma receptor-deficient mice. J Immunol 1997;158:5507.
67. Chu CQ, Song Z, Mayton L, et al. IFNgamma deficient C57BL/6 (H-2b) mice develop collagen induced arthritis with predominant usage of T cell receptor Vbeta6 and Vbeta8 in arthritic joints. Ann Rheum Dis 2003;62:983.
68. Chu CQ, Swart D, Alcorn D, et al. Interferon-gamma regulates susceptibility to collagen-induced arthritis through suppression of interleukin-17. Arthritis Rheum 2007;56:1145.
69. Guedez YB, Whittington KB, Clayton JL, et al. Genetic ablation of interferon-gamma up-regulates interleukin-1beta expression and enables the elicitation of collagen-induced arthritis in a nonsusceptible mouse strain. Arthritis Rheum 2001;44:2413.
70. Murphy CA, Langrish CL, Chen Y, et al. Divergent pro- and antiinflammatory roles for IL-23 and IL-12 in joint autoimmune inflammation. J Exp Med 2003;198:1951.
71. Irmler IM, Gajda M, Brauer R. Exacerbation of antigen-induced arthritis in IFN-gamma-deficient mice as a result of unrestricted IL-17 response. J Immunol 2007;179:6228.
72. Nakae S, Nambu A, Sudo K, et al. Suppression of immune induction of collagen-induced arthritis in IL-17-deficient mice. J Immunol 2003;171:6173.
73. Lubberts E, Koenders MI, Oppers-Walgreen B, et al. Treatment with a neutralizing antimurine interleukin-17 antibody after the onset of collagen-induced arthritis reduces joint inflammation, cartilage destruction, and bone erosion. Arthritis Rheum 2004;50:650.
74. Bush KA, Farmer KM, Walker JS, et al. Reduction of joint inflammation and bone erosion in rat adjuvant arthritis by treatment with interleukin-17 receptor IgG1 Fc fusion protein. Arthritis Rheum 2002;46:802.
75. Koenders MI, Kolls JK, Oppers-Walgreen B, et al. Interleukin-17 receptor deficiency results in impaired synovial expression of interleukin-1 and matrix metalloproteinases 3, 9, and 13 and prevents cartilage destruction during chronic reactivated streptococcal cell wall-induced arthritis. Arthritis Rheum 2005;52:3239.
76. Lubberts E, Schwarzenberger P, Huang W, et al. Requirement of IL-17 receptor signaling in radiation-resistant cells in the joint for full progression of destructive synovitis. J Immunol 2005;175:3360.
77. Stolina M, Bolon B, Dwyer D, et al. The evolving systemic and local biomarker milieu at different stages of disease progression in rat collagen-induced arthritis. Biomarkers 2008;13:692.

78. Joosten LA, Abdollahi-Roodsaz S, Heuvelmans-Jacobs M, et al. T cell dependence of chronic destructive murine arthritis induced by repeated local activation of Toll-like receptor-driven pathways: crucial role of both interleukin-1beta and interleukin-17. Arthritis Rheum 2008;58:98.

79. Nakae S, Saijo S, Horai R, et al. IL-17 production from activated T cells is required for the spontaneous development of destructive arthritis in mice deficient in IL-1 receptor antagonist. Proc Natl Acad Sci U S A 2003;100:5986.

80. Hirota K, Hashimoto M, Yoshitomi H, et al. T cell self-reactivity forms a cytokine milieu for spontaneous development of IL-17+ Th cells that cause autoimmune arthritis. J Exp Med 2007;204:41.

81. Boissier MC, Chiocchia G, Bessis N, et al. Biphasic effect of interferon-gamma in murine collagen-induced arthritis. Eur J Immunol 1995;25:1184.

82. Finnegan A, Mikecz K, Tao P, et al. Proteoglycan (aggrecan)-induced arthritis in BALB/c mice is a Th1-type disease regulated by Th2 cytokines. J Immunol 1999;163:5383.

83. Hwang SY, Kim HY. Expression of IL-17 homologs and their receptors in the synovial cells of rheumatoid arthritis patients. Mol Cells 2005;19:180.

84. Chabaud M, Durand JM, Buchs N, et al. Human interleukin-17: A T cell-derived proinflammatory cytokine produced by the rheumatoid synovium. Arthritis Rheum 1999;42:963.

85. Ziolkowska M, Koc A, Luszczykiewicz G, et al. High levels of IL-17 in rheumatoid arthritis patients: IL-15 triggers in vitro IL-17 production via cyclosporin A-sensitive mechanism. J Immunol 2000;164:2832.

86. Shahrara S, Huang Q, Mandelin AM 2nd, et al. TH-17 cells in rheumatoid arthritis. Arthritis Res Ther 2008;10:R93.

87. Raza K, Falciani F, Curnow SJ, et al. Early rheumatoid arthritis is characterized by a distinct and transient synovial fluid cytokine profile of T cell and stromal cell origin. Arthritis Res Ther 2005;7:R784.

88. Kim KW, Cho ML, Park MK, et al. Increased interleukin-17 production via a phosphoinositide 3-kinase/Akt and nuclear factor kappaB-dependent pathway in patients with rheumatoid arthritis. Arthritis Res Ther 2005;7:R139.

89. Lenarczyk A, Helsloot J, Farmer K, et al. Antigen-induced IL-17 response in the peripheral blood mononuclear cells (PBMC) of healthy controls. Clin Exp Immunol 2000;122:41.

90. von Delwig A, Locke J, Robinson JH, et al. Response of Th17 cells to a citrullinated arthritogenic aggrecan peptide in patients with rheumatoid arthritis. Arthritis Rheum 2010;62:143.

91. Kirkham BW, Lassere MN, Edmonds JP, et al. Synovial membrane cytokine expression is predictive of joint damage progression in rheumatoid arthritis: a two-year prospective study (the DAMAGE study cohort). Arthritis Rheum 2006;54:1122.

92. Lundy SK, Sarkar S, Tesmer LA, et al. Cells of the synovium in rheumatoid arthritis. T lymphocytes. Arthritis Res Ther 2007;9:202.

93. Shahrara S, Pickens SR, Dorfleutner A, et al. IL-17 induces monocyte migration in rheumatoid arthritis. J Immunol 2009;182:3884.

94. Ryu S, Lee JH, Kim SI. IL-17 increased the production of vascular endothelial growth factor in rheumatoid arthritis synoviocytes. Clin Rheumatol 2006; 25:16.

95. Numasaki M, Lotze MT, Sasaki H. Interleukin-17 augments tumor necrosis factor-alpha-induced elaboration of proangiogenic factors from fibroblasts. Immunol Lett 2004;93:39.

96. Kotake S, Udagawa N, Takahashi N, et al. IL-17 in synovial fluids from patients with rheumatoid arthritis is a potent stimulator of osteoclastogenesis. J Clin Invest 1999;103:1345.

97. Miranda-Carus ME, Benito-Miguel M, Balsa A, et al. Peripheral blood T lymphocytes from patients with early rheumatoid arthritis express RANKL and interleukin-15 on the cell surface and promote osteoclastogenesis in autologous monocytes. Arthritis Rheum 2006;54:1151.

98. Sato K, Suematsu A, Okamoto K, et al. Th17 functions as an osteoclastogenic helper T cell subset that links T cell activation and bone destruction. J Exp Med 2006;203:2673.

99. Kim KW, Cho ML, Kim HR, et al. Up-regulation of stromal cell-derived factor 1 (CXCL12) production in rheumatoid synovial fibroblasts through interactions with T lymphocytes: role of interleukin-17 and CD40L-CD40 interaction. Arthritis Rheum 2007;56:1076.

100. Cho ML, Kang JW, Moon YM, et al. STAT3 and NF-kappaB signal pathway is required for IL-23-mediated IL-17 production in spontaneous arthritis animal model IL-1 receptor antagonist-deficient mice. J Immunol 2006;176:5652.

101. Caproni M, Antiga E, Melani L, et al. Serum levels of IL-17 and IL-22 are reduced by etanercept, but not by acitretin, in patients with psoriasis: a randomized-controlled trial. J Clin Immunol 2009;29:210.

102. Lubberts E, Koenders MI, van den Berg WB. The role of T-cell interleukin-17 in conducting destructive arthritis: lessons from animal models. Arthritis Res Ther 2005;7:29.

103. Koenders MI, Lubberts E, van de Loo FA, et al. Interleukin-17 acts independently of TNF-alpha under arthritic conditions. J Immunol 2006;176:6262.

104. Chabaud M, Miossec P. The combination of tumor necrosis factor alpha blockade with interleukin-1 and interleukin-17 blockade is more effective for controlling synovial inflammation and bone resorption in an ex vivo model. Arthritis Rheum 2001;44:1293.

105. Jungel A, Distler JH, Kurowska-Stolarska M, et al. Expression of interleukin-21 receptor, but not interleukin-21, in synovial fibroblasts and synovial macrophages of patients with rheumatoid arthritis. Arthritis Rheum 2004;50:1468.

106. Li J, Shen W, Kong K, et al. Interleukin-21 induces T-cell activation and proinflammatory cytokine secretion in rheumatoid arthritis. Scand J Immunol 2006;64:515.

107. Young DA, Hegen M, Ma HL, et al. Blockade of the interleukin-21/interleukin-21 receptor pathway ameliorates disease in animal models of rheumatoid arthritis. Arthritis Rheum 2007;56:1152.

108. Kim HR, Kim HS, Park MK, et al. The clinical role of IL-23p19 in patients with rheumatoid arthritis. Scand J Rheumatol 2007;36:259.

109. Kim HR, Cho ML, Kim KW, et al. Up-regulation of IL-23p19 expression in rheumatoid arthritis synovial fibroblasts by IL-17 through PI3-kinase-, NF-kappaB- and p38 MAPK-dependent signalling pathways. Rheumatology (Oxford) 2007;46:57.

110. Lee HS, Remmers EF, Le JM, et al. Association of STAT4 with rheumatoid arthritis in the Korean population. Mol Med 2007;13:455.

111. Remmers EF, Plenge RM, Lee AT, et al. STAT4 and the risk of rheumatoid arthritis and systemic lupus erythematosus. N Engl J Med 2007;357:977.

112. Hildner KM, Schirmacher P, Atreya I, et al. Targeting of the transcription factor STAT4 by antisense phosphorothioate oligonucleotides suppresses collagen-induced arthritis. J Immunol 2007;178:3427.

113. Ikeuchi H, Kuroiwa T, Hiramatsu N, et al. Expression of interleukin-22 in rheumatoid arthritis: potential role as a proinflammatory cytokine. Arthritis Rheum 2005; 52:1037.
114. Miranda-Carus ME, Balsa A, Benito-Miguel M, et al. IL-15 and the initiation of cell contact-dependent synovial fibroblast-T lymphocyte cross-talk in rheumatoid arthritis: effect of methotrexate. J Immunol 2004;173:1463.
115. Yoshihara K, Yamada H, Hori A, et al. IL-15 exacerbates collagen-induced arthritis with an enhanced CD4+ T cell response to produce IL-17. Eur J Immunol 2007;37:2744.
116. Ferrari-Lacraz S, Zanelli E, Neuberg M, et al. Targeting IL-15 receptor-bearing cells with an antagonist mutant IL-15/Fc protein prevents disease development and progression in murine collagen-induced arthritis. J Immunol 2004;173:5818.
117. Yamamura Y, Gupta R, Morita Y, et al. Effector function of resting T cells: activation of synovial fibroblasts. J Immunol 2001;166:2270.
118. Tran CN, Lundy SK, White PT, et al. Molecular interactions between T cells and fibroblast-like synoviocytes: role of membrane tumor necrosis factor-alpha on cytokine-activated T cells. Am J Pathol 2007;171:1588.
119. Stanley KT, VanDort C, Motyl C, et al. Immunocompetent properties of human osteoblasts: interactions with T lymphocytes. J Bone Miner Res 2006;21:29.
120. Morita Y, Yang J, Gupta R, et al. Dendritic cells genetically engineered to express IL-4 inhibit murine collagen-induced arthritis. J Clin Invest 2001;107: 1275.
121. Sarkar S, Tesmer LA, Hindnavis V, et al. Interleukin-17 as a molecular target in immune-mediated arthritis: immunoregulatory properties of genetically modified murine dendritic cells that secrete interleukin-4. Arthritis Rheum 2007;56:89.
122. Lubberts E, Joosten LA, Chabaud M, et al. IL-4 gene therapy for collagen arthritis suppresses synovial IL-17 and osteoprotegerin ligand and prevents bone erosion. J Clin Invest 2000;105:1697.
123. Kauffman CL, Aria N, Toichi E, et al. A phase I study evaluating the safety, pharmacokinetics, and clinical response of a human IL-12 p40 antibody in subjects with plaque psoriasis. J Invest Dermatol 2004;123:1037.
124. Gottlieb AB, Cooper KD, McCormick TS, et al. A phase 1, double-blind, placebo-controlled study evaluating single subcutaneous administrations of a human interleukin-12/23 monoclonal antibody in subjects with plaque psoriasis. Curr Med Res Opin 2007;23:1081.
125. Krueger GG, Langley RG, Leonardi C, et al. A human interleukin-12/23 monoclonal antibody for the treatment of psoriasis. N Engl J Med 2007;356:580.
126. Leonardi CL, Kimball AB, Papp KA, et al. Efficacy and safety of ustekinumab, a human interleukin-12/23 monoclonal antibody, in patients with psoriasis: 76-week results from a randomised, double-blind, placebo-controlled trial (PHOENIX 1). Lancet 2008;371:1665.
127. Papp KA, Langley RG, Lebwohl M, et al. Efficacy and safety of ustekinumab, a human interleukin-12/23 monoclonal antibody, in patients with psoriasis: 52-week results from a randomised, double-blind, placebo-controlled trial (PHOENIX 2). Lancet 2008;371:1675.
128. Griffiths CE, Strober BE, van de Kerkhof P, et al. Comparison of ustekinumab and etanercept for moderate-to-severe psoriasis. N Engl J Med 2010;362: 118.
129. Gottlieb A, Menter A, Mendelsohn A, et al. Ustekinumab, a human interleukin 12/23 monoclonal antibody, for psoriatic arthritis: randomised, double-blind, placebo-controlled, crossover trial. Lancet 2009;373:633.

130. Sandborn WJ, Feagan BG, Fedorak RN, et al. A randomized trial of Ustekinumab, a human interleukin-12/23 monoclonal antibody, in patients with moderate-to-severe Crohn's disease. Gastroenterology 2008;135:1130.
131. Segal BM, Constantinescu CS, Raychaudhuri A, et al. Repeated subcutaneous injections of IL12/23 p40 neutralising antibody, ustekinumab, in patients with relapsing-remitting multiple sclerosis: a phase II, double-blind, placebo-controlled, randomised, dose-ranging study. Lancet Neurol 2008;7:796.
132. Reddy M, Davis C, Wong J, et al. Modulation of CLA, IL-12R, CD40L, and IL-2Ralpha expression and inhibition of IL-12- and IL-23-induced cytokine secretion by CNTO 1275. Cell Immunol 2007;247:1.
133. Toichi E, Torres G, McCormick TS, et al. An anti-IL-12p40 antibody down-regulates type 1 cytokines, chemokines, and IL-12/IL-23 in psoriasis. J Immunol 2006;177:4917.
134. Takagi N, Mihara M, Moriya Y, et al. Blockage of interleukin-6 receptor ameliorates joint disease in murine collagen-induced arthritis. Arthritis Rheum 1998; 41:2117.
135. Atsumi T, Ishihara K, Kamimura D, et al. A point mutation of Tyr-759 in interleukin 6 family cytokine receptor subunit gp130 causes autoimmune arthritis. J Exp Med 2002;196:979.
136. Guerne PA, Zuraw BL, Vaughan JH, et al. Synovium as a source of interleukin 6 in vitro. Contribution to local and systemic manifestations of arthritis. J Clin Invest 1989;83:585.
137. Houssiau FA, Devogelaer JP, Van Damme J, et al. Interleukin-6 in synovial fluid and serum of patients with rheumatoid arthritis and other inflammatory arthritides. Arthritis Rheum 1988;31:784.
138. Madhok R, Crilly A, Watson J, et al. Serum interleukin 6 levels in rheumatoid arthritis: correlations with clinical and laboratory indices of disease activity. Ann Rheum Dis 1993;52:232.
139. Firestein GS, Alvaro-Gracia JM, Maki R. Quantitative analysis of cytokine gene expression in rheumatoid arthritis. J Immunol 1990;144:3347.
140. Naka T, Kishimoto T. Joint disease caused by defective gp130-mediated STAT signaling. Arthritis Res 2002;4:154.
141. Choy EH, Isenberg DA, Garrood T, et al. Therapeutic benefit of blocking interleukin-6 activity with an anti-interleukin-6 receptor monoclonal antibody in rheumatoid arthritis: a randomized, double-blind, placebo-controlled, dose-escalation trial. Arthritis Rheum 2002;46:3143.
142. Nishimoto N, Yoshizaki K, Miyasaka N, et al. Treatment of rheumatoid arthritis with humanized anti-interleukin-6 receptor antibody: a multicenter, double-blind, placebo-controlled trial. Arthritis Rheum 2004;50:1761.
143. Nishimoto N, Miyasaka N, Yamamoto K, et al. Long-term safety and efficacy of tocilizumab, an anti-IL-6 receptor monoclonal antibody, in monotherapy, in patients with rheumatoid arthritis (the STREAM study): evidence of safety and efficacy in a 5-year extension study. Ann Rheum Dis 2009;68:1580.
144. Maini RN, Taylor PC, Szechinski J, et al. Double-blind randomized controlled clinical trial of the interleukin-6 receptor antagonist, tocilizumab, in European patients with rheumatoid arthritis who had an incomplete response to methotrexate. Arthritis Rheum 2006;54:2817.
145. Smolen JS, Beaulieu A, Rubbert-Roth A, et al. Effect of interleukin-6 receptor inhibition with tocilizumab in patients with rheumatoid arthritis (OPTION study): a double-blind, placebo-controlled, randomised trial. Lancet 2008; 371:987.

146. Genovese MC, McKay JD, Nasonov EL, et al. Interleukin-6 receptor inhibition with tocilizumab reduces disease activity in rheumatoid arthritis with inadequate response to disease-modifying antirheumatic drugs: the tocilizumab in combination with traditional disease-modifying antirheumatic drug therapy study. Arthritis Rheum 2008;58:2968.

147. Emery P, Keystone E, Tony HP, et al. IL-6 receptor inhibition with tocilizumab improves treatment outcomes in patients with rheumatoid arthritis refractory to anti-tumour necrosis factor biologicals: results from a 24-week multicentre randomised placebo-controlled trial. Ann Rheum Dis 2008;67:1516.

148. Jones G, Sebba A, Gu J, et al. Comparison of tocilizumab monotherapy versus methotrexate monotherapy in patients with moderate to severe rheumatoid arthritis: the AMBITION study. Ann Rheum Dis 2010;69:88.

149. Nishimoto N, Hashimoto J, Miyasaka N, et al. Study of active controlled monotherapy used for rheumatoid arthritis, an IL-6 inhibitor (SAMURAI): evidence of clinical and radiographic benefit from an x ray reader-blinded randomised controlled trial of tocilizumab. Ann Rheum Dis 2007;66:1162.

150. Nishimoto N, Miyasaka N, Yamamoto K, et al. Study of active controlled tocilizumab monotherapy for rheumatoid arthritis patients with an inadequate response to methotrexate (SATORI): significant reduction in disease activity and serum vascular endothelial growth factor by IL-6 receptor inhibition therapy. Mod Rheumatol 2009;19:12.

151. Nagashima M, Yoshino S, Ishiwata T, et al. Role of vascular endothelial growth factor in angiogenesis of rheumatoid arthritis. J Rheumatol 1995;22:1624.

152. Kasama T, Kobayashi K, Yajima N, et al. Expression of vascular endothelial growth factor by synovial fluid neutrophils in rheumatoid arthritis (RA). Clin Exp Immunol 2000;121:533.

153. Koch AE, Harlow LA, Haines GK, et al. Vascular endothelial growth factor. A cytokine modulating endothelial function in rheumatoid arthritis. J Immunol 1994;152:4149.

154. Kremer J, Fleischmann R, Brzezicki J, et al. Tocilizumab inhibits structural joint damage, improves physical function, and increases DAS28 remission rates in RA patients who respond inadequately to methotrexate: the Lithe Study. Ann Rheum Dis 2009;68:122.

155. Omata Y, Nakamura I, Matsui T, et al. Neutropenia induced by anti-interleukin-6 receptor antibody, tocilizumab. Ann Rheum Dis 2009;68:582.

156. Genovese M, Van den Bosch F, Roberson S, et al. LY2439821, a Humanized anti-IL-17 monoclonal antibody, in the treatment of patients with rheumatoid arthritis. Arthritis Rheum 2010. [Epub ahead of print].

157. Durez P, Chindalore V, Bittmer B, et al. AIN457, an anti-IL17 antibody, shows good safety and induces clinical responses in patients with active rheumatoid arthritis (RA) despite methotrexate therapy in a randomized, double-blind proof-of-concept trial. Ann Rheum Dis 2009;68:125.

158. Colin EM, Asmawidjaja PS, van Hamburg JP, et al. 1,25-dihydroxyvitamin D(3) modulates Th17 polarization and interleukin-22 expression by memory T cells from patients with early rheumatoid arthritis. Arthritis Rheum 2010;62:132.

159. Kong JS, Yoo SA, Kim HS, et al. Inhibition of synovial hyperplasia, rheumatoid T cell activation, and experimental arthritis in mice by sulforaphane, a naturally occurring isothiocyanate. Arthritis Rheum 2010;62:159.

A Multitude of Kinases—Which are the Best Targets in Treating Rheumatoid Arthritis?

Tamsin M. Lindstrom, PhD[a,b],*, William H. Robinson, MD, PhD[a,b],*

KEYWORDS

- MAPKs • Tyrosine kinases • IKK • Jak
- Syk • Small-molecule inhibitors

The advent of biologic therapeutics, most notably anti–tumor necrosis factor (TNF) agents, has dramatically improved the treatment of rheumatoid arthritis (RA). Nevertheless, the available biologics rarely result in disease remission and provide clinical benefit only in subsets of RA patients. In addition, biologics can be administered only by injection and are expensive. Alternative therapies for RA are needed, and small-molecule kinase inhibitors may fit the bill. Small molecules have several features that give them the edge over other therapeutics: they are orally bioavailable, cell permeable, and inexpensive to manufacture. Insight into intracellular signaling pathways involved in inflammation and immunity has allowed the rational design of small molecules that can counteract aberrant immune responses. Small molecules can exert potent anti-inflammatory effects by inhibiting kinases, many of which lie at the nexus of multiple proinflammatory pathways. The therapeutic potential of kinase inhibitors is showcased by their success in the treatment of cancer.

Adaptive and innate immune responses are involved in the pathogenesis of RA, a systemic autoimmune disease characterized by destruction of the synovial joints. Initiation of the disease involves systemic dysregulation of T- and B-cell responses, which leads to a breach in self-tolerance and eventually to the mounting of an immune response against the synovial joints. During the chronic inflammatory stage of the

This work was supported by NIH NIAMS R01 AR-054822, an American College of Rheumatology Within-Our-Reach grant, and Veterans Affairs Health Care System funding awarded to W.H.R.
[a] Geriatric Research Education and Clinical Center (GRECC), MC154R, VA Palo Alto Health Care System, 3801 Miranda Avenue, Palo Alto, CA 94304, USA
[b] Division of Immunology and Rheumatology, Stanford University School of Medicine, CCSR 4135, 269 Campus Drive, Stanford, CA 94305, USA
* Corresponding author.
E-mail addresses: tlind@stanford.edu (T.M. Lindstrom); wrobins@stanford.edu (W.H. Robinson).

Rheum Dis Clin N Am 36 (2010) 367–383
doi:10.1016/j.rdc.2010.02.005
0889-857X/10/$ – see front matter © 2010 Elsevier Inc. All rights reserved.

disease, mast cells, macrophages, neutrophils, T cells, and B cells all infiltrate the synovium, where they release proinflammatory cytokines and matrix metalloproteinases (MMPs) that erode the synovial cartilage. Inflammation in the joints also triggers the development of apoptosis-resistant, hyperproliferative, fibroblast-like synoviocytes (FLS), which produce further proinflammatory cytokines. The synovial hyperplasia, in turn, leads to the formation of a destructive pannus that invades surrounding cartilage and bone. Finally, inflammation suppresses the formation of bone-forming osteoblasts and augments the formation of bone-resorbing osteoclasts, leading to the erosion of bone. Several kinases have been shown to play important roles in one or more of these pathogenic processes.This article discusses the therapeutic potential of small molecules targeting specific protein kinases in the treatment of RA and provides an overview of the progress to date. Lipid kinases—in particular, the phosphoinositide-3 kinases (PI3Ks)—are also emerging as attractive drug targets in the treatment of inflammation. The therapeutic potential of blocking PI3Ks in RA has been recently reviewed[1] and is not discussed further.

MITOGEN-ACTIVATED PROTEIN KINASES: ADVANCES AND SETBACKS

Mitogen-activated protein kinase (MAPK) signaling comprises 3 interrelated pathways, each mediated by a distinct MAPK: p38, extracellular signal-regulated kinase (ERK), or c-Jun N-terminal kinase (JNK). These pathways involve the sequential activation of multiple kinases, such that the MAPKs are activated by MAPK kinases (MKKs), which are themselves activated by MAPKK kinases (MKKKs). Thus, the p38 kinases (α, β, γ, and δ) are activated by MKK3 and MKK6, the ERKs (1 and 2) by MAPK-ERK kinase (MEK) 1 and MEK2, and the JNKs (1, 2, and 3) by MKK4 and MKK7.[2] JNK, ERK, and p38 are the terminal kinases of these pathways and serve to regulate an array of cellular responses through the phosphorylation of serine/threonine residues in discrete sets of transcription factors. All 3 of these MAPKs are activated in RA synovium[3] and have been proposed as therapeutic targets in the treatment of RA.

P38

Enthusiasm for inhibitors of p38—until recently heralded as one of the most promising classes of oral therapeutics for RA—has finally subsided. Many p38 inhibitors have been developed and tested in preclinical and clinical studies. Although the preclinical data were encouraging, with p38 inhibition shown to suppress inflammation and joint destruction in many different models of RA,[4] these initial successes did not extend to the treatment of RA. The first generation of small-molecule p38 inhibitors, which targeted all 4 isoforms of p38, failed in clinical trials owing to liver, brain, and skin toxicities. Nevertheless, the discovery that p38α is the important isoform in RA, acting to drive the expression of proinflammatory cytokines and the formation of osteoclasts,[5,6] engendered hope that selective inhibition of p38α would avoid the adverse effects of the pan-38 inhibitors. Unfortunately, p38α-specific inhibitors did not perform much better (**Table 1**). For instance, clinical development of SCIO-323 and AMG-548 was terminated because of skin toxicity and liver toxicity, respectively,[7] and the p38α inhibitors that did advance to phase II clinical trials proved ineffective.[8,9]

The toxicity and the inefficacy of p38 inhibitors are most likely target based, rendering the systemic targeting of p38 unviable. Multiple structurally unrelated p38 inhibitors have been shown to be toxic to the liver and skin and to induce only transient reductions in markers of inflammation.[4,7] The pivotal position of p38α in the regulation of inflammation is thought to underlie these phenomena. Although its proinflammatory

Table 1
Small-molecule kinase inhibitors in RA clinical trials

Kinase Target	Inhibitor (Company)	Outcome in RA Clinical Trials
p38α	SCIO-323 (Scios)	Clinical development terminated owing to skin toxicity[7]
	AMG-548 (Amgen)	Clinical development terminated owing to liver toxicity[7]
	Pamapimod (Roche)	Phase II trial comparing efficacy and safety with MTX treatment[8] • ACR20 response rate was higher in the MTX-treated group than in the pamapimod-treated group
	VX-702 (Vertex)	Phase II trial in patients with RA on a background of MTX[9] • Tolerated but no significant increase over placebo in ACR20 response rate
JAKs	INCB18424 (Incyte)	Phase II trial in patients with RA on a background of MTX, SSZ, antimalarials, or prednisone[a] • ACR20, ACR50, ACR70, and ACR90 response rates were 83%, 50%, 25%, and 17%, respectively, in the 15-mg group, compared with 33%, 11%, 0%, and 0% in the placebo group
	CP690550 (Pfizer)	Phase II trial in patients with RA refractory to MTX, etanercept, infliximab, or adalimumab[59] • ACR20 response rates were 70.5%, 81.2%, and 76.8% in the 5-mg, 15-mg, and 30-mg groups, respectively, compared with 29.2% in the placebo group • ACR50 and ACR70 response rates were significantly greater in all treatment groups compared with the placebo group
Syk	R788 (Rigel)	Phase II trial in patients with RA on a background of MTX, SSZ, antimalarials, prednisone, or NSAIDs[64] • ACR20, ACR50, and ACR70 response rates were 72%, 57%, and 40%, respectively, in the 150-mg group compared with 38%, 19%, and 4% in the placebo group
MEK 1/2	ARRY-162 (Array BioPharma)	Phase II trial in patients with RA refractory to MTX[b] • Tolerated but no significant increase over placebo in ACR20 response
c-Kit/PDGFR	AB1010 (AB Science)	Open-label, uncontrolled, phase II trial in patients with RA refractory to MTX or anti-TNF agents[85] • ACR20, ACR50, and ACR70 response rates were 54%, 26%, and 8%, respectively • High rate (37%) of patient withdrawal owing to adverse effects
	Imatinib mesylate (Novartis)	Phase II trial in patients with active RA on a background of MTX[c] • Outcomes not reported

Abbreviations: MTX, methotrexate; SSZ, sulfasalazine.
[a] Incyte press release. Incyte's JAK inhibitor demonstrates marked clinical benefits in phase IIa rheumatoid arthritis study. Available at: http://www.incyte.com/Eular%20PR%206%2012%2008%13-%20Final.pdf. Accessed January 25, 2010.
[b] Array BioPharma. Array BioPharma announces top-line results from rheumatoid arthritis phase 2 trial. Available at: http://www.drugs.com/clinical_trials/array-biopharma-announces-top-line-results-rheumatoid-arthritis-phase-10-trial-7991.html. Accessed January 25, 2010.
[c] Novartis Pharmaceuticals. A study of imatinib 400 mg once daily in combination with methotrexate in the treatment of rheumatoid arthritis. Available at: http://www.clinicaltrials.gov/ct2/show/NCT00154336?term=imatinib-and+rheumatoid&rank=. Accessed January 25, 2010.

role has long been recognized, p38α has more recently been found to play an anti-inflammatory role also. Not only does it drive the expression of important anti-inflammatory genes but also it mediates intracellular feedback loops that constrain the activity of other proinflammatory pathways. For instance, p38α activates mitogen- and stress-activated protein kinase (MSK) 1 and MSK2, which contribute to the resolution of inflammation through the transcriptional activation of anti-inflammatory genes, such as interleukin (IL)-10, IL-1 receptor antagonist, and protein phosphatase dual specificity.[10–12] p38α also reigns in inflammation by phosphorylating TGF-beta-activated kinase (TAK) -associated kinase 1 (TAB1), thereby inhibiting TAK1, which regulates the proinflammatory JNK and inhibitor of κB (IκB) kinase (IKK) pathways, as well as p38α itself.[4] Thus, blockade of p38α would allow inflammation to proceed unchecked. Genetic evidence supports the idea that p38α inhibition underlies the toxicity and inefficacy of p38 inhibitors: myeloid cell-specific ablation of p38α in mice results in increased ERK and JNK activity and in vascular permeability and edema[12]; double deficiency in MSK1 and MSK2 leads to prolonged inflammation in a model of toxic contact eczema[10]; and hepatocyte-specific ablation of p38α in mice results in excessive activation of the proapoptotic JNK in the liver after lipopolysaccharide (LPS) challenge.[13]

Although the death knell may have sounded for inhibitors of p38, components downstream of p38α may yet constitute viable therapeutic targets. MAPK-activated protein kinase 2 (MK2), a kinase downstream of p38α that post-transcriptionally promotes the expression of proinflammatory genes, has been proposed as one such candidate.[4] Targeting of MK2 should spare p38α-mediated anti-inflammatory mechanisms, including the p38α-TAB1 feedback loop and expression of anti-inflammatory genes. Support for such an approach comes from the finding that MK2-deficient mice are protected against collagen-induced arthritis (CIA).[14] One small-molecule MK2 inhibitor has already been shown to reduce LPS-induced TNF production in rats, and many more are being synthesized.[15,16]

MEKs and ERKs

The critical role of MEK-ERK signaling in cell proliferation has led to MEK1 and 2 and ERK1 and 2 being investigated as candidate targets in clinical trials in cancer.[2] MEK-ERK signaling is upregulated in synovial tissues in RA and in CIA[17] and promotes proliferation of RA FLS in vitro.[18] MEK-ERK signaling may thus contribute to the pathogenesis of RA by driving formation of the tumor-like pannus that is characteristic of RA. But the MEK-ERK cascade is not solely a proliferative one—it is also proinflammatory, inducing the production of IL-1β, IL-6, TNF, and MMPs, and itself is activated by proinflammatory cytokines. In addition to promoting inflammation and tissue destruction in the synovial joints, ERK signaling is important in lymphocyte activation and differentiation. ERK mediates B-cell receptor (BCR) and CD40 receptor signaling in B cells and T-cell receptor signaling in T cells.[19,20] Recent data suggest that ERK dysregulation in CD4+ and CD8+ T cells may even contribute to the breakdown of T-cell tolerance in RA by lowering the threshold for T-cell activation.[19]

Several small-molecule inhibitors of MEK 1 and 2 have shown efficacy in animal models of RA (Table 2). Oral administration of PD184352 to mice with CIA suppressed synovitis, pannus formation, and cartilage and bone erosion.[17] These effects correlated closely with the inhibition of ERK phosphorylation in mouse joints. PD184352 also prevented proteoglycan loss in articular cartilage in a rabbit model of IL-1β-induced arthritis.[17] Prophylactic, intraperitoneal administration of subtherapeutic doses of U0126 to SKG mice, which spontaneously develop autoimmune arthritis owing to a mutation in zap70,[21] delayed disease onset and reduced disease severity,

Table 2
Small-molecule kinase inhibitors showing treatment benefit in animal models of RA

Kinase Targeted	Small-Molecule Inhibitor (Company)	RA Model
MEK 1/2	PD184352 (Pfizer)	Mouse CIA; rabbit cytokine-induced cartilage degradation[17]
	U0126 (DuPont Pharmaceuticals)	Mouse SKG[19]
	ARRY-162[a] (Array BioPharma)	Rat CIA and AIA[22]
ERK 1/2	FR180204 (Astellas)	Mouse CIA[23]
JNK 1/2/3	SP600125 (Celgene)	Rat AIA[40]
	AS601245 (EMD Serono)	Mouse CIA[42]
IKK2	BMS-345541 (Bristol-Myers Squibb)	Mouse CIA[95]
	BMS-066 (Bristol-Myers Squibb)	Mouse CIA and rat AIA[96]
	TPCA-1 (GlaxoSmithKline)	Mouse CIA[97]
	PHA-408 (Pfizer)	Rat SCWA[98]
	ML120B (Millenium Pharmaceuticals)	Rat AIA[99]
	IMD-0560 (IMDD)	Mouse CIA[100]
	SPC839 (Celgene)	Rat AIA[101]
c-Fms	GW2580 (GlaxoSmithKline)	Rat AIA[78]; mouse CIA, CAIA, K/BxN[74]
	Ki20227 (Kirin)	Mouse CIA[79]
	Cyanopyrrole 8 (Johnson & Johnson)	Mouse CIA[80]
BTK	Compound 4 (Celera Genomics)	Mouse LPS-induced arthritis[87]
	Cgi1746 (CGI Pharmaceuticals)	Mouse CIA[86]
PI3Kγ	AS-604850, AS-605240 (EMD Serono)	Mouse CAIA[104]

Abbreviations: IMDD, Institute of Medicinal and Molecular Design; PI3Kγ, phosphoinositide-3 kinase γ; SCWA, streptococcal cell wall–induced arthritis.
[a] In clinical trials in RA patients (see **Table 1**).

supporting the concept that ERK dysregulation may contribute to the development of RA.[19] A third MEK1 and 2 inhibitor, ARRY-162, inhibited inflammation and bone resorption in mice with CIA and in rats with adjuvant-induced arthritis (AIA) and exhibited additive efficacy when combined with standard-of-care agents such as anti-TNFs and methotrexate.[22] These promising findings saw ARRY-162 enter clinical development; however, despite being well tolerated, ARRY-162 did not fare any better than placebo in a recent phase II, 12-week trial in patients with active RA on a background of methotrexate treatment (see **Table 1**).

In addition to inhibitors of MEK1 and 2, an inhibitor of the downstream ERKs has been assessed in a mouse model of RA. Intraperitoneal administration of the ERK 1 and 2 inhibitor FR180204 to mice before the induction of CIA reduced the clinical signs of arthritis, the production of anti-collagen type II (CII) antibodies, and CII-specific proliferation of T cells.[23] Conversely, recent studies suggest that targeting components upstream of MEK may also provide efficacy in RA. Tumor progression locus 2 (TPL2) is the MKKK that activates MEK1 and 2 and hence the ERKs.[24,25] Studies using *tpl2*[−/−] mice have shown that TPL2 is required for LPS-induced production of circulating TNF in vivo and for LPS-induced production of TNF by macrophages in vitro.[24,26] Furthermore, TPL2 deficiency has been shown to protect mice from TNF-induced inflammatory bowel disease[27] and arthritis (unpublished data with G. Kollias cited in Das and colleagues[28]). Several small-molecule inhibitors of TPL have been assessed for their ability to suppress TPL2-MEK-ERK–induced inflammation. Compound 1 suppressed LPS- and IL-1β–induced production of TNF by human monocytes as well as IL-1β–induced production of IL-6, IL-8, prostaglandin E2, and MMPs by RA FLS.[29] Compound 44 inhibited the production of TNF in an LPS-induced model of inflammation in rats.[30] Results from the testing of TPL2 inhibitors in animal models of RA have not been described to date.

Thus, small-molecule inhibitors exist for the targeting of the TPL2-MEK-ERK pathway at 3 different levels. The inefficacy of the MEK1 and 2 inhibitor ARRY-162 in a phase II RA trial, however, together with concerns that MEK/ERK inhibition could result in the development of lupus-like disease,[31–33] raise doubts over the potential of MEK/ERK inhibitors for the treatment of RA. Safety might also be an issue with TPL2 inhibitors, but these could potentially provide greater therapeutic efficacy than MEK/ERK inhibitors. Although the signaling defect in TPL2-deficient macrophages and B cells seems restricted to activation of the MEK-ERK pathway,[24,25] TPL2 regulates the activation of JNK and nuclear factor κB (NF-κB), in addition to ERK, in mouse embryonic fibroblasts.[28] Because synovial-fibroblast production of proinflammatory and degradative mediators is important in the pathogenesis of RA, inhibition of TPL2 might provide added benefit by suppressing ERK-driven activation of lymphocytes and ERK-, JNK-, and NF-κB–driven activation of synovial fibroblasts.

JNKS

Activated by stress signals and cytokines, JNKs play important roles in apoptosis, inflammation, and matrix degradation.[34,35] JNKs exist as 3 isoforms: JNK1, JNK2, and JNK3. JNK1 and JNK2 are ubiquitously expressed, and phosphorylation of these isoforms is detected in RA synovium but not in osteoarthritic synovium[36]; JNK3 expression is largely restricted to the brain, heart, and testes, and, therefore, not thought to be involved in RA.[37,38] As discussed later, some of the efficacy of spleen tyrosine kinase (Syk) inhibitors in RA could potentially be attributed to the inhibition of JNKs, because the tyrosine kinase Syk lies upstream of JNK in the MAPK signaling cascade. Syk-activated JNKs drive the expression of IL-6 and MMP-3 in RA FLS.[39] Induction of MMP expression is defective in JNK1- or JNK2-deficient murine FLS, and pharmacologic inhibition of JNK blocks induction of MMP expression in RA FLS.[40] In addition to promoting synoviocyte production of proinflammatory mediators, JNK1 regulates the differentiation of T cells into Th1 cells.[41]

The JNK-driven expression of MMPs seems critical in the destruction of joints in inflammatory arthritis. Subcutaneous administration of SP600125, a small-molecule inhibitor that targets all 3 JNK isoforms, suppressed cartilage and bone erosion in rat AIA, effects associated with inhibition of JNK activity and MMP expression in the joints.[40] Oral administration of another pan-JNK inhibitor, AS601245, attenuated CIA in mice, reducing synovial inflammation and cartilage degradation.[42] JNK1 deficiency, however, does not confer resistance to destructive arthritis in JNK1-deficient, TNF-transgenic mice nor does it reduce the activity of JNK-mediated signaling.[43] In addition, JNK2 deficiency confers only modest protection against the development of anti-collagen antibody-induced arthritis (CAIA).[40] Together, these findings suggest that inhibition of both JNK1 and JNK2 is required for the effective attenuation of inflammatory arthritis.

Although developed as a JNK inhibitor, SP600125 has been shown to inhibit 13 other protein kinases with similar or greater potency and to have an unfavorable pharmacokinetic profile.[36,44] Likewise, AS601245 exhibits only moderate selectivity for JNK.[42] More specific inhibition of the JNK signaling cascade can be achieved by targeting the physical interaction between JNK and other components of the cascade. JNK-interacting protein 1 (JIP1) is a scaffolding protein that promotes JNK activity by facilitating the interaction between JNK and upstream kinases.[45] Overexpression of JIP1, however, suppresses JNK activity (presumably owing to the sequestration of

JNK-interacting components), and a peptide corresponding to the minimal region of JIP1 (pepJIP1) has been developed as an inhibitor of JNK.[46] Although peptide therapeutics are associated with certain disadvantages, such as their rapid degradation in vivo and the need for administration via injection, a small-molecule mimic of pepJIP1, BI-78D3, was recently developed and shown to exert anti-inflammatory effects in vivo, restoring insulin sensitivity in a mouse model of type 2 diabetes.[47] In addition, a small-molecule inhibitor that selectively blocks the DNA-binding activity of AP-1, an important JNK-activated transcription-factor complex, was recently shown to be efficacious in a mouse model of arthritis. Oral administration of the AP-1 inhibitor T-5224 prevented and treated CIA in mice, abrogating joint destruction and suppressing MMP and IL-1β expression.[48]

Although toxicity in animal models treated with inhibitors of the JNK pathway has not been reported, long-term suppression of JNK could potentially have adverse effects due to JNK's role in regulating apoptosis.[35] JNK1-deficient mice spontaneously develop intestinal tumors and are more susceptible to the development of TPA-induced skin tumors.[49,50] Thus, increased tumorigenicity may limit the value of JNK inhibitors for the treatment of chronic inflammatory disorders, such as RA.

TYROSINE KINASES: THE FRONTRUNNERS
Tyrosine Kinases Targeted in RA Clinical Trials

Janus kinases
Janus kinases (Jaks) play important roles in innate and adaptive immune responses, serving to transduce signals from cytokine receptors that lack intrinsic kinase activity. Cytokine receptors containing the common γ-chain subunit signal through Jak1 and Jak3, whereas receptors for hematopoietic growth factors or gp40-containing cytokines signal through Jak2. Jak1 and Jak2 are ubiquitously expressed and are essential for lymphopoiesis and hematopoiesis, respectively.[51] Jak3 is expressed primarily in cells of the immune system and is critical in lymphocyte activation, function, and proliferation[52]; accordingly, the defect in Jak3-deficient mice seems to be restricted to T cells, B cells, and natural killer cells.[53,54]

Given their multifarious roles in innate and adaptive immunity, it might be expected that Jaks are involved in the pathogenesis of RA. It was not until recently, however, that Jaks began to be explored as candidate therapeutic targets in RA. Progress has since been rapid. The finding that inhibition of Jak3 ameliorates clinical signs of inflammatory arthritis by greater than 90% and protects against joint damage in rodent models of RA[55] was swiftly followed by assessment of the therapeutic efficacy of 2 small-molecule Jak inhibitors—CP690550 and INCB18424—in patients with RA. CP690550 was developed as a Jak3 inhibitor but also inhibits Jak2, albeit less potently; its selectivity for the Jaks has been confirmed by testing against a panel of 317 kinases.[56] INCB18424 is an inhibitor primarily of Jak1 and 2. High hopes are now pinned on these Jak inhibitors. They are arguably the best-performing investigational small-molecule drugs in RA at present, with CP690550 and INCB18424 proving efficacious and well tolerated in initial phase II clinical trials (CP690550, 6-week trial; INCB18424, 28-day trial) (see **Table 1**). Which of these 2 Jak inhibitors will prove to be safer in the long term remains to be seen. On the one hand, the restriction of Jak3 expression to hematopoietic cells might mean that a Jak3 inhibitor will have fewer target-based adverse effects than a Jak1 and 2 inhibitor; on the other hand, *Jak3* mutations in humans are known to cause severe immunodeficiency syndrome.[57,58] In addition, the nature of the adverse effects seen with CP690550 suggest that therapeutically efficacious doses of this compound result in inhibition of Jak2 in addition to Jak3.[59] Conversely, Jak3 signaling may be indirectly affected by inhibitors of Jak1, because Jak1 and Jak3 cooperate in the transduction of multiple signals.[60] The outcomes of phase IIb trials of CP690550 and INCB18424 are eagerly awaited.

Syk

Another prime therapeutic contender is R788, the prodrug for the R406 small-molecule inhibitor of Syk. Syk is expressed in all hematopoietic cells, mediating immunoreceptor signaling, such as BCR signaling in B cells and FcγR signaling in mast cells, macrophages, neutrophils, and basophils.[61] It is also expressed in nonhematopoietic cells, in which it transduces signals from receptors for TNF, IL-1, and LPS. Syk activity is upregulated in RA synovium compared with control osteoarthritic synovium and mediates the production of IL-6 and MMP-3—major culprits in joint destruction—in TNF-stimulated RA FLS.[39] Syk also promotes osteoclast activity.[61] Thus, Syk may promote both the adaptive immune responses and the destructive effector processes that underlie RA, making it an attractive therapeutic target.

The R406 Syk inhibitor suppressed inflammation and joint destruction in 2 antibody-mediated models of RA in mice[62] as well as in a T-cell–mediated model of RA in rats.[63] In a preliminary 12-week phase II trial in RA, R788 (which is rapidly converted to R406 after oral administration) proved efficacious and generally well tolerated.[64] R788 administration resulted in a rapid and sustained decrease in serum IL-6 and MMP-3 levels, an indication that Syk inhibition may be able to halt joint damage. The long-term efficacy and safety of R788 is the focus of an ongoing open-label study of the RA patients who completed the initial R788 phase II trial. Although relatively specific for Syk,[62] R788 did cause hypertension in a few RA patients, which may reflect off-target inhibition of the vascular-endothelial growth factor receptor (VEGFR).[64] This observation has raised some concern about the safety of R788 in RA, a disease associated with increased cardiovascular complications.[65] As for target-mediated adverse effects, the ubiquity of Syk may be an issue, but its nonredundant functions in adulthood may not be as widespread as its expression.[61] Syk has been shown to signal upstream of JNK in mast cells[66] and in RA FLS[39]; therefore, Syk inhibition could potentially share some of the advantages and disadvantages of JNK inhibition (discussed previously).

Tyrosine Kinases Targeted in Animal Models of RA

Several other tyrosine kinases have been implicated in RA, partly on the basis of observations in cancer patients treated with imatinib mesylate (imatinib). Imatinib, the first kinase inhibitor introduced into clinical practice, targets several tyrosine kinases, including BCR-ABL, platelet-derived growth factor (PDGFR), c-Fms, c-Kit, Syk, and leukocyte-specific kinase. Case studies documented the alleviation of RA symptoms in patients administered imatinib for the treatment of chronic myelogenous leukemias or c-Kit–expressing gastrointestinal stromal tumors,[67,68] suggesting that one or more of the imatinib-targeted kinases are important in the pathogenesis of RA. Prompted by these findings, Eklund and Joensuu[69] administered imatinib to 3 patients with treatment-refractory RA. All 3 patients showed some degree of clinical improvement; 1 patient continued treatment for 24 months and showed marked and long-lasting clinical improvement.[70] Two of the 3 patients in this study, however, discontinued imatinib treatment at 2 and at 4 months, owing to adverse events. Furthermore, the outcomes of a double-blind, placebo-controlled, 3-month, phase II trial conducted by Novartis, in which imatinib was administered to patients with active RA despite methotrexate treatment, were never reported. Although toxicities—including cardiotoxicity due to inhibition of Abl[71]—may limit the use of imatinib in nononcologic chronic diseases, selectively inhibiting the imatinib-targeted kinases that are important in RA may provide a more favorable risk-to-benefit ratio. In mouse studies, imatinib-induced attenuation of CIA was associated with suppression of c-Fms activation in synovial macrophages, of PDGFR activation in FLS, and of c-Kit activation in mast cells.[72] The involvement of each of these tyrosine kinases in RA has been independently investigated.

Accumulating evidence suggests that c-Fms and its ligand, macrophage colony-stimulating factor (M-CSF), are involved in the pathogenesis of RA. M-CSF–c-Fms signaling is integral to macrophage and osteoclast formation, as evidenced by the osteopetrosis and the reduction in tissue macrophages in M-CSF– and in c-Fms–deficient mice.[73] M-CSF levels are elevated in the synovial fluid and serum of RA patients,[74,75] and administration of exogenous M-CSF to mice exacerbates submaximal CIA.[76] Conversely, M-CSF–deficient mice are resistant to the development of CIA, and neutralizing antibodies against M-CSF or c-Fms attenuate mouse CIA.[76,77] Several small-molecule inhibitors of c-Fms have been developed and tested in models of RA. In parallel experiments, the c-Fms–specific inhibitor GW2580 was as efficacious as imatinib in attenuating inflammatory arthritis in antibody-mediated and T-cell–mediated mouse models of RA.[74] In these models, prophylactic, oral administration of GW2580 reduced synovitis, pannus formation, and cartilage and bone erosion; GW2580 was also able to treat established arthritis. The amelioration of arthritis was associated with reduced macrophage infiltration and c-Fms expression in the synovial joints. In vitro, GW2580 inhibited the differentiation of monocytes into macrophages and osteoclasts; the resorption of bone by osteoclasts; and the priming of TNF production in Fc receptor (FcR)-stimulated macrophages.[74] Thus, c-Fms inhibitors may have potential in the treatment of RA through the mitigation of the non–antigen-specific processes that underpin the chronic inflammatory stage of RA. GW2580 has also been shown to attenuate tissue and bone destruction in the joints of rats with AIA, although no effects on joint inflammation were detected in this model.[78] Two other orally bioavailable c-Fms inhibitors, Ki20027 and cyanopyrrole 8, have been shown to reduce joint inflammation and bone destruction in rodent models of RA, but these compounds are less selective than GW2580.[79,80] Tested against a panel of 179 kinases, GW2580 proved relatively selective, inhibiting only c-Fms (IC_{50} of 0.03 µM) and TrkA (IC_{50} of 0.88 µM).[78] The restriction of c-Fms expression to monocyte-lineage cells might mean that c-Fms inhibitors are relatively safe and well tolerated. Nevertheless, elevations in levels of liver enzymes in arthritic mice treated with GW2580, although not associated with histologic evidence of pathology, could indicate potential toxicities of GW2580.[78]

Although PDGFR and c-Kit have been implicated in RA, small-molecule inhibitors that selectively inhibit either one of these kinases are not currently available. PDGFR is a ubiquitous tyrosine kinase that plays a key role in fibroblast proliferation, and imatinib has been shown to inhibit PDGFR-mediated proliferation of FLS derived from arthritic mice or from RA patients.[72,81] Therefore, PDGFR is thought to contribute to RA pathogenesis by promoting synovial hyperplasia and, thus, pannus formation. c-Kit has been proposed as contributing by mediating the aberrant activation of mast cells. c-Kit is essential for the survival and activation of mast cells, and release of proinflammatory mediators from synovial mast cells precedes the onset of clinical signs of inflammation in certain antibody-mediated models of RA.[82] The importance of mast cells in autoimmune arthritis is contentious, however. In initial studies, mouse strains deficient in mast cells—owing to a loss-of-function mutation in the gene encoding the c-Kit ligand (Kit^{Sl}/Kit^{Sl-d} mice) or a mutation in c-Kit ($Kit^{W}Kit^{W-v}$ mice)—were shown to be resistant to arthritis induced by K/BxN serum transfer; moreover, engraftment of mast cells restored susceptibility to arthritis in these mice.[82] These findings cast mast cells as the cellular link between autoantibodies and arthritis.

Subsequent studies, however, showed that Kit^{W-sh} mice, which are mast cell–deficient owing to a mutation that abrogates c-Kit expression specifically in mast cells, develop full-blown CAIA.[83] Thus, c-Kit may contribute to RA through effects in a cell type other than the mast cell. To date, the most potent and specific small-molecule inhibitor of c-Kit is masitinib (AB1010), with an IC_{50} of 200 nM for inhibition of recombinant c-Kit.[84] Masitinib, however, also inhibits PDGFR and LynB at nanomolar concentrations—although, unlike imatinib, it is a weak inhibitor of c-Fms and Abl. In a small, open-label, dose-ranging, 12-week, phase II trial in RA patients, masitinib exhibited only moderate efficacy (in the absence of a placebo control).[85] Furthermore, patient-withdrawal rate was high, owing to adverse effects. Thus, whether or not inhibiting c-Kit or PDGFR would be of therapeutic value in RA is currently unclear.

Another interesting kinase is Bruton's tyrosine kinase (BTK). It is expressed primarily in B cells, mast cells, platelets, and myeloid cells.[86] Mutations in the BTK gene result in X-linked agammaglobulinemia (XLA), a disease characterized by marked reduction in numbers of mature B cells and by severe immunodeficiency. BTK transduces BCR signaling in B cells, FcεR1 signaling in mast cells, and toll-like receptor (TLR) signaling in monocytes. Monocytes from XLA patients exhibit defective TNF production in response to TLR stimulation, and BTK-deficient mast cells exhibit impairment of degranulation, histamine release, and cytokine production.[86] A relatively selective BTK inhibitor, compound 4, was shown to be efficacious in an LPS-induced mouse model of RA, but its therapeutic use may be limited because it is an irreversible inhibitor.[86,87] Cgi1746, a reversible orally bioavailable BTK inhibitor with good selectivity, showed efficacy in mouse CIA.[86] In addition, the rationally designed BTK inhibitor LFM-A13—an analog of a metabolite of leflunomide (which is used to treat RA)—has been shown to suppress FcεRI-induced release of histamine from rat mast cells.[88] Encouragingly, preclinical studies have demonstrated favorable pharmacokinetic and toxicity profiles of LFM-A13 in mice, rats, and dogs.[89]

The tyrosine kinase VEGFR has also been implicated in RA and is reviewed elsewhere.[90] Therapeutic targeting of VEGFR may be associated, however, with cardiotoxicity and hypertension,[91] which may be of particular concern in RA, a disease that is often accompanied by cardiovascular dysfunction.

INHIBITOR OF κB KINASE 2: RESURGENCE OF AN OLD FAVORITE

The NF-κB pathway is considered the master regulator of inflammation and immunity. It plays a pivotal role in inflammatory and autoimmune diseases—no less so in RA. Several drugs used in the treatment of RA, including sulfasalazine, glucocorticoids, leflunomide, and gold compounds, can inhibit NF-κB. NF-κB is intimately involved in the autoimmune, inflammatory, and destructive processes that underlie RA.[92] It promotes (1) proliferation of T cells, by inducing the expression of IL-2; (2) antibody production and class switching in B cells; (3) recruitment of inflammatory cells, by inducing the expression of adhesion molecules and chemokines; (4) production of proinflammatory cytokines by multiple cell types; and (5) synovial hyperplasia, by driving angiogenesis and FLS proliferation and survival. In addition, NF-κB directly promotes erosion of cartilage and bone by 3 different mechanisms: it induces the expression of the matrix-degrading MMPs; it mediates the survival and differentiation of bone-resorbing osteoclasts; and it inhibits the formation of bone-forming osteoblasts. Underscoring the importance of NF-κB in inflammatory arthritis, mice deficient in the p50 or c-rel NF-κB subunits are resistant to the development of CIA,[93] as are transgenic mice overexpressing a super-repressor form of the NF-κB inhibitor IκBα in the T-cell lineage.[94]

The NF-κB transcription factor is regulated by the upstream IKK complex, consisting of the kinases IKK1 and IKK2 and the regulatory component NF-κB essential modulator (NEMO). IKK2 is the kinase that plays the dominant role in activation of the canonical, proinflammatory NF-κB pathway; thus selective inhibition of IKK2 has been explored as an anti-inflammatory therapeutic approach. Many orally bioavailable, small-molecule inhibitors of IKK2 have been shown to profoundly suppress the development and the progression of inflammatory arthritis in rodent models of RA.[95-101] Confirming that targeting of IKK2 underlies these effects, intra-articular gene transfer of a dominant-negative form of IKK2 was shown to attenuate rat AIA.[102] Although the importance of NF-κB in inflammation and immunity has long been recognized, IKK/NF-κB inhibitors have yet to make it into the clinic. The reason for this is that NF-κB is also important in normal physiology; chronically shutting down NF-κB is expected to incur several serious adverse effects, including increased susceptibility to infection and tissue injury due to generalized apoptosis. Nevertheless, recent findings suggest that IKK/NF-κB inhibitors may have better prospects than once thought. For instance, although NF-κB is indispensable for liver development in the fetus, it seems that inhibition of NF-κB in the developed liver is not hepatotoxic and may even be hepatoprotective.[92] Moreover, approaches allowing partial suppression of NF-κB activity are starting to yield promising results.

One such approach is the use of a cell-permeable peptide corresponding to the NEMO-binding domain (NBD) of IKK2 to disrupt the interaction of IKK2 with NEMO, thereby blocking the formation of the IKK complex. The NBD peptide has been shown to inhibit LPS-induced osteoclastogenesis in vitro and in vivo and to suppress inflammation and bone destruction in the joints of mice with CIA—without inducing any overt toxicity.[103] This favorable therapeutic index has been ascribed to the abrogation of inflammation-induced, but not basal, NF-κB activity. Consistent with this, the NBD peptide reduced serum and joint levels of TNF, IL-1β, and MMP-9 in CIA mice to those seen in naive mice. Because peptide therapeutics are beset by several disadvantages, the full potential of this approach may not be realized until compounds that mimic the effect of the NBD peptide are developed. Another approach to the partial inhibition of NF-κB involves simply administering submaximal doses of a small-molecule inhibitor of IKK2 activity. Periodic, oral administration of the IKK2 inhibitor BMS-066 was recently shown to protect against the development of rat AIA and mouse CIA at doses that only partially and transiently inhibit NF-κB activity.[96] The observed protection was attributed to the cumulative effect of partial inhibition of multiple NF-κB–dependent pathogenic processes. Thus, the scope of NF-κB's role in immunity and inflammation, once thought to preclude the therapeutic targeting of the NF-κB pathway, may be turned to advantage. Dampening, rather than completely blocking, IKK-NF-κB signaling seems to be the way to go.

SUMMARY

The success of small-molecule kinase inhibitors in the treatment of cancer has spurred efforts to identify kinase targets for the treatment of RA. Many kinases have been convincingly implicated in the pathogenesis of RA, and many kinase inhibitors have proved efficacious in the treatment of inflammatory arthritis in animals. Few kinase inhibitors, however, have so far made it into clinical development, let alone survived the rigors of a phase II RA clinical trial. This is partly because the therapeutic index of a therapy needs to be higher for a chronic inflammatory disorder, such as RA, than for cancer. The kinase inhibitors approved for the treatment of cancer are not very selective, and inhibition of multiple kinases heightens the risk of adverse effects.

In selecting suitable therapeutic targets for chronic diseases, not only must potential off-target effects be minimized but also target-based toxicities must be rigorously scrutinized. For instance, the experience with p38α inhibitors highlights the importance of appraising the potential effects of kinase inhibition on feedback loops. Furthermore, the identification of several commonly targeted kinases as important regulators of cardiac function underscores the need for careful selection of kinase targets to preclude cardiotoxicity.[91] Finally, caution should be exerted in assigning culpability to a specific kinase on the basis of the effects of small-molecule inhibitors, most of which lack specificity.

Despite these hurdles, the treatment of RA with oral kinase inhibitors seems within reach. Attaining the fine line between therapeutic efficacy and toxicity is crucial and tricky, but it may be possible. Unlike cancer, which is frequently driven by mutations in kinases and thus requires treatment with high doses of kinase inhibitors, inflammatory diseases are driven by aberrant activation of wild-type kinases, against which low doses of inhibitor may be effective. Lower doses of kinase inhibitors should result in greater selectivity and reduced toxicity. Moreover, as recently illustrated for IKK, inhibition of an essential kinase—if not absolute—may be tolerated. Such partial sparing of target kinase activity may well underlie the tolerability of many of the kinase inhibitors tested and should perhaps be an overt goal in the development of new kinase inhibitors. Emergent kinome-profiling technologies are expected to facilitate the discovery of additional kinases involved in RA and the development of more-selective kinase inhibitors. Greater specificity may also be achieved by targeting substrate- or scaffold-protein-specific docking sites on kinases rather than the highly conserved ATP-binding sites, as illustrated by the pepJIP1 and its small-molecule mimic, T-5224. Finally, the burgeoning efforts at biomarker discovery in RA may one day mean that even those kinase inhibitors now relegated to the scrap heap can be used as effective and safe therapy in specific patient subsets.

REFERENCES

1. Rommel C, Camps M, Ji H. PI3K delta and PI3K gamma: partners in crime in inflammation in rheumatoid arthritis and beyond? Nat Rev Immunol 2007;7:191.
2. Roberts PJ, Der CJ. Targeting the Raf-MEK-ERK mitogen-activated protein kinase cascade for the treatment of cancer. Oncogene 2007;26:3291.
3. Schett G, Tohidast-Akrad M, Smolen JS, et al. Activation, differential localization, and regulation of the stress-activated protein kinases, extracellular signal-regulated kinase, c-JUN N-terminal kinase, and p38 mitogen-activated protein kinase, in synovial tissue and cells in rheumatoid arthritis. Arthritis Rheum 2000;43:2501.
4. Gaestel M, Kotlyarov A, Kracht M. Targeting innate immunity protein kinase signalling in inflammation. Nat Rev Drug Discov 2009;8:480.
5. Bohm C, Hayer S, Kilian A, et al. The alpha-isoform of p38 MAPK specifically regulates arthritic bone loss. J Immunol 2009;183:5938.
6. Schett G, Zwerina J, Firestein G. The p38 mitogen-activated protein kinase (MAPK) pathway in rheumatoid arthritis. Ann Rheum Dis 2008;67:909.
7. Genovese MC. Inhibition of p38: has the fat lady sung? Arthritis Rheum 2009; 60:317.
8. Cohen SB, Cheng TT, Chindalore V, et al. Evaluation of the efficacy and safety of pamapimod, a p38 MAP kinase inhibitor, in a double-blind, methotrexate-controlled study of patients with active rheumatoid arthritis. Arthritis Rheum 2009;60:335.

9. Damjanov N, Kauffman RS, Spencer-Green GT. Efficacy, pharmacodynamics, and safety of VX-702, a novel p38 MAPK inhibitor, in rheumatoid arthritis: results of two randomized, double-blind, placebo-controlled clinical studies. Arthritis Rheum 2009;60:1232.

10. Ananieva O, Darragh J, Johansen C, et al. The kinases MSK1 and MSK2 act as negative regulators of Toll-like receptor signaling. Nat Immunol 2008;9:1028.

11. Darragh J, Ananieva O, Courtney A, et al. MSK1 regulates the transcription of IL-1ra in response to TLR activation in macrophages. Biochem J 2010;425:595.

12. Kim C, Sano Y, Todorova K, et al. The kinase p38 alpha serves cell type-specific inflammatory functions in skin injury and coordinates pro- and anti-inflammatory gene expression. Nat Immunol 2008;9:1019.

13. Heinrichsdorff J, Luedde T, Perdiguero E, et al. p38 alpha MAPK inhibits JNK activation and collaborates with IkappaB kinase 2 to prevent endotoxin-induced liver failure. EMBO Rep 2008;9:1048.

14. Hegen M, Gaestel M, Nickerson-Nutter CL, et al. MAPKAP kinase 2-deficient mice are resistant to collagen-induced arthritis. J Immunol 2006;177:1913.

15. Anderson DR, Hegde S, Reinhard E, et al. Aminocyanopyridine inhibitors of mitogen activated protein kinase-activated protein kinase 2 (MK-2). Bioorg Med Chem Lett 2005;15:1587.

16. Keminer O, Kraemer J, Kahmann J, et al. Novel MK2 inhibitors by fragment screening. Comb Chem High Throughput Screen 2009;12:697.

17. Thiel MJ, Schaefer CJ, Lesch ME, et al. Central role of the MEK/ERK MAP kinase pathway in a mouse model of rheumatoid arthritis: potential proinflammatory mechanisms. Arthritis Rheum 2007;56:3347.

18. Morel J, Audo R, Hahne M, et al. Tumor necrosis factor-related apoptosis-inducing ligand (TRAIL) induces rheumatoid arthritis synovial fibroblast proliferation through mitogen-activated protein kinases and phosphatidylinositol 3-kinase/Akt. J Biol Chem 2005;280:15709.

19. Singh K, Deshpande P, Pryshchep S, et al. ERK-dependent T cell receptor threshold calibration in rheumatoid arthritis. J Immunol 2009;183:8258.

20. Mizuno T, Rothstein TL. B cell receptor (BCR) cross-talk: CD40 engagement enhances BCR-induced ERK activation. J Immunol 2005;174:3369.

21. Sakaguchi N, Takahashi T, Hata H, et al. Altered thymic T-cell selection due to a mutation of the ZAP-70 gene causes autoimmune arthritis in mice. Nature 2003;426:454.

22. Winkler J, Wright D, Pheneger J, et al. ARRY-162, a potent and selective inhibitor of Mek 1/2: preclinical and clinical evidence of activity in arthritis. Proceeding of 9th World Congress on Inflammation. 2009.

23. Ohori M, Takeuchi M, Maruki R, et al. FR180204, a novel and selective inhibitor of extracellular signal-regulated kinase, ameliorates collagen-induced arthritis in mice. Naunyn Schmiedebergs Arch Pharmacol 2007;374:311.

24. Dumitru CD, Ceci JD, Tsatsanis C, et al. TNF-alpha induction by LPS is regulated posttranscriptionally via a Tpl2/ERK-dependent pathway. Cell 2000;103:1071.

25. Eliopoulos AG, Wang CC, Dumitru CD, et al. Tpl2 transduces CD40 and TNF signals that activate ERK and regulates IgE induction by CD40. EMBO J 2003;22:3855.

26. Sugimoto K, Ohata M, Miyoshi J, et al. A serine/threonine kinase, Cot/Tpl2, modulates bacterial DNA-induced IL-12 production and Th cell differentiation. J Clin Invest 2004;114:857.

27. Kontoyiannis D, Boulougouris G, Manoloukos M, et al. Genetic dissection of the cellular pathways and signaling mechanisms in modeled tumor necrosis factor-induced Crohn's-like inflammatory bowel disease. J Exp Med 2002;196:1563.

28. Das S, Cho J, Lambertz I, et al. Tpl2/cot signals activate ERK, JNK, and NF-kappaB in a cell-type and stimulus-specific manner. J Biol Chem 2005;280:23748.

29. Hall JP, Kurdi Y, Hsu S, et al. Pharmacologic inhibition of tpl2 blocks inflammatory responses in primary human monocytes, synoviocytes, and blood. J Biol Chem 2007;282:33295.

30. Green N, Hu Y, Janz K, et al. Inhibitors of tumor progression loci-2 (Tpl2) kinase and tumor necrosis factor alpha (TNF-alpha) production: selectivity and in vivo antiinflammatory activity of novel 8-substituted-4-anilino-6-aminoquinoline-3-carbonitriles. J Med Chem 2007;50:4728.

31. Deng C, Kaplan MJ, Yang J, et al. Decreased Ras-mitogen-activated protein kinase signaling may cause DNA hypomethylation in T lymphocytes from lupus patients. Arthritis Rheum 2001;44:397.

32. Deng C, Lu Q, Zhang Z, et al. Hydralazine may induce autoimmunity by inhibiting extracellular signal-regulated kinase pathway signaling. Arthritis Rheum 2003;48:746.

33. Sawalha AH, Richardson B. MEK/ERK pathway inhibitors as a treatment for inflammatory arthritis might result in the development of lupus. comment on the article by Thiel et al. Arthritis Rheum 2008;58:1203.

34. Kyriakis JM, Avruch J. Sounding the alarm: protein kinase cascades activated by stress and inflammation. J Biol Chem 1996;271:24313.

35. Tournier C, Hess P, Yang DD, et al. Requirement of JNK for stress-induced activation of the cytochrome c-mediated death pathway. Science 2000; 288:870.

36. Sweeney SE, Firestein GS. Mitogen activated protein kinase inhibitors: where are we now and where are we going? Ann Rheum Dis 2006;65(Suppl 3):iii83.

37. Gupta S, Barrett T, Whitmarsh AJ, et al. Selective interaction of JNK protein kinase isoforms with transcription factors. EMBO J 1996;15:2760.

38. Martin JH, Mohit AA, Miller CA. Developmental expression in the mouse nervous system of the p493F12 SAP kinase. Brain Res Mol Brain Res 1996;35:47.

39. Cha HS, Boyle DL, Inoue T, et al. A novel spleen tyrosine kinase inhibitor blocks c-Jun N-terminal kinase-mediated gene expression in synoviocytes. J Pharmacol Exp Ther 2006;317:571.

40. Han Z, Chang L, Yamanishi Y, et al. Joint damage and inflammation in c-Jun N-terminal kinase 2 knockout mice with passive murine collagen-induced arthritis. Arthritis Rheum 2002;46:818–23.

41. Dong C, Yang DD, Wysk M, et al. Defective T cell differentiation in the absence of Jnk1. Science 1998;282:2092.

42. Gaillard P, Jeanclaude-Etter I, Ardissone V, et al. Design and synthesis of the first generation of novel potent, selective, and in vivo active (benzothiazol-2-yl) acetonitrile inhibitors of the c-Jun N-terminal kinase. J Med Chem 2005;48:4596.

43. Koller M, Hayer S, Redlich K, et al. JNK1 is not essential for TNF-mediated joint disease. Arthritis Res Ther 2005;7:R166.

44. Bain J, McLauchlan H, Elliott M, et al. The specificities of protein kinase inhibitors: an update. Biochem J 2003;371:199.

45. Whitmarsh AJ, Cavanagh J, Tournier C, et al. A mammalian scaffold complex that selectively mediates MAP kinase activation. Science 1998;281:1671.

46. Heo YS, Kim SK, Seo CI, et al. Structural basis for the selective inhibition of JNK1 by the scaffolding protein JIP1 and SP600125. EMBO J 2004;23:2185.

47. Stebbins JL, De SK, Machleidt T, et al. Identification of a new JNK inhibitor targeting the JNK-JIP interaction site. Proc Natl Acad Sci U S A 2008;105: 16809.

48. Aikawa Y, Morimoto K, Yamamoto T, et al. Treatment of arthritis with a selective inhibitor of c-Fos/activator protein-1. Nat Biotechnol 2008;26:817.
49. She QB, Chen N, Bode AM, et al. Deficiency of c-Jun-NH(2)-terminal kinase-1 in mice enhances skin tumor development by 12-O-tetradecanoylphorbol-13-acetate. Cancer Res 2002;62:1343.
50. Tong C, Yin Z, Song Z, et al. c-Jun NH2-terminal kinase 1 plays a critical role in intestinal homeostasis and tumor suppression. Am J Pathol 2007;171:297.
51. Ghoreschi K, Laurence A, O'Shea JJ. Janus kinases in immune cell signaling. Immunol Rev 2009;228:273.
52. Kawamura M, McVicar DW, Johnston JA, et al. Molecular cloning of L-JAK, a Janus family protein-tyrosine kinase expressed in natural killer cells and activated leukocytes. Proc Natl Acad Sci U S A 1994;91:6374.
53. Nosaka T, van Deursen JM, Tripp RA, et al. Defective lymphoid development in mice lacking Jak3. Science 1995;270:800.
54. Thomis DC, Gurniak CB, Tivol E, et al. Defects in B lymphocyte maturation and T lymphocyte activation in mice lacking Jak3. Science 1995;270:794.
55. Milici AJ, Kudlacz EM, Audoly L, et al. Cartilage preservation by inhibition of Janus kinase 3 in two rodent models of rheumatoid arthritis. Arthritis Res Ther 2008;10:R14.
56. Karaman MW, Herrgard S, Treiber DK, et al. A quantitative analysis of kinase inhibitor selectivity. Nat Biotechnol 2008;26:127.
57. Macchi P, Villa A, Giliani S, et al. Mutations of Jak-3 gene in patients with autosomal severe combined immune deficiency (SCID). Nature 1995;377:65.
58. Russell SM, Tayebi N, Nakajima H, et al. Mutation of Jak3 in a patient with SCID: essential role of Jak3 in lymphoid development. Science 1995;270:797.
59. Kremer JM, Bloom BJ, Breedveld FC, et al. The safety and efficacy of a JAK inhibitor in patients with active rheumatoid arthritis: results of a double-blind, placebo-controlled phase IIa trial of three dosage levels of CP-690,550 versus placebo. Arthritis Rheum 2009;60:1895.
60. Waldburger JM, Firestein GS. Garden of therapeutic delights: new targets in rheumatic diseases. Arthritis Res Ther 2009;11:206.
61. Bajpai M, Chopra P, Dastidar SG, et al. Spleen tyrosine kinase: a novel target for therapeutic intervention of rheumatoid arthritis. Expert Opin Investig Drugs 2008;17:641.
62. Braselmann S, Taylor V, Zhao H, et al. R406, an orally available spleen tyrosine kinase inhibitor blocks fc receptor signaling and reduces immune complex-mediated inflammation. J Pharmacol Exp Ther 2006;319:998.
63. Pine PR, Chang B, Schoettler N, et al. Inflammation and bone erosion are suppressed in models of rheumatoid arthritis following treatment with a novel Syk inhibitor. Clin Immunol 2007;124:244.
64. Weinblatt ME, Kavanaugh A, Burgos-Vargas R, et al. Treatment of rheumatoid arthritis with a Syk kinase inhibitor: a twelve-week, randomized, placebo-controlled trial. Arthritis Rheum 2008;58:3309.
65. Hueber AJ, McInnes IB. Is spleen tyrosine kinase inhibition an effective therapy for patients with RA? Nat Clin Pract Rheumatol 2009;5:130.
66. Matsubara S, Li G, Takeda K, et al. Inhibition of spleen tyrosine kinase prevents mast cell activation and airway hyperresponsiveness. Am J Respir Crit Care Med 2006;173:56.
67. Demetri GD, von Mehren M, Blanke CD, et al. Efficacy and safety of imatinib mesylate in advanced gastrointestinal stromal tumors. N Engl J Med 2002;347:472.

68. Druker BJ, Talpaz M, Resta DJ, et al. Efficacy and safety of a specific inhibitor of the BCR-ABL tyrosine kinase in chronic myeloid leukemia. N Engl J Med 2001; 344:1031.
69. Eklund KK, Joensuu H. Treatment of rheumatoid arthritis with imatinib mesylate: clinical improvement in three refractory cases. Ann Med 2003;35:362.
70. Eklund KK, Lindstedt K, Sandler C, et al. Maintained efficacy of the tyrosine kinase inhibitor imatinib mesylate in a patient with rheumatoid arthritis. J Clin Rheumatol 2008;14:294.
71. Kerkela R, Grazette L, Yacobi R, et al. Cardiotoxicity of the cancer therapeutic agent imatinib mesylate. Nat Med 2006;12:908.
72. Paniagua RT, Sharpe O, Ho PP, et al. Selective tyrosine kinase inhibition by imatinib mesylate for the treatment of autoimmune arthritis. J Clin Invest 2006; 116:2633.
73. Dai XM, Ryan GR, Hapel AJ, et al. Targeted disruption of the mouse colony-stimulating factor 1 receptor gene results in osteopetrosis, mononuclear phagocyte deficiency, increased primitive progenitor cell frequencies, and reproductive defects. Blood 2002;99:111.
74. Paniagua RT, Chang A, Mariano M, et al. c-Fms-mediated differentiation and priming of monocyte lineage cells plays a central role in autoimmune arthritis. Arthritis Res Ther 2010;12(1):R32.
75. Yang PT, Kasai H, Xiao WG, et al. Increased expression of macrophage colony-stimulating factor in ankylosing spondylitis and rheumatoid arthritis. Ann Rheum Dis 2006;65:1671.
76. Campbell IK, Rich MJ, Bischof RJ, et al. The colony-stimulating factors and collagen-induced arthritis: exacerbation of disease by M-CSF and G-CSF and requirement for endogenous M-CSF. J Leukoc Biol 2000;68:144.
77. Kitaura H, Zhou P, Kim HJ, et al. M-CSF mediates TNF-induced inflammatory osteolysis. J Clin Invest 2005;115:3418.
78. Conway JG, Pink H, Bergquist ML, et al. Effects of the cFMS kinase inhibitor 5-(3-methoxy-4-((4-methoxybenzyl)oxy)benzyl)pyrimidine-2,4-diamine (GW2580) in normal and arthritic rats. J Pharmacol Exp Ther 2008;326:41.
79. Ohno H, Uemura Y, Murooka H, et al. The orally-active and selective c-Fms tyrosine kinase inhibitor Ki20227 inhibits disease progression in a collagen-induced arthritis mouse model. Eur J Immunol 2008;38:283.
80. Illig CR, Chen J, Wall MJ, et al. Discovery of novel FMS kinase inhibitors as anti-inflammatory agents. Bioorg Med Chem Lett 2008;18:1642.
81. Sandler C, Joutsiniemi S, Lindstedt KA, et al. Imatinib mesylate inhibits platelet derived growth factor stimulated proliferation of rheumatoid synovial fibroblasts. Biochem Biophys Res Commun 2006;347:31.
82. Lee DM, Friend DS, Gurish MF, et al. Mast cells: a cellular link between autoantibodies and inflammatory arthritis. Science 2002;297:1689.
83. Zhou JS, Xing W, Friend DS, et al. Mast cell deficiency in Kit(W-sh) mice does not impair antibody-mediated arthritis. J Exp Med 2007;204:2797.
84. Dubreuil P, Letard S, Ciufolini M, et al. Masitinib (AB1010), a potent and selective tyrosine kinase inhibitor targeting KIT. PLoS One 2009;4:e7258.
85. Tebib J, Mariette X, Bourgeois P, et al. Masitinib in the treatment of active rheumatoid arthritis: results of a multicentre, open-label, dose-ranging, phase 2a study. Arthritis Res Ther 2009;11:R95.
86. Rokosz LL, Beasley JR, Carroll CD, et al. Kinase inhibitors as drugs for chronic inflammatory and immunological diseases: progress and challenges. Expert Opin Ther Targets 2008;12:883.

87. Pan Z, Scheerens H, Li SJ, et al. Discovery of selective irreversible inhibitors for Bruton's tyrosine kinase. ChemMedChem 2007;2:58.

88. Heinonen JE, Smith CI, Nore BF. Silencing of Bruton's tyrosine kinase (Btk) using short interfering RNA duplexes (siRNA). FEBS Lett 2002;527:274.

89. Uckun FM, Tibbles H, Venkatachalam T, et al. Preclinical toxicity and pharmaco-kinetics of the Bruton's tyrosine kinase-targeting anti-leukemic drug candidate, alpha-cyano-beta-hydroxy-beta-methyl-N- (2,5-dibromophenyl) propenamide (LFM-A13). Arzneimittelforschung 2007;57:31.

90. D'Aura Swanson C, Paniagua RT, Lindstrom TM, et al. Tyrosine kinases as targets for the treatment of rheumatoid arthritis. Nat Rev Rheumatol 2009;5:317.

91. Force T, Krause DS, Van Etten RA. Molecular mechanisms of cardiotoxicity of tyrosine kinase inhibition. Nat Rev Cancer 2007;7:332.

92. Strnad J, Burke JR. IkappaB kinase inhibitors for treating autoimmune and inflam-matory disorders: potential and challenges. Trends Pharmacol Sci 2007;28:142.

93. Campbell IK, Gerondakis S, O'Donnell K, et al. Distinct roles for the NF-kappaB1 (p50) and c-Rel transcription factors in inflammatory arthritis. J Clin Invest 2000; 105:1799.

94. Seetharaman R, Mora AL, Nabozny G, et al. Essential role of T cell NF-kappa B activation in collagen-induced arthritis. J Immunol 1999;163:1577.

95. McIntyre KW, Shuster DJ, Gillooly KM, et al. A highly selective inhibitor of I kappa B kinase, BMS-345541, blocks both joint inflammation and destruction in collagen-induced arthritis in mice. Arthritis Rheum 2003;48:2652.

96. Gillooly KM, Pattoli MA, Taylor TL, et al. Periodic, partial inhibition of IkappaB Kinase beta-mediated signaling yields therapeutic benefit in preclinical models of rheumatoid arthritis. J Pharmacol Exp Ther 2009;331:349.

97. Podolin PL, Callahan JF, Bolognese BJ, et al. Attenuation of murine collagen-induced arthritis by a novel, potent, selective small molecule inhibitor of IkappaB Kinase 2, TPCA-1 (2-[(aminocarbonyl)amino]-5-(4-fluorophenyl)-3-thio-phenecarboxamide), occurs via reduction of proinflammatory cytokines and antigen-induced T cell Proliferation. J Pharmacol Exp Ther 2005;312:373.

98. Mbalaviele G, Sommers CD, Bonar SL, et al. A novel, highly selective, tight binding IkappaB kinase-2 (IKK-2) inhibitor: a tool to correlate IKK-2 activity to the fate and functions of the components of the nuclear factor-kappaB pathway in arthritis-relevant cells and animal models. J Pharmacol Exp Ther 2009;329:14.

99. Schopf L, Savinainen A, Anderson K, et al. IKKbeta inhibition protects against bone and cartilage destruction in a rat model of rheumatoid arthritis. Arthritis Rheum 2006;54:3163.

100. Okazaki Y, Sawada T, Nagatani K, et al. Effect of nuclear factor-kappaB inhibi-tion on rheumatoid fibroblast-like synoviocytes and collagen induced arthritis. J Rheumatol 2005;32:1440.

101. Hammaker D, Sweeney S, Firestein GS. Signal transduction networks in rheu-matoid arthritis. Ann Rheum Dis 2003;62(Suppl 2):ii86.

102. Tak PP, Gerlag DM, Aupperle KR, et al. Inhibitor of nuclear factor kappaB kinase beta is a key regulator of synovial inflammation. Arthritis Rheum 2001;44:1897.

103. Jimi E, Aoki K, Saito H, et al. Selective inhibition of NF-kappa B blocks osteo-clastogenesis and prevents inflammatory bone destruction in vivo. Nat Med 2004;10:617.

104. Camps M, Ruckle T, Ji H, et al. Blockade of PI3Kgamma suppresses joint inflam-mation and damage in mouse models of rheumatoid arthritis. Nat Med 2005; 11:936.

Bone Damage in Rheumatoid Arthritis: Mechanistic Insights and Approaches to Prevention

Sougata Karmakar, PhD, Jonathan Kay, MD,
Ellen M. Gravallese, MD*

KEYWORDS

- Rheumatoid arthritis • Therapy • Osteoclasts • Osteoblasts
- Wnt • cytokines

Rheumatoid arthritis (RA) is a systemic disease process that is characterized by inflammation of the synovial tissues lining the joints. Proliferation of synovial lining cells and infiltration of inflammatory cells, including monocytes and activated leukocytes, into the joint tissues results in formation of pannus tissue that covers the surfaces of articular cartilage and bone[1] and produces proinflammatory factors that lead to destruction of cartilage and bone matrix.

A common and characteristic feature of RA is focal articular bone loss, or erosion, that becomes evident early in the disease process.[2] In RA, inflamed joints are also often associated with periarticular bone loss, which precedes focal bone erosion. Erosions occur at sites where pannus invades cortical and subchondral bone and the adjacent marrow spaces. Ultimately, trabecular bone is also lost. Systemic bone loss also commonly affects the appendicular and axial skeleton in RA and, with time, results in increased fracture risk.[3,4] When RA is not detected and treated early, focal bone erosions progress rapidly and result in joint deformity and functional disability.[2,5] Thus, early treatment to prevent focal bone erosions is a critical objective in caring for patients with RA. In this review, the authors summarize the mechanisms, cell types, and proinflammatory factors implicated in the pathogenesis of focal

Division of Rheumatology, Department of Medicine, University of Massachusetts Medical School, UMass Memorial Medical Center, Lazare Research Building, Suite 223, 364 Plantation Street, Worcester, MA 01605, USA
* Corresponding author.
E-mail address: ellen.gravallese@umassmed.edu

Rheum Dis Clin N Am 36 (2010) 385–404
doi:10.1016/j.rdc.2010.03.003
0889-857X/10/$ – see front matter © 2010 Elsevier Inc. All rights reserved.

rheumatic.theclinics.com

articular bone loss and review recent advances in targeted biologic therapies to prevent progression of structural damage in RA.

ROLE OF OSTEOCLASTS IN FOCAL ARTICULAR BONE LOSS IN RA

Osteoclasts are specialized multinucleated cells that arise from cells of monocyte-macrophage lineage. After attaching to bone matrix proteins, osteoclasts secrete proteinases and create a local acidic environment that mediates bone destruction. During physiologic bone remodeling, bone loss mediated by osteoclasts is balanced by bone formation mediated by osteoblasts. Focal bone loss in RA is mediated by osteoclasts located at the pannus-bone interface and in subchondral locations.[6,7] These cells express typical markers of the osteoclast lineage, including cathepsin K and tartrate-resistant acid phosphatase (TRAP), as well as the calcitonin receptor, a marker of terminal osteoclast differentiation.[7,8]

The receptor activator of NF-κB (RANK) ligand (RANKL) pathway regulates osteoclast differentiation and function during normal physiologic bone remodeling. RANKL promotes osteoclastogenesis by binding to its cognate receptor RANK on osteoclast precursor cells. Osteoprotegerin (OPG) is a soluble decoy receptor for RANKL that blocks the pro-osteoclastogenic activity of RANKL. In inflammatory arthritis, the RANK/RANKL pathway is activated, resulting in dysregulated bone remodeling. RA synovial tissues exhibit an increased ratio of RANKL/OPG mRNA expression, indicating that pro-osteo-clastogenic conditions dominate within the microenvironment of the RA joint.[9]

Support for the critical role of osteoclasts in the process of bone erosion in RA is provided by studies using mice deficient in RANKL, an essential factor for osteoclast differentiation. These mice are devoid of osteoclasts and thus have an osteopetrotic bone phenotype.[10] Induction of serum transfer arthritis in RANKL-deficient mice resulted in full-blown arthritis, but these osteoclast-deficient mice were protected from focal articular bone loss.[11] This finding was confirmed in transgenic mice express-ing human tumor necrosis factor (hTNF.tg) that develop a spontaneous, severe, and destructive polyarthritis resulting in extensive focal articular bone erosion.[12] When crossed with osteopetrotic c-fos–deficient mice that have no osteoclasts, the resulting mutant mice developed TNF-dependent arthritis without focal articular bone loss, despite developing inflammation comparable with that of littermate controls express-ing c-fos.[13] In a T-cell–dependent model of rat adjuvant arthritis characterized by severe joint inflammation accompanied by bone and cartilage destruction, administra-tion of OPG prevented bone and cartilage destruction but not inflammation, indicating the ability of OPG to block RANK signaling and focal bone erosion.[14,15] Further support for a critical role of osteoclasts in mediating focal bone erosion in RA has arisen from murine studies that used bisphosphonates to block osteoclast-mediated bone resorption. hTNF.Tg mice treated with pamidronate or zolendronic acid showed inhibi-tion of focal articular bone loss without any significant change in inflammation.[16] This was also shown with zolendronic acid treatment of mice with collagen-induced arthritis,[17] a model of RA that is driven by T cells and antibodies.

In addition to RANKL, macrophage colony-stimulating factor (M-CSF) is required for osteoclastogenesis and amplifies the pool of osteoclast cellular precursors.[18] RANKL and M-CSF are synthesized mainly by cells of the osteoblast lineage in the setting of physiologic bone remodeling.[19] In human disease and animal models of RA, activated CD4+ T cells and synovial fibroblasts are alternative sources of RANKL that can drive osteoclastogenesis.[8,14]

OPG, the decoy receptor for RANKL that is synthesized by osteoblast-lineage cells, acts as a key negative regulator of osteoclastogenesis by binding soluble RANKL and preventing its binding to its receptor RANK, thereby inhibiting osteoclast differentia-tion.[10,20] In RA, the balance between RANKL and OPG expression levels is a funda-mental regulator of osteoclast differentiation and function.[21,22] Thus, targeting the RANKL/RANK/OPG pathway to inhibit osteoclast differentiation represents an impor-tant potential therapeutic strategy to prevent bone erosion in inflammatory arthritis. However, even with aggressive treatment of RA to stop the progression of articular bone destruction, erosive lesions are not typically repaired; only a limited amount of new bone forms at sites of erosion. This suggests that osteoblast-mediated bone formation may also be compromised at sites where inflammation and erosion occur, thereby contributing to the net loss of bone.

ROLE OF OSTEOBLASTS IN FOCAL ARTICULAR BONE LOSS IN RA

The role of osteoblasts in focal articular bone loss in RA has received less attention than that of osteoclasts. Osteoblasts are important regulators of bone remodeling. These cells produce and mineralize bone matrix and modulate osteoclast differentia-tion and function by producing RANKL and OPG.[23] Osteoblasts arise from mesen-chymal stem cells and undergo maturation and differentiation toward cells with the capacity to produce and mineralize bone matrix.[24] As osteoblasts mature toward functional bone-forming cells, they diminish their expression of RANKL and increase their expression of OPG, thereby creating a microenvironment that favors bone forma-tion over bone loss.[25]

Although patients with RA receiving disease-modifying antirheumatic drug (DMARD) therapy demonstrate slowing or inhibition of progression of articular bone erosions on plain radiographs in clinical trials and long-term observational studies,[26] healing of erosions has been considered to occur only infrequently. However, in recent years, repair of bone erosions with formation of new bone has been documented in patients with RA treated with DMARDs.[27–30] Based on results of 2 studies conducted by the OMERACT Subcommittee on Healing of Erosions, Sharp and colleagues[31] confirmed that repair of erosions does occur in RA. Additional studies reported a strong association between clinical remission of disease and radiographic evidence of repair of erosions,[32,33] suggesting that joint inflammation may play an important role in suppress-ing the functional capacity of osteoblasts to produce bone and thereby repair erosions.

These observations are supported by a recent study from our laboratory in a murine model of arthritis that showed that mineralized bone formation was compromised at sites of erosion in areas of bone where there was local inflammation.[34] It would be expected that bone formation rates would be increased at sites of erosion where bone has been lost. However, using dynamic bone histomorphometry, no differences were observed in the rate of mineralized bone formation at bone surfaces in inflamed areas, compared with similar areas without arthritis. In addition, there was a notable paucity of osteoblast-lineage cells expressing markers of cell maturity at bone surfaces adjacent to inflammation, but there were abundant immature osteoblast-lineage cells expressing Runx2, a marker of early osteoblast-lineage cells. Further-more, cellular expression of alkaline phosphatase, a marker of the mineralization phase of bone formation, was minimal at sites of bone erosion. These observations support the hypothesis that inflammation may inhibit the functional capacity of osteoblasts to repair erosions in RA.

WNT SIGNALING PATHWAY IN RA

To elucidate the effect of inflammation on osteoblasts and bone formation, investiga-tors have focused on the Wingless (Wnt) family of proteins. The Wnt signaling pathway plays an important regulatory role in embryonic development, tissue homeostasis and cancer.[35] Wnt proteins are secreted glycoproteins that bind and activate the receptor complex of a 7-transmembrane domain-spanning frizzled receptor and the low-density lipoprotein receptor-related protein 5 and 6 (LRP5/6) coreceptors present on mesenchymal cells. Binding of Wnt proteins to the receptor complex induces the differentiation of osteoblast-lineage cells into mature osteoblasts, leading to bone formation.[36] The importance of the Wnt signaling pathway in bone homeostasis is shown by the abnormal bone phenotypes that result from receptor mutations. Mutations inducing loss of function in the Lrp5 gene, which encodes the LRP5 receptor, decrease bone formation in humans and mice.[37] In contrast, gain-of-function mutations in the Lrp5 gene result in increased bone mass.[38]

β-Catenin plays a critical role in bone remodeling. Modulation of Wnt signaling alters β-catenin expression and activity, thereby affecting bone formation and osteoclast-mediated bone resorption. Mice that do not express β-catenin in differentiated osteoblasts develop severe osteopenia associated with increased numbers of activated osteoclasts resulting from an increased RANKL/OPG ratio.[39,40] In contrast, mice expressing constitutively active β-catenin–mediated Wnt signaling in differentiated osteoblasts have increased OPG expression and exhibit a decrease in bone resorption and an osteopetrotic phenotype.[39,40] The functional dysregulation of osteoblasts seen in mice deficient in β-catenin signaling resembles the osteoblast phenotype found at sites of focal bone loss in inflammatory arthritis, suggesting that inhibition of Wnt signaling may be a mechanism whereby bone formation is compromised in inflammatory states.

Several families of endogenous inhibitors of the Wnt signaling pathway have been identified; these function by limiting the effects of Wnt signaling. The Dickkopf (DKK) and secreted frizzled-related protein (sFRP) family members are the best characterized. Diarra and colleagues[41] showed that DKK1, a member of the DKK family of Wnt antagonists, plays a central role in regulating bone remodeling in RA. Administration of a neutralizing antibody specific to DKK1 protected against focal bone erosion in the hTNF.Tg RA mouse model. In the setting of DKK1 blockade, new bone formation was observed at sites where erosion would typically occur. However, these effects were due, at least in part, to up-regulation of OPG expression, which would result in inhibition of bone resorption; the effect of inhibition of Wnt signaling on osteoblast function at sites of erosion was not directly assessed in this study.

The possible role of DKK1 in promoting bone loss is supported by the finding of increased serum levels of DKK1 in patients with RA[41] and in postmenopausal women with established osteoporosis,[42] and evidence for a role for DKK1 in ankylosing spondylitis.[43] Recently, Uderhardt and colleagues[44] showed that blocking TNFα in hTNF.Tg mice did not promote ankylosis of sacroiliac joints. In contrast, blocking DKK1 promoted cartilage formation and ankylosis of sacroiliac joints but had no effect on inflammation, indicating a potential role of DKK1 in the anabolic pattern of axial skeletal remodeling that is observed in ankylosing spondylitis. These results indicate that DKK1 may be one of many factors regulating bone remodeling in the rheumatic diseases. In a recent study from our laboratory, the authors found that several members of the DKK and sFRP families of Wnt signaling inhibitors were expressed at sites of inflammation-induced bone erosion in arthritic mice,[34] indicating their putative roles in regulating bone erosion at arthritic sites.

PROINFLAMMATORY CYTOKINES IN RA, AND THEIR EFFECTS ON BONE

Synovial tissue in inflamed joints, infiltrated with activated macrophages and leukocytes, is a rich source of proinflammatory cytokines, including TNFα, interleukin

(IL)-1, IL-6 and IL-17, and of growth factors, such as M-CSF, that affect bone remodeling within the RA bone microenvironment.[23] The proinflammatory cytokines expressed in the microenvironment of the arthritic joint exert their influence on osteoclast differentiation and activation and on osteoblasts, thereby contributing to progressive joint destruction in RA. Several key cytokines that mediate inflammation in RA and likely play a role in bone remodeling are discussed in the following section.

Tumor Necrosis Factor-alpha

Within the inflamed bone microenvironment in RA, TNFα is a dominant proinflammatory cytokine with pleiotropic effects. Among its diverse pathologic effects, TNFα induces the production of other proinflammatory cytokines (IL-1, IL-6, IL-8),[45] stimulates synovial fibroblast cells to express adhesion molecules that attract leukocytes into affected joints,[46] increases the rate of synthesis of metalloproteinases by synovial macrophages and fibroblasts,[47] and inhibits the synthesis of proteoglycans in cartilage.[48] TNFα is synthesized mainly by macrophages and synovial lining cells, as well as by activated T cells, within the microenvironment of the RA joint.[49,50] TNFα also exerts important effects on bone remodeling; it regulates the abundance of osteoclast precursors in the bone marrow directly by up-regulating c-Fms expression[51] and activates osteoclasts by enhancing RANKL signaling mechanisms.[52]

TNFα also indirectly influences osteoclastogenesis by inducing expression of RANKL and M-CSF by bone marrow stromal cells of the osteoblast lineage.[53] TNFα is considered to be an upstream, dominant proinflammatory cytokine, based on the observation that anti-TNFα antibodies significantly reduce IL-1 production in cultures of synovial cells from patients with RA.[54] TNFα also affects osteoblasts by inhibiting osteoblast differentiation[55] and maturation,[56,57] with an associated decrease in alkaline phosphatase and osteocalcin expression. Addition of TNFα to fetal calvarial precursor cells or MC3T3-E1 pre-osteoblastic cell cultures led to a dose-dependent suppression of mRNA for the critical osteoblast transcription factor, Runx2.[58] TNFα also induced apoptosis of MC3T3-E1 cells when added to cell cultures.[59]

The role of TNFα in inflammatory arthritis and bone erosion has been studied in detail, using the hTNF.tg mouse model. hTNF.tg mice and wild-type mice treated with exogenous TNFα have increased numbers of CD11b$^+$ osteoclast precursor cells,[60,61] an effect of TNFα that is independent of RANKL. Differentiation of CD11b$^+$ osteoclast precursors into activated osteoclasts requires the presence of functional RANKL/RANK signaling.[60] Blocking either TNFα (using anti-TNFα antibodies) or RANKL (using OPG.Fc) signaling in the hTNF.tg murine model results in reduced osteoclastogenesis and reduced bone erosion.[62] However, blocking both cytokines together (using anti-TNFα antibodies and OPG.Fc) did not result in a synergistic reduction of osteoclastogenesis.[63] In human disease, data from clinical trials confirm that inhibiting TNFα activity in RA effectively protects against bone erosion.[64] Although this is due in large part to the antiinflammatory effects of TNF inhibition, direct reduction of osteoclast-mediated bone loss and augmentation of osteoblast-mediated bone formation are potential mechanisms by which TNF inhibition reduces structural damage in RA.

Interleukin-1

The proinflammatory cytokine IL-1 belongs to a family of cytokines that includes IL-1α, IL-1β, the soluble antagonist IL-1Ra, and IL-18. Activated macrophages and synovial fibroblasts present within the inflamed joint are the main sources of IL-1 in RA.[49] IL-1 signals through its cognate receptor, IL-1R1. IL-1Ra competes with IL-1 for binding to the IL-1R1 receptor. More than 95% occupancy of the IL-1R1 receptor by IL-1Ra is required to effectively block IL-1 signaling; however, this may be difficult to achieve in patients with RA.[65]

Data from various animal models suggest an important role for IL-1 in the pathogenesis of inflammatory arthritis. Overexpression of IL-1α or IL-1β or deficiency of the soluble IL-1 receptor antagonist (IL-1Ra) in murine RA models resulted in the development of arthritis with associated bone and cartilage destruction.[66–68] Blocking IL-1 in the hTNF.tg mouse model of RA using recombinant IL-1Ra was not as effective in reducing numbers of osteoclasts or bone erosions as was blocking TNFα, although IL-1Ra effectively reduced inflammation.[63] Blocking IL-1 and TNFα resulted in almost complete suppression of osteoclast differentiation, inflammation, and bone destruction, indicating that the biologic effects of these two proinflammatory cytokines are additive in vivo.[63] In vitro studies have shown that addition of IL-1Ra inhibited TNFα-mediated induction of RANKL expression in bone marrow stromal cells.[53] Furthermore, the addition of TNFα to these stromal cells induced the expression of IL-1, whereas the addition of IL-1 and TNFα resulted in up-regulation of IL-1R1 expression on these cells, indicating a positive feedback loop. Similarly, treating osteoclast precursor cells with TNFα induced the expression of IL-1 and IL-1R1 in these cells and, in turn, IL-1 augmented RANKL-mediated osteoclast differentiation. Also, treating mice deficient in IL-1R1 expression with TNFα resulted in almost 50% reduction in osteoclastogenesis, indicating the existence of IL-1-independent signaling pathways.[53] These studies provide evidence that IL-1 may be downstream of TNFα in RA.

Addition of IL-1 decreased the apoptotic rate of osteoclast-like cells in vitro.[69] In addition, IL-1 has been shown to affect osteoblasts/osteoblast lineage cells in vitro. Addition of IL-1α to rat osteoblast cultures decreased formation of mineralized nodules.[70] Fetal rat calvarial cell cultures treated with IL-1β resulted in potent inhibition of mineralized nodule formation.[71] These in vitro effects may also be relevant in inflammatory arthritis, although this has not been shown directly.

Interleukin-6

IL-6 belongs to the family of cytokines that signal via a gp130-dependent mechanism that also includes IL-11, leukemia inhibitory factor (LIF), and oncostatin M (OSM). These cytokines share common receptor subunits and signaling pathways. IL-6 is a pleiotropic proinflammatory cytokine produced by a variety of cell types in the inflamed RA bone microenvironment including macrophages, fibroblast-like synoviocytes, and chondrocytes.[72] Synovial fluid levels of IL-6 are increased in patients with RA and circulating levels of IL-6 correlate with progressive joint damage in RA,[73,74] indicating an important role for IL-6 in the pathogenesis of RA. Furthermore, in patients with RA, levels of IL-6 and its soluble receptor (sIL-6R) have been correlated with the degree of bone loss evident on plain radiographs.[75]

IL-6 modulates osteoclast differentiation by modulating its interaction with the sIL-6R complex that is present on osteoblast lineage cells, resulting in up-regulation of cyclooxygenase (COX)-2-dependent prostaglandin E_2 (PGE$_2$) synthesis. This, in turn, up-regulates RANKL expression while down-regulating OPG expression, leading to enhanced osteoclastogenesis.[76] In a recent study, in vitro blocking of IL-6R reduced osteoclast formation in mouse monocyte cells stimulated with either RANKL or RANKL plus TNF.[77] Addition of IL-6 also stimulated osteoclast-like multinucleated cell formation in long-term human bone marrow cultures by inducing synthesis of IL-1β.[78] Furthermore, administration of blocking antibodies directed against IL-6R in hTNF.tg mice significantly reduced osteoclast formation and bone erosion, although not reducing joint inflammation, indicating that IL-6 exerts a specific and direct inhibitory effect on osteoclastogenesis in vitro and in vivo.[77] That IL-6 is an important effector of inflammation in arthritis is supported by the observation that mice deficient in IL-6 were protected against inflammation and bone destruction in an antigen-induced arthritis model.[79,80] Blocking the IL-6 receptor in a murine collagen-induced arthritis (CIA) model delayed the onset of inflammation and reduced joint destruction. In addition, administration of IL-6R neutralizing antibody at the time of CIA induction completely abolished the inflammatory response,[81] indicating that IL-6 plays an important role in the initiation of arthritis. Accordingly, blockade of the interaction between IL-6 and its cognate receptor has been developed as a treatment of RA.

Interleukin-17

The IL-17 cytokine family, which has at least 6 members, plays an important role in the pathogenesis of RA.[82] IL-17 is synthesized by Th17 cells, a novel population of T helper cells that is distinct from the previously described Th1 and Th2 cell populations and that has a unique pattern of cytokine expression.[83] High levels of IL-17 have been detected in synovial fluid specimens obtained from patients with RA.[84] In RA synovium, IL-17 is expressed in areas that are rich in T cells.[85] The addition of IL-17 to osteoblast-lineage cells induces the expression of RANKL and down-regulates OPG expression.[84] Furthermore, in cultured RA synoviocytes, the addition of exogenous IL-17 synergized with IL-1 and TNFα to induce the expression of IL-1, IL-6, and TNFα in vitro.[86] IL-17 promoted bone erosion in a murine CIA model by up-regulating the expression of RANKL and RANK, thereby enhancing osteoclastogenesis.[87] In mice, blocking IL-17 after the onset of CIA reduced joint inflammation and bone erosion,[88] whereas blocking IL-17 during reactivation of antigen-induced arthritis reduced joint inflammation and bone erosion by suppressing RANKL, IL-1, and TNFα production.[89] The development of spontaneous arthritis was completely suppressed in the progeny of IL-1Ra-deficient mice crossed with IL-17 deficient mice, indicating that IL-17 and IL-1 are necessary for this spontaneous development of arthritis.[90] IL-17 has also been shown to affect osteoblast lineage cells. Addition of IL-17 enhanced TNFα-stimulated IL-6 synthesis in osteoblast-like cells via activation of the p38 mitogen-activated protein[91] and induced the expression of RANKL mRNA in mouse osteoblasts.[84] Because blocking IL-17 attenuates inflammation and bone erosion in murine models of inflammatory arthritis, IL-17 inhibition has emerged as an approach to treat RA. **Table 1** lists the reported effects of proinflammatory cytokines on osteoclasts and osteoblasts.

EFFECTS OF THERAPEUTIC INTERVENTIONS ON BONE REMODELING IN RA

In the past decade, the introduction of targeted biologic therapy has resulted in significantly improved clinical and structural outcomes for patients with RA. These therapeutic agents have specific mechanisms of action, including inhibiting the action of individual cytokines, blocking cell-cell interactions, and depleting certain cell types. Observations of the effect of each targeted therapy on bone loss in patients with RA has provided further information about the role of each of these pathways in the pathophysiology of bone destruction in this disease.

RANKL Blockade

The therapeutic potential of blocking of the biologic actions of RANKL was initially reported in postmenopausal women.[92] A single injection of OPG.Fc resulted in a rapid and sustained reduction in urinary cross-linked amino-terminal telopeptide of type I

Table 1
Reported effects of proinflammatory cytokines on cells within bone

Cytokine	Effects on Osteoclasts (OC)	Effects on Osteoblasts (OB)
RANKL	Required for OC activation and differentiation[10]	
TNF	Stimulates OC precursor differentiation; synergistic with RANKL in OC differentiation[52] Increases CD11b high osteoclast precursors[61] Increases osteoclast precursor numbers through up-regulation of c-Fms expression[51]	Inhibits OB differentiation[55] Inhibits Runx2, OB differentiation factor[58] Induces expression of RANKL in OB-lineage cells[53] Induces OB apoptosis[59]
IL-1 (α and β)	Increases osteoclastogenesis, along with TNF[53] Decreases apoptotic rate of OCs[69]	IL-1α: inhibits differentiation, matrix formation in vitro[70] IL-1β: inhibits bone collagen synthesis in vitro[71]
IL-6	Blocking of IL-6R reduces OC formation[77] Stimulates OC-like multinucleated cell formation in long-term human marrow culture[78]	Indirectly increases osteoclastogenesis by stimulating PGE$_2$ synthesis, increasing RANKL/OPG in OBs[76]
IL-17	Increases osteoclastogenesis; induces RANKL and RANK[84,87]	Indirectly up-regulates IL-6 via TNFα[91] Increases RANKL in OB-lineage cells in vitro[84]

collagen (NTx), an indicator of bone resorption. In a subsequent phase I study conducted on patients with multiple myeloma (MM) or breast cancer-related bone metastases, administration of a recombinant OPG.Fc construct also resulted in a rapid, sustained, dose-dependent reduction in urinary NTx.[93] These results suggested the therapeutic potential of blocking RANKL to prevent further bone loss in patients with osteoporosis and bone malignancies. However, because OPG.Fc is a complex protein that requires frequent dosing in patients, further development of OPG.Fc as a therapeutic agent was curtailed in favor of the development of antibodies that directly target RANKL. Denosumab (formerly known as AMG162), is a fully humanized IgG2 monoclonal antibody that inhibits the biologic activity of RANKL and has been studied in clinical trials in patients with RA and focal bone loss as well as in patients with osteoporosis.

In a study of 412 postmenopausal women with low bone mineral density, denosumab administration increased bone mineral density and decreased bone resorption.[94] This finding was confirmed in the recently concluded Fracture Reduction Evaluation of Denosumab in Osteoporosis Every 6 Months (FREEDOM) study, which enrolled 7868 women between the ages of 60 and 90 years. Blockade of RANKL with denosumab reduced the risk of spinal and hip fractures by 68% and 40%, respectively, in postmenopausal women with osteoporosis compared with subjects treated with placebo.[95] In a phase II clinical trial, administration of denosumab to patients with RA inhibited the development of structural damage evident on magnetic resonance imaging, produced a sustained decrease in markers of bone turnover, and resulted in increased bone mineral density.[96] Radiographic progression of structural damage for a period of 12 months was also significantly decreased among patients with RA who received denosumab, compared with those who received placebo. These studies suggest the promise of osteoclast inhibition as a therapeutic modality to protect against focal and systemic bone loss in RA, osteoporosis, and other diseases in which bone is destroyed.

TARGETING PROINFLAMMATORY CYTOKINES
Anti-TNF Biologic Agents

TNFα is a dominant proinflammatory cytokine in the pathophysiology of RA and is the target of 5 biologic agents now used to treat RA: adalimumab, certolizumab pegol, etanercept, golimumab, and infliximab. The efficacy of these TNFα antagonists has been shown primarily in 2 different populations of patients with RA: individuals with active early RA who had not yet been treated with methotrexate and those with RA of longer disease duration who were inadequately responsive to methotrexate. The administration of adalimumab,[97] etanercept,[98,99] golimumab,[100] and infliximab[101] to patients with active early RA significantly reduced clinical signs of disease activity and effected clinical remission in some patients. Among these patients, adalimumab,[97] etanercept,[102,103] and infliximab[64] each also slowed progression of structural damage, more so when administered in combination with methotrexate than when used as monotherapy.[97,103] Among patients with active RA of longer duration, adalimumab,[104] etanercept,[105] and infliximab,[106,107] each administered in combination with methotrexate, have provided long-term sustained improvement in clinical signs and symptoms of RA and slowed progression of structural damage. Both of the newer TNF antagonists, certolizumab pegol[108–110] and golimumab,[100,111] when administered either alone or in combination with methotrexate, have also significantly reduced clinical evidence of disease activity and effected clinical remission in some patients.

The goal of RA treatment is to achieve complete remission of disease activity and halt progression of structural damage. Despite tight control of clinical disease activity, treating to the target of a low disease activity state, progressive joint destruction becomes evident on radiographs of patients not receiving TNF antagonist therapy.[112,113] The addition of a TNF antagonist to the therapeutic regimen decreases the rate at which structural damage progresses among patients with active RA.[97,103,113] The combination of methotrexate and TNF antagonist therapy slows this radiographic progression more than treatment with methotrexate alone, at any level of clinical response.[97,103,114] In a study comparing methotrexate and etanercept monotherapy with the combination of etanercept plus methotrexate in patients with active RA, erosions did not progress over 2 years in 86% of patients treated with combination therapy, compared with 75% of patients receiving etanercept alone and 66% of those receiving methotrexate alone. The combination of etanercept plus methotrexate resulted in a negative mean change in the total Sharp score over 2 years, suggesting that structural damage improves when a TNF antagonist is used in combination with methotrexate therapy.[103] In another study that compared the combination of infliximab plus methotrexate to methotrexate monotherapy, structural damage progressed less among patients with RA treated with infliximab plus methotrexate than among those treated with methotrexate alone, regardless of disease activity. Among those patients treated with methotrexate alone, progression of structural damage was associated with increased levels of acute phase reactants or persistent disease activity.[64] Patients with RA may demonstrate slowing of radiographic progression with etanercept or infliximab therapy, despite experiencing a suboptimal clinical response.[106,115] Thus, the effect of TNF antagonist therapy on reducing the progression of structural damage may be dissociated from the effect of these agents on decreasing signs and symptoms of RA. This is likely because of the independent effects of TNFα on osteoclast differentiation and function.

Inhibition of IL-1

Interleukin-1 (IL-1) plays an important role in the progression of structural damage in RA by contributing to destruction of cartilage, bone, and periarticular tissues. Recombinant human IL-1Ra (anakinra) reduces the rate of radiographic progression of RA, compared with treatment with placebo.[116] However, anakinra provides only modest benefit in improving signs and symptoms of active RA as monotherapy[117] or in combination with methotrexate.[118] Treatment with anakinra in combination with etanercept was no more effective in controlling signs and symptoms of RA than treatment with etanercept alone. Because the incidence of serious infections, injection site reactions, and neutropenia was higher among patients treated with combination therapy, the use of anakinra together with other biologic therapies is not recommended.[119]

Anti-IL-6 Receptor Biologic Agent

Tocilizumab is a humanized anti-IL-6 receptor monoclonal antibody that binds to the membrane-bound and soluble forms of the IL-6 receptor and blocks binding of IL-6 to its receptor, thereby preventing signaling. The combination of tocilizumab and methotrexate[120,121] or of tocilizumab and DMARD therapy[122] was superior to methotrexate or DMARD monotherapy in controlling signs and symptoms of active RA among patients inadequately responsive to either methotrexate or DMARDs, respectively. The combination of tocilizumab and methotrexate was also more effective than methotrexate monotherapy in controlling the signs and symptoms of RA among patients who previously had been exposed to a TNF antagonist.[123] Among patients with active RA who were naive to methotrexate or had discontinued methotrexate for reasons other than lack of efficacy or toxicity[124] and among patients with active RA who were inadequately responsive to methotrexate monotherapy,[120] tocilizumab monotherapy was superior to methotrexate monotherapy in improving the signs and symptoms of disease. Based on the results of these clinical trials, tocilizumab has been approved for the treatment of patients with active RA.

In a study of Japanese patients with RA inadequately responsive to DMARDs, including low-dose weekly methotrexate, tocilizumab monotherapy improved the signs and symptoms of disease and reduced progression of bone erosion and joint cartilage space narrowing on plain radiographs significantly more than did continuation of DMARD therapy alone.[125] Similarly, in a multinational clinical trial that enrolled patients with active RA who were inadequately responsive to methotrexate monotherapy, tocilizumab in combination with methotrexate was superior to methotrexate alone in improving the signs and symptoms of RA and in slowing the progression of radiographic evidence of structural damage.[126] These findings support a significant role for IL-6 in the pathogenesis of joint destruction in RA.

Anti-IL-17 Biologic Agents

Initial results of phase II clinical trials of 2 monoclonal antibodies that neutralize IL-17 suggest that treatment with anti-IL-17 antibodies reduces the signs and symptoms of RA without notable adverse effects. In a randomized placebo-controlled study of 77 patients with RA treated with the monoclonal anti-IL-17 antibody, LY2439821, clinical improvement was evident within a week of beginning drug therapy and persisted for 8 weeks.[127] In another randomized placebo-controlled study of 52 patients with RA treated with the monoclonal anti-IL-17 antibody AIN457 for 6 weeks, the signs and symptoms of RA also improved.[128] However, both of these studies were of inadequate duration to assess progression of structural damage. Larger and longer multicenter, placebo-controlled clinical trials of these antibodies are needed to confirm these promising initial results.

TARGETING B AND T CELLS
B-cell–depleting Monoclonal Antibody

Rituximab is a chimeric monoclonal anti-CD20 monoclonal antibody that depletes B cells. Rituximab improved the signs and symptoms of RA significantly better than placebo, 24 weeks after 2 intravenous infusions of 1000 mg administered 14 days apart in combination with background methotrexate therapy, in patients who had responded inadequately to treatment with a TNF antagonist[129] and in those who had responded inadequately to methotrexate therapy.[130] Among patients inadequately responsive to TNF antagonist therapy, treatment with rituximab and methotrexate was superior to methotrexate alone in slowing the progression of bone erosion and joint cartilage space narrowing on plain radiographs.[131] This finding supports a significant role for B cells in the pathogenesis of bone and joint destruction in RA. However, the occurrence of the rare, usually fatal, central nervous system demyelinating disease, progressive multifocal leukoencephalopathy, in some patients with RA who were treated with rituximab may limit its widespread use, especially in patients with early disease who have not yet failed treatment with other medications.[132]

Inhibition of T-cell Costimulation

Abatacept is a fusion protein of recombinant, dimerized cytotoxic T-lymphocyte antigen 4 (CTLA-4), a natural inhibitor of T-cell activation, and the hinge, CH2, and CH3 domains of IgG1. By blocking the interaction of CD28 on a T cell with B7 on an antigen-presenting cell, abatacept interferes with T-cell costimulation. In patients with active RA inadequately responsive to a TNF antagonist, abatacept in combination with background DMARD therapy was more effective than background DMARD therapy alone in reducing the signs and symptoms of RA and improving physical function.[133] The combination of abatacept and methotrexate was also more effective than methotrexate monotherapy in controlling the signs and symptoms of RA and in improving physical function among patients with RA active despite methotrexate therapy.[134] In combination with background methotrexate therapy, abatacept slowed significantly the progression of bone erosion and joint cartilage space narrowing on plain radiographs.[134,135] These findings support a role for activated T cells in the pathogenesis of joint destruction in RA.

SUMMARY

The current understanding of pathogenic mechanisms of focal articular bone damage in RA and current therapeutic approaches to prevent this damage are reviewed. In RA, cells within the inflamed synovium and pannus elaborate a variety of cytokines and factors that affect osteoclast-mediated bone erosion and osteoblast-mediated bone repair. The RANKL/RANK/OPG pathway plays a critical role in regulating osteoclastogenesis in RA. Proinflammatory cytokines, including TNF-α, IL-1, IL-6, and IL-17, are expressed by various cell types in the inflamed synovium and exert effects on osteoclastogenesis as well as on osteoclast function and survival. The results of clinical trials of targeted biologic therapies for RA indicate that multiple cytokines and cell types contribute to the pathogenesis of inflammation, and suggest possible direct effects on destruction of bone. Further study of these and additional novel targeted therapies in animal models and in human subjects will clarify the molecular mechanisms of this important pathologic process.

ACKNOWLEDGMENTS

Dr Karmakar's work was funded by the Arthritis National Research Foundation and The Sontag Foundation. Dr Gravallese's work was funded by the American College of Rheumatology Research and Education Foundation Within Our Reach grant, and by AR047665 and AR055952 from the NIH.

REFERENCES

1. Gravallese EM, Monach PA. Rheumatoid synovitis and pannus. In: Hochberg M, Smolen J, Weinblatt M, et al, editors. Rheumatology. 4th edition. London: Elsevier Ltd; 2008. p. 841–65.
2. Scott DL. Radiological progression in established rheumatoid arthritis. J Rheumatol Suppl 2004;69:55–65.
3. Sambrook PN. The skeleton in rheumatoid arthritis: common mechanisms for bone erosion and osteoporosis? J Rheumatol 2000;27(11):2541–2.
4. Joffe I, Epstein S. Osteoporosis associated with rheumatoid arthritis: pathogenesis and management. Semin Arthritis Rheum 1991;20(4):256–72.
5. Wollheim FA. Established and new biochemical tools for diagnosis and monitoring of rheumatoid arthritis. Curr Opin Rheumatol 1996;8(3):221–5.
6. Bromley M, Woolley DE. Chondroclasts and osteoclasts at subchondral sites of erosion in the rheumatoid joint. Arthritis Rheum 1984;27(9):968–75.
7. Gravallese EM, Harada Y, Wang JT, et al. Identification of cell types responsible for bone resorption in rheumatoid arthritis and juvenile rheumatoid arthritis. Am J Pathol 1998;152(4):943–51.
8. Gravallese EM, Manning C, Tsay A, et al. Synovial tissue in rheumatoid arthritis is a source of osteoclast differentiation factor. Arthritis Rheum 2000; 43(2):250–8.
9. Haynes DR, Crotti TN, Loric M, et al. Osteoprotegerin and receptor activator of nuclear factor kappaB ligand (RANKL) regulate osteoclast formation by cells in the human rheumatoid arthritic joint. Rheumatology (Oxford) 2001;40(6):623–30.
10. Kong YY, Yoshida H, Sarosi I, et al. OPGL is a key regulator of osteoclastogenesis, lymphocyte development and lymph-node organogenesis. Nature 1999; 397(6717):315–23.
11. Pettit AR, Ji H, von Stechow D, et al. TRANCE/RANKL knockout mice are protected from bone erosion in a serum transfer model of arthritis. Am J Pathol 2001;159(5):1689–99.
12. Keffer J, Probert L, Cazlaris H, et al. Transgenic mice expressing human tumour necrosis factor: a predictive genetic model of arthritis. EMBO J 1991;10(13): 4025–31.
13. Redlich K, Hayer S, Ricci R, et al. Osteoclasts are essential for TNF-alpha-mediated joint destruction. J Clin Invest 2002;110(10):1419–27.
14. Kong YY, Feige U, Sarosi I, et al. Activated T cells regulate bone loss and joint destruction in adjuvant arthritis through osteoprotegerin ligand. Nature 1999; 402(6759):304–9.
15. Schett G, Redlich K, Hayer S, et al. Osteoprotegerin protects against generalized bone loss in tumor necrosis factor-transgenic mice. Arthritis Rheum 2003;48(7):2042–51.

16. Herrak P, Gortz B, Hayer S, et al. Zoledronic acid protects against local and systemic bone loss in tumor necrosis factor-mediated arthritis. Arthritis Rheum 2004;50(7):2327–37.
17. Sims NA, Green JR, Glatt M, et al. Targeting osteoclasts with zoledronic acid prevents bone destruction in collagen-induced arthritis. Arthritis Rheum 2004; 50(7):2338–46.
18. Tsurukai T, Udagawa N, Matsuzaki K, et al. Roles of macrophage-colony stimulating factor and osteoclast differentiation factor in osteoclastogenesis. J Bone Miner Metab 2000;18(4):177–84.
19. Tanaka S, Takahashi N, Udagawa N, et al. Macrophage colony-stimulating factor is indispensable for both proliferation and differentiation of osteoclast progenitors. J Clin Invest 1993;91(1):257–63.
20. Simonet WS, Lacey DL, Dunstan CR, et al. Osteoprotegerin: a novel secreted protein involved in the regulation of bone density. Cell 1997;89(2):309–19.
21. Skoumal M, Kolarz G, Haberhauer G, et al. Osteoprotegerin and the receptor activator of NF-kappa B ligand in the serum and synovial fluid. A comparison of patients with longstanding rheumatoid arthritis and osteoarthritis. Rheumatol Int 2005;26(1):63–9.
22. Geusens PP, Landewe RB, Garnero P, et al. The ratio of circulating osteoprotegerin to RANKL in early rheumatoid arthritis predicts later joint destruction. Arthritis Rheum 2006;54(6):1772–7.
23. Lorenzo J, Horowitz M, Choi Y. Osteoimmunology: interactions of the bone and immune system. Endocr Rev 2008;29(4):403–40.
24. Aubin JE. Bone stem cells. J Cell Biochem Suppl 1998;30-31:73–82.
25. Atkins GJ, Kostakis P, Pan B, et al. RANKL expression is related to the differentiation state of human osteoblasts. J Bone Miner Res 2003;18(6):1088–98.
26. Pincus T, Ferraccioli G, Sokka T, et al. Evidence from clinical trials and long-term observational studies that disease-modifying anti-rheumatic drugs slow radiographic progression in rheumatoid arthritis: updating a 1983 review. Rheumatology (Oxford) 2002;41(12):1346–56.
27. Menninger H, Meixner C, Sondgen W. Progression and repair in radiographs of hands and forefeet in early rheumatoid arthritis. J Rheumatol 1995;22(6): 1048–54.
28. Rau R, Wassenberg S, Herborn G, et al. Identification of radiologic healing phenomena in patients with rheumatoid arthritis. J Rheumatol 2001;28(12): 2608–15.
29. Sokka T, Hannonen P. Healing of erosions in rheumatoid arthritis. Ann Rheum Dis 2000;59(8):647–9.
30. Ideguchi H, Ohno S, Hattori H, et al. Bone erosions in rheumatoid arthritis can be repaired through reduction in disease activity with conventional disease-modifying antirheumatic drugs. Arthritis Res Ther 2006;8(3):R76.
31. Sharp JT, Van Der Heijde D, Boers M, et al. Repair of erosions in rheumatoid arthritis does occur. Results from 2 studies by the OMERACT Subcommittee on Healing of Erosions. J Rheumatol 2003;30(5):1102–7.
32. Voskuyl AE, Dijkmans BA. Remission and radiographic progression in rheumatoid arthritis. Clin Exp Rheumatol 2006;24(6 Suppl 43):S37–40.
33. Rau R. Is remission in rheumatoid arthritis associated with radiographic healing? Clin Exp Rheumatol 2006;24(6 Suppl 43):S41–4.
34. Walsh NC, Reinwald S, Manning CA, et al. Osteoblast function is compromised at sites of focal bone erosion in inflammatory arthritis. J Bone Miner Res 2009; 24(9):1572–85.

35. Clevers H. Wnt/beta-catenin signaling in development and disease. Cell 2006; 127(3):469–80.
36. Schett G, Zwerina J, David JP. The role of Wnt proteins in arthritis. Nat Clin Pract Rheumatol 2008;4(9):473–80.
37. Gong Y, Slee RB, Fukai N, et al. LDL receptor-related protein 5 (LRP5) affects bone accrual and eye development. Cell 2001;107(4):513–23.
38. Johnson ML. The high bone mass family–the role of Wnt/Lrp5 signaling in the regulation of bone mass. J Musculoskelet Neuronal Interact 2004;4(2):135–8.
39. Glass DA 2nd, Bialek P, Ahn JD, et al. Canonical Wnt signaling in differentiated osteoblasts controls osteoclast differentiation. Dev Cell 2005;8(5):751–64.
40. Holmen SL, Zylstra CR, Mukherjee A, et al. Essential role of beta-catenin in post-natal bone acquisition. J Biol Chem 2005;280(22):21162–8.
41. Diarra D, Stolina M, Polzer K, et al. Dickkopf-1 is a master regulator of joint remodeling. Nat Med 2007;13(2):156–63.
42. Anastasilakis AD, Polyzos SA, Avramidis A, et al. The effect of teriparatide on serum Dickkopf-1 levels in postmenopausal women with established osteoporosis. Clin Endocrinol (Oxf) 2009. [Epub ahead of print].
43. Daoussis D, Liossis SN, Solomou EE, et al. Evidence that Dkk-1 is dysfunctional in ankylosing spondylitis. Arthritis Rheum 2010;62(1):150–8.
44. Uderhardt S, Diarra D, Katzenbeisser J, et al. Blockade of Dickkopf-1 induces fusion of sacroiliac joints. Ann Rheum Dis 2010;69(3):592–7.
45. Butler DM, Maini RN, Feldmann M, et al. Modulation of proinflammatory cytokine release in rheumatoid synovial membrane cell cultures. Comparison of monoclonal anti TNF-alpha antibody with the interleukin-1 receptor antagonist. Eur Cytokine Netw 1995;6(4):225–30.
46. Chin JE, Winterrowd GE, Krzesicki RF, et al. Role of cytokines in inflammatory synovitis. The coordinate regulation of intercellular adhesion molecule 1 and HLA class I and class II antigens in rheumatoid synovial fibroblasts. Arthritis Rheum 1990;33(12):1776–86.
47. Burrage PS, Mix KS, Brinckerhoff CE. Matrix metalloproteinases: role in arthritis. Front Biosci 2006;11:529–43.
48. Hardingham TE, Bayliss MT, Rayan V, et al. Effects of growth factors and cytokines on proteoglycan turnover in articular cartilage. Br J Rheumatol 1992; 31(Suppl 1):1–6.
49. MacNaul KL, Hutchinson NI, Parsons JN, et al. Analysis of IL-1 and TNF-alpha gene expression in human rheumatoid synoviocytes and normal monocytes by in situ hybridization. J Immunol 1990;145(12):4154–66.
50. Choy EH, Panayi GS. Cytokine pathways and joint inflammation in rheumatoid arthritis. N Engl J Med 2001;344(12):907–16.
51. Yao Z, Li P, Zhang Q, et al. Tumor necrosis factor-alpha increases circulating osteoclast precursor numbers by promoting their proliferation and differentiation in the bone marrow through up-regulation of c-Fms expression. J Biol Chem 2006;281(17):11846–55.
52. Lam J, Takeshita S, Barker JE, et al. TNF-alpha induces osteoclastogenesis by direct stimulation of macrophages exposed to permissive levels of RANK ligand. J Clin Invest 2000;106(12):1481–8.
53. Wei S, Kitaura H, Zhou P, et al. IL-1 mediates TNF-induced osteoclastogenesis. J Clin Invest 2005;115(2):282–90.
54. Brennan FM, Chantry D, Jackson A, et al. Inhibitory effect of TNF alpha antibodies on synovial cell interleukin-1 production in rheumatoid arthritis. Lancet 1989;2(8657):244–7.

55. Gilbert L, He X, Farmer P, et al. Inhibition of osteoblast differentiation by tumor necrosis factor-alpha. Endocrinology 2000;141(11):3956–64.

56. Kuroki T, Shingu M, Koshihara Y, et al. Effects of cytokines on alkaline phosphatase and osteocalcin production, calcification and calcium release by human osteoblastic cells. Br J Rheumatol 1994;33(3):224–30.

57. Panagakos FS, Hinojosa LP, Kumar S. Formation and mineralization of extracellular matrix secreted by an immortal human osteoblastic cell line: modulation by tumor necrosis factor-alpha. Inflammation 1994;18(3):267–84.

58. Gilbert L, He X, Farmer P, et al. Expression of the osteoblast differentiation factor RUNX2 (Cbfa1/AML3/Pebp2alpha A) is inhibited by tumor necrosis factor-alpha. J Biol Chem 2002;277(4):2695–701.

59. Jilka RL, Weinstein RS, Bellido T, et al. Osteoblast programmed cell death (apoptosis): modulation by growth factors and cytokines. J Bone Miner Res 1998;13(5):793–802.

60. Li P, Schwarz EM, O'Keefe RJ, et al. RANK signaling is not required for TNFalpha-mediated increase in CD11(hi) osteoclast precursors but is essential for mature osteoclast formation in TNFalpha-mediated inflammatory arthritis. J Bone Miner Res 2004;19(2):207–13.

61. Li P, Schwarz EM, O'Keefe RJ, et al. Systemic tumor necrosis factor alpha mediates an increase in peripheral CD11bhigh osteoclast precursors in tumor necrosis factor alpha-transgenic mice. Arthritis Rheum 2004;50(1):265–76.

62. Redlich K, Hayer S, Maier A, et al. Tumor necrosis factor alpha-mediated joint destruction is inhibited by targeting osteoclasts with osteoprotegerin. Arthritis Rheum 2002;46(3):785–92.

63. Zwerina J, Hayer S, Tohidast-Akrad M, et al. Single and combined inhibition of tumor necrosis factor, interleukin-1, and RANKL pathways in tumor necrosis factor-induced arthritis: effects on synovial inflammation, bone erosion, and cartilage destruction. Arthritis Rheum 2004;50(1):277–90.

64. Smolen JS, Van Der Heijde DM, St Clair EW, et al. Predictors of joint damage in patients with early rheumatoid arthritis treated with high-dose methotrexate with or without concomitant infliximab: results from the ASPIRE trial. Arthritis Rheum 2006;54(3):702–10.

65. Abramson SB, Amin A. Blocking the effects of IL-1 in rheumatoid arthritis protects bone and cartilage. Rheumatology (Oxford) 2002;41(9):972–80.

66. Niki Y, Yamada H, Kikuchi T, et al. Membrane-associated IL-1 contributes to chronic synovitis and cartilage destruction in human IL-1 alpha transgenic mice. J Immunol 2004;172(1):577–84.

67. Ghivizzani SC, Kang R, Georgescu HI, et al. Constitutive intra-articular expression of human IL-1 beta following gene transfer to rabbit synovium produces all major pathologies of human rheumatoid arthritis. J Immunol 1997;159(7): 3604–12.

68. Horai R, Saijo S, Tanioka H, et al. Development of chronic inflammatory arthropathy resembling rheumatoid arthritis in interleukin 1 receptor antagonist-deficient mice. J Exp Med 2000;191(2):313–20.

69. Jimi E, Shuto T, Koga T. Macrophage colony-stimulating factor and interleukin-1 alpha maintain the survival of osteoclast-like cells. Endocrinology 1995;136(2): 808–11.

70. Tanabe N, Ito-Kato E, Suzuki N, et al. IL-1alpha affects mineralized nodule formation by rat osteoblasts. Life Sci 2004;75(19):2317–27.

71. Stashenko P, Dewhirst FE, Rooney ML, et al. Interleukin-1 beta is a potent inhibitor of bone formation in vitro. J Bone Miner Res 1987;2(6):559–65.

72. Okamoto H, Yamamura M, Morita Y, et al. The synovial expression and serum levels of interleukin-6, interleukin-11, leukemia inhibitory factor, and oncostatin M in rheumatoid arthritis. Arthritis Rheum 1997;40(6):1096–105.

73. Hirano T, Matsuda T, Turner M, et al. Excessive production of interleukin 6/B cell stimulatory factor-2 in rheumatoid arthritis. Eur J Immunol 1988;18(11): 1797–801.

74. Dasgupta B, Corkill M, Kirkham B, et al. Serial estimation of interleukin 6 as a measure of systemic disease in rheumatoid arthritis. J Rheumatol 1992; 19(1):22–5.

75. Kotake S, Sato K, Kim KJ, et al. Interleukin-6 and soluble interleukin-6 receptors in the synovial fluids from rheumatoid arthritis patients are responsible for osteoclast-like cell formation. J Bone Miner Res 1996;11(1):88–95.

76. Liu XH, Kirschenbaum A, Yao S, et al. Cross-talk between the interleukin-6 and prostaglandin E(2) signaling systems results in enhancement of osteoclastogenesis through effects on the osteoprotegerin/receptor activator of nuclear factor-{kappa}B (RANK) ligand/RANK system. Endocrinology 2005;146(4):1991–8.

77. Axmann R, Bohm C, Kronke G, et al. Inhibition of interleukin-6 receptor directly blocks osteoclast formation in vitro and in vivo. Arthritis Rheum 2009;60(9): 2747–56.

78. Kurihara N, Bertolini D, Suda T, et al. IL-6 stimulates osteoclast-like multinucleated cell formation in long term human marrow cultures by inducing IL-1 release. J Immunol 1990;144(11):4226–30.

79. Boe A, Baiocchi M, Carbonatto M, et al. Interleukin 6 knock-out mice are resistant to antigen-induced experimental arthritis. Cytokine 1999;11(12):1057–64.

80. Ohshima S, Saeki Y, Mima T, et al. Interleukin 6 plays a key role in the development of antigen-induced arthritis. Proc Natl Acad Sci U S A 1998;95(14):8222–6.

81. Takagi N, Mihara M, Moriya Y, et al. Blockage of interleukin-6 receptor ameliorates joint disease in murine collagen-induced arthritis. Arthritis Rheum 1998; 41(12):2117–21.

82. Lubberts E. IL-17/Th17 targeting: on the road to prevent chronic destructive arthritis? Cytokine 2008;41(2):84–91.

83. Harrington LE, Hatton RD, Mangan PR, et al. Interleukin 17-producing CD4+ effector T cells develop via a lineage distinct from the T helper type 1 and 2 lineages. Nat Immunol 2005;6(11):1123–32.

84. Kotake S, Udagawa N, Takahashi N, et al. IL-17 in synovial fluids from patients with rheumatoid arthritis is a potent stimulator of osteoclastogenesis. J Clin Invest 1999;103(9):1345–52.

85. Chabaud M, Durand JM, Buchs N, et al. Human interleukin-17: a T cell-derived proinflammatory cytokine produced by the rheumatoid synovium. Arthritis Rheum 1999;42(5):963–70.

86. Kehlen A, Pachnio A, Thiele K, et al. Gene expression induced by interleukin-17 in fibroblast-like synoviocytes of patients with rheumatoid arthritis: upregulation of hyaluronan-binding protein TSG-6. Arthritis Res Ther 2003;5(4):R186–92.

87. Lubberts E, van den Bersselaar L, Oppers-Walgreen B, et al. IL-17 promotes bone erosion in murine collagen-induced arthritis through loss of the receptor activator of NF-kappa B ligand/osteoprotegerin balance. J Immunol 2003; 170(5):2655–62.

88. Lubberts E, Koenders MI, Oppers-Walgreen B, et al. Treatment with a neutralizing anti-murine interleukin-17 antibody after the onset of collagen-induced arthritis reduces joint inflammation, cartilage destruction, and bone erosion. Arthritis Rheum 2004;50(2):650–9.

89. Koenders MI, Lubberts E, Oppers-Walgreen B, et al. Blocking of interleukin-17 during reactivation of experimental arthritis prevents joint inflammation and bone erosion by decreasing RANKL and interleukin-1. Am J Pathol 2005;167(1): 141–9.

90. Nakae S, Saijo S, Horai R, et al. IL-17 production from activated T cells is required for the spontaneous development of destructive arthritis in mice deficient in IL-1 receptor antagonist. Proc Natl Acad Sci U S A 2003;100(10): 5986–90.

91. Tokuda H, Kanno Y, Ishisaki A, et al. Interleukin (IL)-17 enhances tumor necrosis factor-alpha-stimulated IL-6 synthesis via p38 mitogen-activated protein kinase in osteoblasts. J Cell Biochem 2004;91(5):1053–61.

92. Bekker PJ, Holloway D, Nakanishi A, et al. The effect of a single dose of osteoprotegerin in postmenopausal women. J Bone Miner Res 2001;16(2):348–60.

93. Body JJ, Greipp P, Coleman RE, et al. A phase I study of AMGN-0007, a recombinant osteoprotegerin construct, in patients with multiple myeloma or breast carcinoma related bone metastases. Cancer 2003;97(Suppl 3):887–92.

94. McClung MR, Lewiecki EM, Cohen SB, et al. Denosumab in postmenopausal women with low bone mineral density. N Engl J Med 2006;354(8):821–31.

95. Cummings SR, San Martin J, McClung MR, et al. Denosumab for prevention of fractures in postmenopausal women with osteoporosis. N Engl J Med 2009; 361(8):756–65.

96. Cohen SB, Dore RK, Lane NE, et al. Denosumab treatment effects on structural damage, bone mineral density, and bone turnover in rheumatoid arthritis: a twelve-month, multicenter, randomized, double-blind, placebo-controlled, phase II clinical trial. Arthritis Rheum 2008;58(5):1299–309.

97. Breedveld FC, Weisman MH, Kavanaugh AF, et al. The PREMIER study: a multicenter, randomized, double-blind clinical trial of combination therapy with adalimumab plus methotrexate versus methotrexate alone or adalimumab alone in patients with early, aggressive rheumatoid arthritis who had not had previous methotrexate treatment. Arthritis Rheum 2006;54(1):26–37.

98. Bathon JM, Martin RW, Fleischmann RM, et al. A comparison of etanercept and methotrexate in patients with early rheumatoid arthritis. N Engl J Med 2000; 343(22):1586–93.

99. Klareskog L, van der Heijde D, de Jager JP, et al. Therapeutic effect of the combination of etanercept and methotrexate compared with each treatment alone in patients with rheumatoid arthritis: double-blind randomised controlled trial. Lancet 2004;363(9410):675–81.

100. Emery P, Fleischmann RM, Moreland LW, et al. Golimumab, a human anti-tumor necrosis factor alpha monoclonal antibody, injected subcutaneously every four weeks in methotrexate-naive patients with active rheumatoid arthritis: twenty-four-week results of a phase III, multicenter, randomized, double-blind, placebo-controlled study of golimumab before methotrexate as first-line therapy for early-onset rheumatoid arthritis. Arthritis Rheum 2009;60(8):2272–83.

101. St Clair EW, van der Heijde DM, Smolen JS, et al. Combination of infliximab and methotrexate therapy for early rheumatoid arthritis: a randomized, controlled trial. Arthritis Rheum 2004;50(11):3432–43.

102. Genovese MC, Bathon JM, Fleischmann RM, et al. Longterm safety, efficacy, and radiographic outcome with etanercept treatment in patients with early rheumatoid arthritis. J Rheumatol 2005;32(7):1232–42.

103. van der Heijde D, Klareskog L, Rodriguez-Valverde V, et al. Comparison of etanercept and methotrexate, alone and combined, in the treatment of rheumatoid

arthritis: two-year clinical and radiographic results from the TEMPO study, a double-blind, randomized trial. Arthritis Rheum 2006;54(4):1063–74.

104. Weinblatt ME, Keystone EC, Furst DE, et al. Adalimumab, a fully human anti-tumor necrosis factor alpha monoclonal antibody, for the treatment of rheumatoid arthritis in patients taking concomitant methotrexate: the ARMADA trial. Arthritis Rheum 2003;48(1):35–45.

105. Weinblatt ME, Kremer JM, Bankhurst AD, et al. A trial of etanercept, a recombinant tumor necrosis factor receptor:Fc fusion protein, in patients with rheumatoid arthritis receiving methotrexate. N Engl J Med 1999;340(4):253–9.

106. Smolen JS, Han C, Bala M, et al. Evidence of radiographic benefit of treatment with infliximab plus methotrexate in rheumatoid arthritis patients who had no clinical improvement: a detailed subanalysis of data from the anti-tumor necrosis factor trial in rheumatoid arthritis with concomitant therapy study. Arthritis Rheum 2005;52(4):1020–30.

107. Maini RN, Breedveld FC, Kalden JR, et al. Sustained improvement over two years in physical function, structural damage, and signs and symptoms among patients with rheumatoid arthritis treated with infliximab and methotrexate. Arthritis Rheum 2004;50(4):1051–65.

108. Fleischmann R, Vencovsky J, van Vollenhoven RF, et al. Efficacy and safety of certolizumab pegol monotherapy every 4 weeks in patients with rheumatoid arthritis failing previous disease-modifying antirheumatic therapy: the FAST4-WARD study. Ann Rheum Dis 2009;68(6):805–11.

109. Keystone E, Heijde D, Mason D Jr, et al. Certolizumab pegol plus methotrexate is significantly more effective than placebo plus methotrexate in active rheumatoid arthritis: findings of a fifty-two-week, phase III, multicenter, randomized, double-blind, placebo-controlled, parallel-group study. Arthritis Rheum 2008; 58(11):3319–29.

110. Smolen J, Landewe RB, Mease P, et al. Efficacy and safety of certolizumab pegol plus methotrexate in active rheumatoid arthritis: the RAPID 2 study. A randomised controlled trial. Ann Rheum Dis 2009;68(6):797–804.

111. Kay J, Matteson EL, Dasgupta B, et al. Golimumab in patients with active rheumatoid arthritis despite treatment with methotrexate: a randomized, double-blind, placebo-controlled, dose-ranging study. Arthritis Rheum 2008;58(4): 964–75.

112. Grigor C, Capell H, Stirling A, et al. Effect of a treatment strategy of tight control for rheumatoid arthritis (the TICORA study): a single-blind randomised controlled trial. Lancet 2004;364(9430):263–9.

113. Goekoop-Ruiterman YP, de Vries-Bouwstra JK, Allaart CF, et al. Clinical and radiographic outcomes of four different treatment strategies in patients with early rheumatoid arthritis (the BeSt study): a randomized, controlled trial. Arthritis Rheum 2008;58(Suppl 2):S126–35.

114. Lipsky PE, van der Heijde DM, St Clair EW, et al. Infliximab and methotrexate in the treatment of rheumatoid arthritis. Anti-Tumor Necrosis Factor Trial in Rheumatoid Arthritis with Concomitant Therapy Study Group. N Engl J Med 2000; 343(22):1594–602.

115. Landewe R, van der Heijde D, Klareskog L, et al. Disconnect between inflammation and joint destruction after treatment with etanercept plus methotrexate: results from the trial of etanercept and methotrexate with radiographic and patient outcomes. Arthritis Rheum 2006;54(10):3119–25.

116. Jiang Y, Genant HK, Watt I, et al. A multicenter, double-blind, dose-ranging, randomized, placebo-controlled study of recombinant human interleukin-1

receptor antagonist in patients with rheumatoid arthritis: radiologic progression and correlation of Genant and Larsen scores. Arthritis Rheum 2000;43(5): 1001–9.

117. Bresnihan B, Alvaro-Gracia JM, Cobby M, et al. Treatment of rheumatoid arthritis with recombinant human interleukin-1 receptor antagonist. Arthritis Rheum 1998;41(12):2196–204.

118. Cohen S, Hurd E, Cush J, et al. Treatment of rheumatoid arthritis with anakinra, a recombinant human interleukin-1 receptor antagonist, in combination with methotrexate: results of a twenty-four-week, multicenter, randomized, double-blind, placebo-controlled trial. Arthritis Rheum 2002;46(3):614–24.

119. Genovese MC, Cohen S, Moreland L, et al. Combination therapy with etanercept and anakinra in the treatment of patients with rheumatoid arthritis who have been treated unsuccessfully with methotrexate. Arthritis Rheum 2004;50(5):1412–9.

120. Maini RN, Taylor PC, Szechinski J, et al. Double-blind randomized controlled clinical trial of the interleukin-6 receptor antagonist, tocilizumab, in European patients with rheumatoid arthritis who had an incomplete response to metho-trexate. Arthritis Rheum 2006;54(9):2817–29.

121. Smolen JS, Beaulieu A, Rubbert-Roth A, et al. Effect of interleukin-6 receptor inhibition with tocilizumab in patients with rheumatoid arthritis (OPTION study): a double-blind, placebo-controlled, randomised trial. Lancet 2008;371(9617): 987–97.

122. Genovese MC, McKay JD, Nasonov EL, et al. Interleukin-6 receptor inhibition with tocilizumab reduces disease activity in rheumatoid arthritis with inadequate response to disease-modifying antirheumatic drugs: the tocilizumab in combi-nation with traditional disease-modifying antirheumatic drug therapy study. Arthritis Rheum 2008;58(10):2968–80.

123. Emery P, Keystone E, Tony HP, et al. IL-6 receptor inhibition with tocilizumab improves treatment outcomes in patients with rheumatoid arthritis refractory to anti-tumour necrosis factor biologicals: results from a 24-week multicentre rand-omised placebo-controlled trial. Ann Rheum Dis 2008;67(11):1516–23.

124. Jones G, Sebba A, Gu J, et al. Comparison of tocilizumab monotherapy versus methotrexate monotherapy in patients with moderate to severe rheumatoid arthritis: the AMBITION study. Ann Rheum Dis 2010;69(1):88–96.

125. Nishimoto N, Hashimoto J, Miyasaka N, et al. Study of active controlled mono-therapy used for rheumatoid arthritis, an IL-6 inhibitor (SAMURAI): evidence of clinical and radiographic benefit from an x ray reader-blinded randomised controlled trial of tocilizumab. Ann Rheum Dis 2007;66(9):1162–7.

126. Fleischmann R, Burgos-Vargas R, Ambs P, et al. Tocilizumab inhibits radio-graphic progression and improves physical function in rheumatoid arthritis (RA) patients (Pts) at 2 yrs with increasing clinical efficacy over time [abstract]. Arthritis Rheum 2009;60(Suppl 10):637.

127. Genovese MC, Van den Bosch F, Roberson SA, et al. LY2439821, a humanized anti-interleukin-17 monoclonal antibody, in the treatment of patients with rheu-matoid arthritis: a phase I randomized, double-blind, placebo-controlled, proof-of-concept study. Arthritis Rheum 2010;62(4):929–39.

128. Tak PP, Durez P, Gomez-Reino JJ, et al. AIN457 shows a good safety profile and clinical benefit in patients with active rheumatoid arthritis (RA) despite metho-trexate therapy: 16-weeks results from a randomized proof-of-concept trial [abstract]. Arthritis Rheum 2009;60(Suppl 10):1922.

129. Cohen SB, Emery P, Greenwald MW, et al. Rituximab for rheumatoid arthritis refractory to anti-tumor necrosis factor therapy: results of a multicenter,

randomized, double-blind, placebo-controlled, phase III trial evaluating primary efficacy and safety at twenty-four weeks. Arthritis Rheum 2006;54(9):2793–806.

130. Emery P, Fleischmann R, Filipowicz-Sosnowska A, et al. The efficacy and safety of rituximab in patients with active rheumatoid arthritis despite methotrexate treatment: results of a phase IIB randomized, double-blind, placebo-controlled, dose-ranging trial. Arthritis Rheum 2006;54(5):1390–400.

131. Keystone E, Emery P, Peterfy CG, et al. Rituximab inhibits structural joint damage in patients with rheumatoid arthritis with an inadequate response to tumour necrosis factor inhibitor therapies. Ann Rheum Dis 2009;68(2):216–21.

132. Fleischmann RM. Progressive multifocal leukoencephalopathy following rituximab treatment in a patient with rheumatoid arthritis. Arthritis Rheum 2009; 60(11):3225–8.

133. Genovese MC, Becker JC, Schiff M, et al. Abatacept for rheumatoid arthritis refractory to tumor necrosis factor alpha inhibition. N Engl J Med 2005; 353(11):1114–23.

134. Kremer JM, Genant HK, Moreland LW, et al. Effects of abatacept in patients with methotrexate-resistant active rheumatoid arthritis: a randomized trial. Ann Intern Med 2006;144(12):865–76.

135. Kremer JM, Genant HK, Moreland LW, et al. Results of a two-year followup study of patients with rheumatoid arthritis who received a combination of abatacept and methotrexate. Arthritis Rheum 2008;58(4):953–63.

Cardiovascular Complications of Rheumatoid Arthritis: Assessment, Prevention, and Treatment

Mariana J. Kaplan, MD

KEYWORDS
- Rheumatoid arthritis • Atherosclerosis • Heart failure
- Inflammation • Cardiovascular • Cytokines

THE IMPACT OF CARDIOVASCULAR DISEASE IN THE PROGNOSIS OF PATIENTS WITH RHEUMATOID ARTHRITIS

Rheumatoid arthritis (RA), a chronic inflammatory disease that affects approximately 1% of the general population, is associated with increased mortality and reduced life expectancy, with standardized mortality rates ranging from 1.28 to 3.0.[1–7] Despite remarkable improvements in RA treatment, there is evidence indicating that the mortality gap between patients with this disease and the general population is not closing. When patients in the Rochester RA cohort were grouped by the decade of disease incidence when they first met American College of Rheumatology criteria, no significant differences in survival were observed over four decades.[8] Because the control population showed decreases in mortality rate, these observations support the notion that the mortality gap between patients with RA and healthy controls is actually widening, particularly in patients who are seropositive for the rheumatoid factor (RF).[9]

This increase in mortality in RA is predominantly caused by accelerated coronary artery and cerebrovascular atherosclerosis, and to other cardiovascular (CV) complications, including heart failure.[10–12] Indeed, cardiovascular disease (CVD)-associated mortality risk is increased in men and women with seropositive RA.[13] A recent meta-analysis indicated that the risk for CVD-associated death could be as much as 50% higher among patients with RA compared with controls, with the risk for ischemic

Funding support: This work was supported by the National Institutes of Health through PHS grant R01 HL086553.
Division of Rheumatology, Department of Internal Medicine, University of Michigan Medical School, 1150 West Medical Center Drive, 5520 MSRBI, Box 5680, Ann Arbor, MI 48109, USA
E-mail address: makaplan@med.umich.edu

Rheum Dis Clin N Am 36 (2010) 405–426
doi:10.1016/j.rdc.2010.02.002
0889-857X/10/$ – see front matter
rheumatic.theclinics.com

heart disease and cerebrovascular diseases being elevated to a similar degree.[14] RA is an independent risk factor for multi-vessel coronary artery disease.[15] The enhanced vascular risk is not restricted to individuals with established RA, because increased mortality in patients who are positive for the RF and have early inflammatory polyarthritis has been reported.[13,16]

In men and women with RA with disease onset in the 1980s and 1990s, CVD mortality was significantly increased (standardized mortality rates of 1.36 and 1.93, respectively). However, standardized admission rates for CV complications were not raised in these patients, suggesting either that vascular disease in RA has a higher case fatality than in the general population or that it often goes unrecognized before the fatal event.[17] Patients with RA also have substantially increased 30-day mortality from all causes and from CVD following a first acute vascular event,[18] and more frequent recurrent ischemic events after acute coronary syndrome.[19] RA extra-articular manifestations, usually related to uncontrolled inflammation, are also associated with increased CV mortality,[20] suggesting that processes intrinsic to RA pathogenesis play important roles in CV damage and its clinical consequences.

CVD does not only impact mortality in RA but also leads to significant morbidity. CV events occur approximately a decade earlier in RA than in controls[21] and patients with RA are twice as likely to suffer a myocardial infarction[6,8,16] with the increased relative risk for CV events being concentrated in younger patients with RA and individuals without known prior CV events.[22] However, in a population of male United States' veterans older than 50 years, RA has also been associated with a higher risk for major adverse CV events, particularly in patients with increased disease activity independent of traditional risk factors.[23]

Patients with prolonged arthritis have more atherosclerosis than patients of the same age with more recent disease onset, suggesting that atherogenesis accelerates after the onset of RA.[24,25] The odds ratio for the likelihood of having more severe coronary artery calcification in established RA has been determined at 3.42, after adjusting for traditional CV risk factors.[26] Further, an increased prevalence of severe subclinical atherosclerotic findings in long-term treated patients who have RA without clinical evidence of atherosclerotic disease has been reported.[27] However, even patients with early RA show evidence of increased subclinical atherosclerosis,[28] as assessed by carotid plaque, carotid intima media thickness, and coronary calcification. Patients with RA also exhibit significantly increased arterial stiffness[29] and young to middle-aged patients who have RA with low disease activity and free from traditional CV risk factors and overt CVD have altered endothelial reactivity.[30]

In many ways, CVD in RA shares similarities with CVD in diabetes mellitus (DM). Preclinical atherosclerosis and the risk for CVD appears to be of equal frequency and severity in RA and DM of similar duration.[31] Compared with non-diabetic controls, patients who are non-diabetic with RA and those with type 2 DM have comparable hazard ratios for CVD: 2.16 (95% CI 1.28–3.63, $P = .004$) and 2.04 (95% CI 1.12–3.67, $P = .019$), respectively.[32] Further, similar to what occurs in DM, patients with RA are less likely to report symptoms of angina and more likely to experience unrecognized myocardial infarction and sudden cardiac death.[33] However, despite the increased risk for vascular events, strategies to prevent CVD are similar among women with and those without RA.[34]

Patients with RA are also at significantly higher risk for congestive heart failure (CHF) compared with those without the disease. CHF risk precedes the diagnosis of RA and cannot be explained by an increased incidence of traditional CV risk factors.[35] RA is associated with increased left ventricular mass, which is independently related to disease duration, whereas systolic function is typically preserved.[36] Abnormalities of transmitral and pulmonary venous flow have been proposed as markers of altered diastolic function in patients who have long-standing RA with normal systolic function.[37] The clinical presentation and the outcome of CHF differ significantly between RA and control individuals. In the former, CHF presentation may be more subtle but mortality from this complication is significantly higher.[38] Even after adjusting for CV risk factors and ischemic heart disease, patients with RA have almost twice the risk for developing CHF than patients without arthritis. Again, this increase has been seen primarily in patients who are seropositive for the RF.[35] In addition, patients with RA are at increased risk for death in the period immediately after CHF develops and this risk remains elevated for 6 months.[38]

Previous studies have suggested that traditional CV risk factors do not fully account for the increased propensity to vascular complications in RA[39] and that immune dysregulation, inflammation, and metabolic disturbances observed in RA could play an important role in accelerated atherogenesis and mortality. Indeed, histologic examination of coronary arteries in RA has revealed less atherosclerosis but greater evidence of inflammation and instability.[40]

PATHOGENIC MECHANISMS INVOLVED IN PREMATURE CARDIOVASCULAR DISEASE IN PATIENTS WITH RHEUMATOID ARTHRITIS

Over the past few years, striking similarities in the inflammatory and immunologic responses in atherosclerosis and RA have been described.[41] Although chronic inflammation can promote endothelial cell activation and vascular dysfunction, which leads to decreased blood vessel compliance and atheroma formation, the reasons for the dramatic increase in atherosclerotic disease in RA are not totally understood and appear to be fairly complex (**Fig. 1**). It appears that variables that increase CV mortality in RA are present very early during the natural history of the disease, because patients with new onset RF positive inflammatory arthritis exhibit evidence of abnormal endothelial function, which is considered a good predictor of future development of atherosclerosis.[42] RF as an independent risk factor for ischemic heart disease in the general population has been suggested by some studies. Indeed, RF has been associated

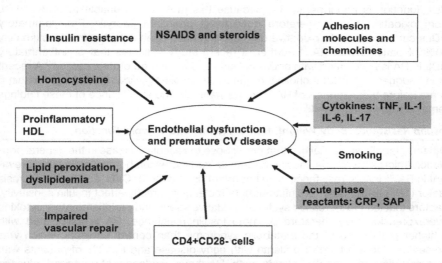

Fig. 1. Putative mechanisms leading to endothelial dysfunction and vascular damage in RA.

with increased all-cause mortality and CV mortality after adjustment for traditional risk factors, even among subjects without joint symptoms.[43,44] Further, preliminary evidence indicates that patients with RA who are positive for anti-cyclic citrullinated peptide antibodies (Abs) (anti-CCP) have higher subclinical atherosclerosis than those who are not.[45] A recent study indicated that anti-CCP Abs in RA are independently associated with the development of ischemic heart disease (odds ratio[OR] 2.8; 95% CI 1.19–6.56; $P = .009$).[46] The precise role that autoantibodies (autoAbs) play in premature CVD in RA, however, remains to be determined.

Traditional Cardiovascular Risk Factors

RA is associated with traditional and nontraditional CV risk factors.[39,47–53] Therefore, assessments based only on traditional risk factors are insufficient to capture the extent of CV risk in RA. A higher Framingham risk score is independently associated to coronary calcification in RA.[54] Age and hypertension correlate with increased CV risk RA, but so do factors associated with inflammation, including neutrophil count and radiographic score.[13] It also appears that physically inactive patients with RA have significantly worse CVD risk profile compared with those who are physically active.[55] Although smoking is associated with RF and anti-CCP Abs production and is now recognized as an independent risk factor for RA development,[56,57] it does not appear to predict CV events or cardiac-associated mortality in seropositive patients with inflammatory arthritis.[13,58] However, the prevalence and severity of coronary calcification in established RA has been linked in part to tobacco use.[26] Indeed, a personal history of ischemic heart disease, smoking, hypertension, and diabetes mellitus has been found to contribute to CV death in RA.[59]

A proatherogenic lipid profile has been reported in patients with RA.[60] Beyond the abnormalities in plasma lipids, increased levels of small, dense LDL are common in patients who are drug-naïve with early RA. The role that these particles may play in the atherogenic process in this disease is still unclear.[61] AutoAbs recognizing oxidized LDL are associated with atherosclerosis in the general population. These antibodies are present in RA and correlate with inflammation but their role in CVD in RA remains to be determined.[62] Serum lipoprotein A is significantly increased and high-density lipoprotein cholesterol (HDL) significantly decreased in women with RA. In addition, HDL function is abnormal in RA, because this molecule is unable to protect LDL from oxidation and is therefore considered proinflammatory.[63] Proinflammatory HDLs can contribute to oxidative damage and have been reported in approximately 20% of patients with RA.[64] Further, a recent study indicates that proinflammatory HDL in RA is associated with active disease and an altered protein cargo.[65] A recent study suggests that total cholesterol and LDL levels significantly decrease within 5 years before the diagnosis of RA. The mechanisms and significance of these findings remains to be determined.[66]

Insulin Resistance, Body Weight, Homocysteine, and Thyroid Function

Other metabolic abnormalities that predispose to vascular disease in the general population (microalbuminuria, insulin resistance, and increased homocysteine) are prevalent in RA.[67] Insulin resistance is an important risk factor for CVD, and tumor necrosis factor (TNF)-α and other proinflammatory molecules directly affect insulin sensitivity. Factors that lead to increased systemic oxidative stress and proinflammatory cytokine overexpression may therefore promote insulin resistance. RA is associated with a higher prevalence of the metabolic syndrome than control subjects, which was present in about a third of patients with early disease and in 42% of patients with long-standing disease.[68] Patients with RA have evidence of impaired glucose handling, which is secondary to peripheral insulin resistance mediated by the inflammatory response. Further, patients who have RA with carotid plaque have higher insulin resistance.[69] The precise role that corticosteroids play in insulin resistance development in RA remains to be determined.[70] Insulin resistance has been shown to improve with the use of disease-modifying antirheumatic drugs (DMARDs) and biologics in RA.[71,72] Increased trunk fat has been significantly and independently associated with increased arterial stiffness in patients who are postmenopausal with RA.[73]

High homocysteine levels have been linked to atherothrombosis in RA.[67] A potential role of thyroid function in the development of subclinical atherosclerosis in this disease has also been proposed, because hypothyroidism in RA is an independent association with carotid plaque and this is enhanced in patients who also have other traditional CV risk factors or neutrophilia.[74]

Family History

A parental history of death from CVD is associated with a 70% increase in risk for fatal CVD in RA and an increase in 10-year mortality from CVD from 5% to 10% in men and from 2% to 4% in women aged 50 to 67 years.[75]

Genetic Influences

Functional polymorphisms that relate to major histocompatibility complex (MHC) expression are associated with increased susceptibility to RA, myocardial infarction, and multiple sclerosis.[76] A $-168A \rightarrow G$ polymorphism in the type III promoter of the MHC class II transactivator (MHC2TA) has been associated with increased susceptibility to these three diseases and with lower expression of MHC2TA after leukocyte stimulation with interferon-γ. These polymorphisms may result in differential MHC molecule expression and could potentially be associated with susceptibility to common complex diseases with inflammatory components.[76] Shared epitope alleles (HLA-DRB1 genotype), particularly compound heterozygotes, are associated with death from all causes and from CVD, independently of autoAb status in RA. However, the combination of shared epitope, smoking, and anti-CCP antibodies is associated with a higher risk for premature death in patients with inflammatory polyarthritis and RA.[77] Other studies have also linked the shared epitope to ischemic heart disease in RA.[78,79] The exact mechanisms by which the presence of the shared epitope may enhance premature vascular damage in RA remain to be determined.

A recent study suggests that the IL-6-174C-allele may associate with CVD in RA and possibly exerts its effect via increased inflammation.[80] Patients with RA who carry the TNF-α-1031 T/C polymorphism have smaller LDL particles that have greater affinity for extracellular matrix and higher susceptibility for oxidation.[81] Other genetic polymorphisms that have been proposed to be associated to the development of CVD in RA include plasminogen activator inhibitor I (PAI-1) and coagulation factor XIII.[82] Polymorphisms in TNF receptor type II are associated with hypertension in Scandinavian subjects with RA.[83] In another recent Scandinavian study, no increased occurrence of CVD before the onset of RA was detected. The authors then concluded that shared risk factors or susceptibilities for RA and CVD likely contributed less than RA-related factors to the increased occurrence of vascular complications in this disease.[84]

The Role of Inflammation in Cardiovascular Disease in Rheumatoid Arthritis

Recent evidence indicates that there is a close temporal correlation between inflammation and morphologic features of rapidly progressive carotid atherosclerosis, which suggests that elevations in inflammatory biomarkers might help in predicting the presence of atherosclerosis.[85] Markers of systemic inflammation confer a statistically significant additional risk for CV death among patients with RA, even after controlling for traditional CV risk factors and comorbidities.[59,86] Increased levels of proinflammatory mediators, including TNF; interleukin-6 (IL-6); interleukin-17 (IL-17); and others, could be detrimental to the endothelium and myocardium and promote insulin resistance. Levels of these cytokines are increased in RA.[87-89] The C-reactive protein (CRP) concentration at baseline is an important predictor of subsequent death from CVD in patients with new onset inflammatory polyarthritis, and is independent of other factors of disease severity.[90] High levels of CRP also correlate with carotid intima media thickness.[91] High sensitivity CRP and lower glomerular filtration rate have been independently predictive of endothelial dysfunction in RA.[92] Higher erythrocyte sedimentation rate, small and large joint swelling, rheumatoid nodules, vasculitis and rheumatoid lung have been independently associated with increased risk for CV death.[59] In a recent study comparing subjects with RA and controls, TNF-α and IL-6 were significantly associated with the severity of coronary artery calcification in RA, independent of Framingham risk score.[93] Enhanced arterial stiffness in RA correlates with CRP and IL-6 levels.[29] Similarly, in those subjects experiencing new onset CHF, the proportion of subjects with high sedimentation rate was greatest in the 6 months preceding the diagnosis of cardiac dysfunction. This finding indicates that an enhanced inflammatory process may promote the development of heart dysfunction in inflammatory arthritis[94] The magnitude and chronicity of the inflammatory response, as measured by circulating levels of inflammatory markers, correlates with carotid atherosclerosis development in RA.[91] Levels of adhesion molecules linked to vascular damage, including soluble vascular cell adhesion molecule-1 (VCAM-1); intercellular adhesion molecule-1; and endothelial–leukocyte adhesion molecule, were higher in RA. VCAM-1 levels have been associated with carotid atherosclerosis in RA.[92]

Although the exact role of IL-17 in premature vascular damage in RA remains to be determined, recent work indicates that this cytokine may play a role in atherosclerosis development in murine models of vascular disease[95,96] and elevated circulating levels of IL-17 have been reported in patients with acute coronary syndromes.[97] IL-17 is produced concomitantly with IFN-γ by coronary artery-infiltrating T cells and these cytokines act synergistically to induce proinflammatory responses in vascular smooth muscle cells.[98] IL-17 accelerates myocardial fibrosis in animal models of heart injury.[99] However, there is recent evidence that IL-17 may also play a regulatory role in atherosclerosis[100] and future studies should determine whether this cytokine plays a pivotal role in vascular damage in RA.

T Cells

An expanded population of CD4+CD28− T cells has been demonstrated in the peripheral blood of patients with RA,[101] and clonal expansion of a similar T-cell subset has been reported in the blood and atherosclerotic plaques of patients with unstable angina.[102] These cells can injure the endothelium and cause vascular damage. Patients who have RA with persistent CD4+CD28− expansion have presented with increased preclinical atherosclerotic changes, including endothelial dysfunction and carotid atherosclerosis, compared with those without expansion.[102,103] TNF-α induces downregulation of the CD28 molecule in CD4+ T cells, suggesting a pathogenic mechanism for the development of these cells.[104] Treatment with anti-TNF agents has been found to downregulate this cell subset in patients with RA and in patients with unstable angina and no RA.[104,105] The precise role that these cells play in the development of acute coronary events in RA requires further investigation.

Abnormalities in Vasculogenesis

An adequate balance between endothelium destruction and regeneration is needed to maintain vascular health. Endothelial progenitor cells (EPCs) are present in the circulation of patients with different forms of vascular damage and are released from the bone marrow during acute vascular injury.[106] EPCs appear to be crucial in normal revascularization after endothelium damage occurs. Furthermore, reduced EPC numbers and abnormal EPC function correlate with increased incidence of atherosclerosis, impaired vasculogenesis after ischemia, and future CV events.[106,107] Recent reports [108,109] suggest that EPC numbers are decreased in the systemic circulation of patients with active RA and that their functions are impaired. Potentially, this phenomenon could contribute to atherosclerosis but further studies correlating abnormal EPCs with functional markers of endothelial dysfunction in RA are needed. Endothelial dysfunction in patients who have RA with low-grade inflammation was associated with decreased EPC numbers and low-grade dysfunction of these cells.[109] A single dose of infliximab significantly increases EPC numbers and improves their functional properties in RA.[110] Others have proposed that asymmetric dimethylarginine, a major endogenous inhibitor of nitric oxide synthase associated with atherosclerosis risk in the general population,[111] may contribute to EPC depletion in RA via depressed NO-dependent mobilization or survival of these cells.[112]

EPCs can contribute to synovial neovascularization in RA.[113] Proinflammatory cytokines upregulate vascular endothelial growth factor, which increases synovial EPCs and is essential to the pro-angiogenic process. The discrepancy observed between decreased angiogenic responses in RA peripheral blood and enhanced angiogenesis at the level of the synovium has not been clarified but may be related to differences in EPC homing, perhaps driven by the proinflammatory milieu of the joint.[113]

EFFECT OF RHEUMATOID ARTHRITIS TREATMENT ON CARDIOVASCULAR DISEASE RISK

The lack of a unifying explanation for accelerated CVD in RA is reflected by the confusion that still exists regarding possible preventive measures aimed at decreasing atherogenic risk. There is still considerable uncertainty on how to manage patients with RA effectively to reduce their risk for future CV events, because some of the medications used to treat RA might have dual effects on risk for CV morbidity. This risk is exemplified by the use of corticosteroids, which on one hand may decrease CV complications in RA by decreasing inflammation but on the other hand increase it by promoting pro-atherosclerotic lipid profiles, hypertension, and insulin resistance.[114] Methotrexate can promote hyperhomocysteinemia (usually corrected by folic acid supplementation)[115] and cause endothelial damage.[116] However, long-term follow-up of patients with RA has suggested that methotrexate significantly reduces overall and CV mortality.[117] Furthermore, use of DMARDs is associated with reductions in risk for hospitalization for congestive heart failure in RA.[118] The author will now discuss the role that various medications may play in CV risk or prevention in RA.

Nonsteroidal Antiinflammatory Drugs and Cardiovascular Complications in Rheumatoid Arthritis

Current and new users of all classes of non-aspirin nonsteroidal antiinflammatory drugs (NSAIDS), including patients with RA, have an elevated relative risk estimate for myocardial infarction.[119] Several patient characteristics increase the risk for CV events among users of some NSAIDS, including increased age, hypertension, previous myocardial infarction and CVD, chronic renal disease, chronic obstructive pulmonary disease, and RA. This finding indicates that patients who have RA with various comorbidities and advanced age may be particularly prone to developed CV complications while on specific NSAIDS.[120] However, a large case-control analysis found that the risk for first-time myocardial infarction is increased for several weeks after the cessation of NSAID therapy, an effect that is more pronounced in patients with RA or lupus and in individuals who discontinue NSAID therapy after previous long-term use.[121] These findings suggest that NSAIDs might have a role in suppressing the risk for myocardial infarction in patients with RA and other inflammatory conditions and that, ideally, abrupt discontinuation of NSAIDS in these populations should be avoided.

Role of Corticosteroids in Cardiovascular Disease in Rheumatoid Arthritis

Corticosteroids can induce hypertension, insulin resistance, and disturbances in blood lipids; they induce obesity and may enhance hypercoagulability.[122] As mentioned earlier, whether glucocorticoids promote accelerated atherogenesis in RA is still a matter of debate. In one study, subjects exposed to glucocorticoids had higher incidence of carotid plaque and arterial incompressibility, independent of CV risk factors and RA clinical manifestations.[123] A Scandinavian study reported that treatment with low-dose prednisolone did not influence endothelial function or carotid intima media thickness in RA, although it promoted higher levels of total cholesterol.[124] An increased risk for CV events with high cumulative exposure to corticosteroids has been found in patients with RA who are seropositive for RF, but not on the patients who are seronegative.[125] However, in patients who have RA with a history of ischemic heart disease, use of corticosteroids attenuated the risk for CV death.[59]

Disease-Modifying Antirheumatic Drugs

A recent study indicated that prolonged exposure to various DMARDS, including methotrexate, leflunomide, and sulfasalazine, was associated with a reduction of CV risk in RA, and similar trends were observed with corticosteroid use.[126] Further supporting a beneficial effect of methotrexate treatment in CVD prevention, this drug reduced the incidence of vascular disease in veterans with psoriasis or RA.[127] Low to moderate cumulative doses appeared to be more beneficial than higher doses. In addition, a combination of methotrexate and folic acid led to a further reduction in the incidence of CVD, suggesting that the latter did not decrease the efficacy of methotrexate. Furthermore, methotrexate use was associated with a significantly lower risk for CV events in patients with RA compared with patients who had never used DMARDs (OR 0.16). Methotrexate use has also been associated with a decreased incidence of the metabolic syndrome, whereas corticosteroids or other DMARDS did not show a protective effect.[72] Adding additional DMARDS, such as sulfasalazine and hydroxychloroquine, appears to provide additional CV protection.[128] In a Canadian study, DMARD use was associated with a reduction in myocardial infarction risk in patients with RA, whereas corticosteroids showed an increased risk and coxibs did not change risk.[129] In a recent cross-sectional analysis, drugs used to treat RA did not have major adverse effects on CV risk factors and use of antimalarials was actually associated with beneficial lipid profiles and lower blood pressure.[130] As a potential antiatherogenic mechanism of methotrexate (MTX), Reiss and colleagues[131] have shown that through adenosine A2A receptor activation, MTX promotes reverse cholesterol transport and limits foam cell formation in macrophages.

Anti-tumor Necrosis Factor Therapy

The effects of TNF-α blockers on CVD in RA are complex because these drugs may promote CHF and decrease heart compliance while controlling inflammation and decreasing risk for plaque formation.[132] Infliximab can improve endothelial function in RA after 12 weeks of therapy,[89] and anti-TNF therapy also reduces aortic stiffness to a level comparable to that of healthy individuals by 4 and 12 weeks of treatment.[133] Prolonged effects on endothelial function (18 months of therapy) were recently reported with infliximab and adalimumab.[134] It appears that the risk to develop first CV events in RA is lower in patients treated with TNF blockers.[135] However, prospective, long-term, longitudinal studies are required to evaluate the precise role of anti-TNF therapy in atherosclerosis prevention. Anti-TNF therapy can also improve other risk factors for accelerated atherosclerosis, including promoting a decrease in insulin resistance,[71] CRP, IL-6 and $CD4^+CD28^-$ T cells, and an increase in HDL.[132,136] However, it appears that at least some of the beneficial effects of anti-TNF agents on endothelial function are not sustained, have not been reported in all studies, and are not seen in all patient populations (eg, in the case of patients with diabetes treated with etanercept).[137-139] In one study, although an initial improvement in RA endothelial function was observed with infliximab, values returned to baseline 4 weeks after the infusion in subjects followed for 1 year.[138] Another report found that, although infliximab induces a transient increase in flow-mediated dilatation (FMD), the drug also induces vasoconstriction and increases in wall shear stress.[140] There is also evidence that biologics may induce elevations in blood lipids with a deleterious shift in the atherogenic index in RA.[140] It is possible that the various TNF antagonists have different effects on endothelial and smooth muscle cells and on vascular function. Animal studies suggest a negative influence of TNF-α inhibitors on collateral artery growth, and this observation deserves further investigation into the potential role of this therapy in decreasing alternative mechanisms of cardiac perfusion in individuals with impaired coronary circulation.[141]

Previous studies in the general population have shown that short-term TNF-α antagonism with infliximab does not improve and high doses (10 mg/kg) adversely affect the clinical condition of patients with moderate-to-severe chronic heart failure.[142] Despite contraindication to the use of these agents in patients with moderate-severe heart failure, epidemiologic studies in RA have not consistently substantiated this association.[143,144] In fact, a recent German study has concluded that inhibition of TNF that effectively reduces inflammatory activity in RA is more likely to be beneficial than harmful with regards to CHF risk, especially when not combined with corticosteroids of coxibs.[145] Similarly, a recent study indicates that blocking TNF in patients who have RA without evident heart failure decreases N-terminal pro-brain natriuretic peptide pointing at no treatment-induced deterioration in cardiac function, and a potential CV risk benefit.[146] However, TNF-inhibitors may increase the risk for first hospitalization and exacerbation of CHF in elderly patients with RA.[147] A recent study indicates that, when compared with patients who have RA receiving MTX monotherapy, those receiving biologic immunosuppressive agents had no changes in the risk for experiencing a CV event, whereas use of oral glucocorticoids and other cytotoxic immunosuppressive agents (leflunomide, azathioprine) was associated with significant increases in the risk for CV events.[148]

Rituximab and Other Biologics

Preliminary data from various groups suggests that rituximab infusions exert early and sustained favorable effects on endothelial dysfunction and plasma lipids.[149,150] The role of abatacept and anakinra in CV prevention in RA remains to be determined, although there is some preliminary evidence that chronic inhibition of IL-1 actions with anakinra improves left ventricle deformation in parallel with endothelial function and nitro-oxidative stress in RA.[151]

RISK ASSESSMENT AND PREVENTION OF CARDIOVASCULAR DISEASE IN RHEUMATOID ARTHRITIS

Ideally, preventive strategies to decrease CV risk in RA should start shortly after its diagnosis. This statement is supported by observations that the factors that promote premature CV mortality in this disease are present early on, maybe even before overt clinical manifestations manifest. Clearly, a significant proportion of patients with RA have suboptimal management of CV risk factors. Depending on the risk stratification method used, it is considered that 2% to 26% of patients who have RA without overt CVD have sufficiently high risk for requiring statin therapy, yet most of them remain untreated.[152] There is also evidence that target organ damage is highly prevalent in patients with RA and associates independently with hypertension, arterial stiffness, and heart rate.[153] These observations indicate an urgent need for CV reduction strategies. However, specific guidelines that address the management of CV risk factors in RA are not available and several important questions with regards to prevention remain unanswered. It is unknown which levels of lipids or blood pressure should prompt pharmacologic intervention in RA and whether these interventions can modify CV risk. Although RA and DM have a comparable enhanced CV risk, it is unclear whether guidelines similar to the ones developed for diabetes would lead to significant CV risk reduction in RA. Similarly, it is unknown which patients with RA should be considered as candidates for subclinical and clinical coronary artery and carotid artery disease screening or for heart function screening.

The author suggests that CV assessment in RA should start by considering and detecting the presence of other major comorbidities, including hypertension, tobacco use, hyperglycemia, dyslipidemia, increased body mass index, central obesity, physical inactivity, and family history of CV disease. Proper identification of these factors is crucial as a first step toward developing a plan for CV risk reduction in RA. It is unclear whether the presence of RA should be used as an additional risk factor during stratification; however, there are strong indications from the literature that this should be the case. Given the high prevalence of silent ischemia and decreased CV symptoms in RA, future prospective studies should investigate whether effective strategies for earlier detection of clinical CV disease will reduce morbidity and mortality in these patients. For patients that are deemed to be at high risk (seropositive for RF or anti-CCP Abs, aggressive erosive disease, extra-articular RA manifestations, and high inflammatory markers) or for those with specific CV risk factors in addition to the arthritis, specialized testing, including 24-hour monitoring of ambulatory blood pressure, stress test, or echocardiography, may be warranted. However, until clear guidelines are developed for CV prevention in this and other systemic autoimmune diseases, the justification for these tests remains unclear.

Targeting Traditional Cardiovascular Risk Factors in Rheumatoid Arthritis

Optimal blood pressure should be targeted with weight maintenance, physical activity, sodium control, judicious use of corticosteroids, and when indicated antihypertensive drugs (**Table 1**). A recent study suggested that 10 mg/day of ramipril for 8 weeks in combination with standard of care markedly improved endothelial function in patients with RA[154] and ACE inhibitors may be considered a good antihypertensive strategy in this disease. Intensive strategies for smoking cessation should be initiated early and aggressively. Weight loss and increased exercise are first-line strategies for reducing insulin resistance and hyperglycemia and should be attempted in conjunction with good control of the inflammatory response. The role of thiazolidinediones in the improvement of insulin resistance and CVD in RA remains to be determined and is

Table 1
Managing cardiovascular risk factors in rheumatoid arthritis

Risk Factor	Cardiovascular Prevention Strategies
Smoking	Counseling, nicotine patches or gum, bupropion, varenicline
Hypertension	Frequent blood pressure monitoring, diet, exercise, stress management, antihypertensives, minimize NSAID and corticosteroid use
Hyperlipidemia	Diet, exercise, moderate alcohol use,[a] statins, minimize corticosteroid use, antimalarials[a]
Diabetes	Counseling, diet, exercise, oral hypoglycemic agents or insulin
Insulin resistance	Counseling, diet, control of inflammation (DMARDS/biologics), PPAR-agonists[a]
Obesity	Counseling, diet, exercise, minimize corticosteroid use
High homocysteine	Folic acid supplementation with methotrexate/sulfasalazine use
Family history of CVD	Counseling, monitoring risk factors
Inflammation	DMARDS, biologics, NSAIDS, statins,[a] PPAR-agonists[a]
Thrombotic risk	Low dose aspirin, consider anticoagulation when other risk factors for thrombosis are present

Abbreviation: PPAR, peroxisome proliferator activated receptor.
[a] Not enough evidence to suggest as standard of care.

currently being investigated in controlled clinical trials. These drugs have pleiotropic effects on the endothelium that go beyond glucose control and may prove to have a dual beneficial effect in CV prevention and control of joint inflammation. There are hypothetical concerns with regards to thiazolidinedione use, specifically CHF and increased risk for fracture in RA, that should be explored.

Statins can mediate modest but clinically apparent antiinflammatory effects in RA.[155] Atorvastatin, 20 mg/day for 12 weeks, resulted in significant improvements in arterial stiffness in subjects with RA, particularly in subjects with active disease.[156] Similarly, subjects with RA treated with 40 mg simvastatin for 4 weeks had a reduction in proatherogenic lipids and markers of oxidative stress, and improvement in FMD.[157] In another recent study, simvastatin 20 mg/day also improved FMD in RA. The drug also lowered CRP and TNF-α concentrations.[158] Ezetimibe and simvastatin treatment for 6 weeks similarly reduced disease activity and inflammatory markers in RA, and also reduced aortic pulse wave velocity and improved endothelial function.[159] Although it is still unclear which levels of lipids are ideal for CV prevention in RA, optimal LDL and HDL cholesterol levels should be sought. A recommended LDL level of less than 100 mg/dL and HDL over 40 mg/dL, similar to what is recommended for patients with other CV risk factors, is warranted until more specific information becomes available for RA. Maximal dietary therapy should be tried with the addition of drug therapy when necessary. The benefit of use of antiplatelet agents in RA is unclear. A recent study indicated that statins may be protective for RA development in individuals with dyslipidemia.[160]

Current and Future Strategies for Targeting Disease-Specific Cardiovascular Risk Factors in Rheumatoid Arthritis

As mentioned earlier, various therapies used in the management of RA may have a protective CV risk effect. In addition, patients with RA and prolonged exposure to hydroxychloroquine have a reduced risk for developing diabetes.[161] Studies have also suggested that antimalarials could have a vasculoprotective effect in inflammatory diseases, at least in part mediated by beneficial effects on lipids.[162] Further investigation is required to determine whether specific doses or duration of corticosteroid use is beneficial or harmful to the vasculature in RA. The deleterious adverse effects on the vasculature might be prominent in patients receiving over 7.5 mg per day of prednisone for at least 6 months.[163] There is some evidence that low-dose corticosteroids could have a beneficial effect on lipid profiles.[48] Overall, as mentioned earlier, exposure to DMARDS appears to be associated with decreased CV morbidity and with decreased hospitalizations for heart failure.[118,128] However, because the mortality gap between RA and the general population appears to be widening, it is unclear that the current use of DMARDS and biologics is effectively reducing CV risk. As new biologics become more widely available for use in clinical practice, assessment of their role in CV prevention or damage in RA should become possible. These strategies include anti-IL-6, anti-IL-17, other anti-B cell therapies, and so forth. Certainly, a better understanding of the mechanisms that promote RA development and severity may provide additional light into the most effective preventive strategies for vascular damage in this disease.

SUMMARY

Given the serious impact of the increased risk for atherosclerosis in RA, future work should focus on understanding the precise molecular mechanisms that lead to premature vascular damage in inflammatory arthritides and on assessing the individual effects of various treatments on CVD in these patients by performance of rigorous studies. Future studies should also focus on the development of effective screening methods for the identification of those patients who are at the highest cardiovascular risk and who would benefit from early intervention. Clearly, the development of guidelines for the management of CV risk factors in RA, similar to those that have been developed for diabetes, is greatly needed. In the meantime, a combination of strategies that include appropriate control of the inflammatory cascade, immunologic diatheses, and metabolic changes observed in RA should be sought. Finally, an increased awareness of the increased risk for silent ischemia, early myocardial infarction, heart failure, and sudden death is warranted in this patient population.

REFERENCES

1. Wong JB, Ramey DR, Singh G. Long-term morbidity, mortality, and economics of rheumatoid arthritis. Arthritis Rheum 2001;44(12):2746–9.
2. Symmons DP, Jones MA, Scott DL, et al. Long-term mortality outcome in patients with rheumatoid arthritis: early presenters continue to do well. J Rheumatol 1998;25(6):1072–7.
3. Myllykangas-Luosujarvi R, Aho K, Kautiainen H, et al. Shortening of life span and causes of excess mortality in a population-based series of subjects with rheumatoid arthritis. Clin Exp Rheumatol 1995;13(2):149–53.
4. Myllykangas-Luosujarvi R, Aho K, Kautiainen H, et al. Cardiovascular mortality in women with rheumatoid arthritis. J Rheumatol 1995;22(6):1065–7.
5. Prior P, Symmons DP, Scott DL, et al. Cause of death in rheumatoid arthritis. Br J Rheumatol 1984;23(2):92–9.
6. Jacobsson LT, Knowler WC, Pillemer S, et al. Rheumatoid arthritis and mortality. A longitudinal study in Pima Indians. Arthritis Rheum 1993;36(8):1045–53.
7. Book C, Saxne T, Jacobsson LT. Prediction of mortality in rheumatoid arthritis based on disease activity markers. J Rheumatol 2005;32(3):430–4.

8. Gabriel SE, Crowson CS, Kremers HM, et al. Survival in rheumatoid arthritis: a population-based analysis of trends over 40 years. Arthritis Rheum 2003; 48(1):54–8.
9. Gonzalez A, Maradit Kremers H, Crowson CS, et al. The widening mortality gap between rheumatoid arthritis patients and the general population. Arthritis Rheum 2007;56(11):3583–7.
10. Goodson N, Symmons D. Rheumatoid arthritis in women: still associated with an increased mortality. Ann Rheum Dis 2002;61(11):955–6.
11. Riise T, Jacobsen BK, Gran JT, et al. Total mortality is increased in rheumatoid arthritis. A 17-year prospective study. Clin Rheumatol 2001;20(2):123–7.
12. Nicola PJ, Crowson CS, Maradit-Kremers H, et al. Contribution of congestive heart failure and ischemic heart disease to excess mortality in rheumatoid arthritis. Arthritis Rheum 2006;54(1):60–7.
13. Wallberg-Jonsson S, Johansson H, Ohman ML, et al. Extent of inflammation predicts cardiovascular disease and overall mortality in seropositive rheumatoid arthritis. A retrospective cohort study from disease onset. J Rheumatol 1999; 26(12):2562–71.
14. Avina-Zubieta JA, Choi HK, Sadatsafavi M, et al. Risk of cardiovascular mortality in patients with rheumatoid arthritis: a meta-analysis of observational studies. Arthritis Rheum 2008;59(12):1690–7.
15. Warrington KJ, Kent PD, Frye RL, et al. Rheumatoid arthritis is an independent risk factor for multi-vessel coronary artery disease: a case control study. Arthritis Res Ther 2005;7(5):R984–91.
16. Goodson NJ, Wiles NJ, Lunt M, et al. Mortality in early inflammatory polyarthritis: cardiovascular mortality is increased in seropositive patients. Arthritis Rheum 2002;46(8):2010–9.
17. Goodson N, Marks J, Lunt M, et al. Cardiovascular admissions and mortality in an inception cohort of patients with rheumatoid arthritis with onset in the 1980s and 1990s. Ann Rheum Dis 2005;64(11):1595–601.
18. Van Doornum S, Brand C, King B, et al. Increased case fatality rates following a first acute cardiovascular event in patients with rheumatoid arthritis. Arthritis Rheum 2006;54(7):2061–8.
19. Douglas KM, Pace AV, Treharne GJ, et al. Excess recurrent cardiac events in rheumatoid arthritis patients with acute coronary syndrome. Ann Rheum Dis 2006;65(3):348–53.
20. Van Doornum S, McColl G, Wicks IP. Accelerated atherosclerosis: an extra-articular feature of rheumatoid arthritis? Arthritis Rheum 2002;46:862–73.
21. Bacon PA, Stevens RJ, Carruthers DM, et al. Accelerated atherogenesis in autoimmune rheumatic diseases. Autoimmun Rev 2002;1(6):338–47.
22. Solomon DH, Goodson NJ, Katz JN, et al. Patterns of cardiovascular risk in rheumatoid arthritis. Ann Rheum Dis 2006;65(12):1608–12.
23. Banerjee S, Compton AP, Hooker RS, et al. Cardiovascular outcomes in male veterans with rheumatoid arthritis. Am J Cardiol 2008;101(8):1201–5.
24. Del Rincon I, O'Leary DH, Freeman GL, et al. Acceleration of atherosclerosis during the course of rheumatoid arthritis. Atherosclerosis 2007;195(2):354–60.
25. Kao AH, Krishnaswami S, Cunningham A, et al. Subclinical coronary artery calcification and relationship to disease duration in women with rheumatoid arthritis. J Rheumatol 2008;35(1):61–9.
26. Chung CP, Oeser A, Raggi P, et al. Increased coronary-artery atherosclerosis in rheumatoid arthritis: relationship to disease duration and cardiovascular risk factors. Arthritis Rheum 2005;52(10):3045–53.

27. Gonzalez-Juanatey C, Llorca J, Testa A, et al. Increased prevalence of severe subclinical atherosclerotic findings in long-term treated rheumatoid arthritis patients without clinically evident atherosclerotic disease. Medicine (Baltimore) 2003;82(6):407–13.
28. Hannawi S, Haluska B, Marwick TH, et al. Atherosclerotic disease is increased in recent-onset rheumatoid arthritis: a critical role for inflammation. Arthritis Res Ther 2007;9(6):R116.
29. Roman MJ, Devereux RB, Schwartz JE, et al. Arterial stiffness in chronic inflammatory diseases. Hypertension 2005;46(1):194–9.
30. Vaudo G, Marchesi S, Gerli R, et al. Endothelial dysfunction in young patients with rheumatoid arthritis and low disease activity. Ann Rheum Dis 2004;63(1):31–5.
31. Stamatelopoulos KS, Kitas GD, Papamichael CM, et al. Atherosclerosis in rheumatoid arthritis versus diabetes: a comparative study. Arterioscler Thromb Vasc Biol 2009;29(10):1702–8.
32. Peters MJ, van Halm VP, Voskuyl AE, et al. Does rheumatoid arthritis equal diabetes mellitus as an independent risk factor for cardiovascular disease? A prospective study. Arthritis Rheum 2009;61(11):1571–9.
33. Maradit-Kremers H, Crowson CS, Nicola PJ, et al. Increased unrecognized coronary heart disease and sudden deaths in rheumatoid arthritis: a population-based cohort study. Arthritis Rheum 2005;52(2):402–11.
34. Solomon DH, Karlson EW, Curhan GC. Cardiovascular care and cancer screening in female nurses with and without rheumatoid arthritis. Arthritis Rheum 2004;51(3):429–32.
35. Nicola PJ, Maradit-Kremers H, Roger VL, et al. The risk of congestive heart failure in rheumatoid arthritis: a population-based study over 46 years. Arthritis Rheum 2005;52(2):412–20.
36. Rudominer RL, Roman MJ, Devereux RB, et al. Independent association of rheumatoid arthritis with increased left ventricular mass but not with reduced ejection fraction. Arthritis Rheum 2009;60(1):22–9.
37. Alpaslan M, Onrat E, Evcik D. Doppler echocardiographic evaluation of ventricular function in patients with rheumatoid arthritis. Clin Rheumatol 2003;22(2):84–8.
38. Davis JM 3rd, Roger VL, Crowson CS, et al. The presentation and outcome of heart failure in patients with rheumatoid arthritis differs from that in the general population. Arthritis Rheum 2008;58(9):2603–11.
39. del Rincon ID, Williams K, Stern MP, et al. High incidence of cardiovascular events in a rheumatoid arthritis cohort not explained by traditional cardiac risk factors. Arthritis Rheum 2001;44(12):2737–45.
40. Aubry MC, Maradit-Kremers H, Reinalda MS, et al. Differences in atherosclerotic coronary heart disease between subjects with and without rheumatoid arthritis. J Rheumatol 2007;34(5):937–42.
41. Pasceri V, Yeh ET. A tale of two diseases: atherosclerosis and rheumatoid arthritis. Circulation 1999;100(21):2124–6.
42. Bergholm R, Leirisalo-Repo M, Vehkavaara S, et al. Impaired responsiveness to NO in newly diagnosed patients with rheumatoid arthritis. Arterioscler Thromb Vasc Biol 2002;22(10):1637–41.
43. Edwards CJ, Syddall H, Goswami R, et al. The autoantibody rheumatoid factor may be an independent risk factor for ischaemic heart disease in men. Heart 2007;93(10):1263–7.

44. Tomasson G, Aspelund T, Jonsson T, et al. The effect of rheumatoid factor on mortality and coronary heart disease. Ann Rheum Dis 2009. [Epub ahead of print].
45. Gerli R, Bartoloni Bocci E, Sherer Y, et al. Association of anti-cyclic citrullinated peptide antibodies with subclinical atherosclerosis in patients with rheumatoid arthritis. Ann Rheum Dis 2008;67(5):724–5.
46. Lopez-Longo FJ, Oliver-Minarro D, de la Torre I, et al. Association between anti-cyclic citrullinated peptide antibodies and ischemic heart disease in patients with rheumatoid arthritis. Arthritis Rheum 2009;61(4):419–24.
47. Dessein PH, Joffe BI, Stanwix AE. Subclinical hypothyroidism is associated with insulin resistance in rheumatoid arthritis. Thyroid 2004;14(6):443–6.
48. Boers M, Nurmohamed MT, Doelman CJ, et al. Influence of glucocorticoids and disease activity on total and high density lipoprotein cholesterol in patients with rheumatoid arthritis. Ann Rheum Dis 2003;62(9):842–5.
49. Dekkers JC, Geenen R, Godaert GL, et al. Elevated sympathetic nervous system activity in patients with recently diagnosed rheumatoid arthritis with active disease. Clin Exp Rheumatol 2004;22(1):63–70.
50. Del Rincon I, Williams K, Stern MP, et al. Association between carotid atherosclerosis and markers of inflammation in rheumatoid arthritis patients and healthy subjects. Arthritis Rheum 2003;48(7):1833–40.
51. Dessein PH, Joffe BI, Stanwix A, et al. The acute phase response does not fully predict the presence of insulin resistance and dyslipidemia in inflammatory arthritis. J Rheumatol 2002;29(3):462–6.
52. Dessein PH, Stanwix AE, Joffe BI. Cardiovascular risk in rheumatoid arthritis versus osteoarthritis: acute phase response related decreased insulin sensitivity and high-density lipoprotein cholesterol as well as clustering of metabolic syndrome features in rheumatoid arthritis. Arthritis Res 2002;4(5):R5.
53. Kim SH, Lee CK, Lee EY, et al. Serum oxidized low-density lipoproteins in rheumatoid arthritis. Rheumatol Int 2004;24(4):230–3.
54. Chung CP, Oeser A, Avalos I, et al. Utility of the Framingham risk score to predict the presence of coronary atherosclerosis in patients with rheumatoid arthritis. Arthritis Res Ther 2006;8(6):R186.
55. Metsios GS, Stavropoulos-Kalinoglou A, Panoulas VF, et al. Association of physical inactivity with increased cardiovascular risk in patients with rheumatoid arthritis. Eur J Cardiovasc Prev Rehabil 2009;16(2):188–94.
56. Wolfe F. The effect of smoking on clinical, laboratory, and radiographic status in rheumatoid arthritis. J Rheumatol 2000;27(3):630–7.
57. Symmons DP, Bankhead CR, Harrison BJ, et al. Blood transfusion, smoking, and obesity as risk factors for the development of rheumatoid arthritis: results from a primary care-based incident case-control study in Norfolk, England. Arthritis Rheum 1997;40(11):1955–61.
58. Wallberg-Jonsson S, Ohman ML, Dahlqvist SR. Cardiovascular morbidity and mortality in patients with seropositive rheumatoid arthritis in Northern Sweden. J Rheumatol 1997;24(3):445–51.
59. Maradit-Kremers H, Nicola PJ, Crowson CS, et al. Cardiovascular death in rheumatoid arthritis: a population-based study. Arthritis Rheum 2005;52(3):722–32.
60. Dursunoglu D, Evrengul H, Polat B, et al. Lp(a) lipoprotein and lipids in patients with rheumatoid arthritis: serum levels and relationship to inflammation. Rheumatol Int 2005;25(4):241–5.

61. Rizzo M, Spinas GA, Cesur M, et al. Atherogenic lipoprotein phenotype and LDL size and subclasses in drug-naive patients with early rheumatoid arthritis. Atherosclerosis 2009;207(2):502–6.
62. Peters MJ, van Halm VP, Nurmohamed MT, et al. Relations between autoantibodies against oxidized low-density lipoprotein, inflammation, subclinical atherosclerosis, and cardiovascular disease in rheumatoid arthritis. J Rheumatol 2008;35(8):1495–9.
63. McMahon M, Grossman J, FitzGerald J, et al. Proinflammatory high-density lipoprotein as a biomarker for atherosclerosis in patients with systemic lupus erythematosus and rheumatoid arthritis. Arthritis Rheum 2006;54(8):2541–9.
64. Hahn BH, Grossman J, Ansell BJ, et al. Altered lipoprotein metabolism in chronic inflammatory states: proinflammatory high-density lipoprotein and accelerated atherosclerosis in systemic lupus erythematosus and rheumatoid arthritis. Arthritis Res Ther 2008;10(4):213.
65. Charles-Schoeman C, Watanabe J, Lee YY, et al. Abnormal function of high-density lipoprotein is associated with poor disease control and an altered protein cargo in rheumatoid arthritis. Arthritis Rheum 2009;60(10):2870–9.
66. Myasoedova E, Crowson CS, Maradit-Kremers H, et al. Total cholesterol and LDL levels decrease before rheumatoid arthritis. Ann Rheum Dis 2009. [Epub ahead of print].
67. Berglund S, Sodergren A, Wallberg Jonsson S, et al. Atherothrombotic events in rheumatoid arthritis are predicted by homocysteine - a six-year follow-up study. Clin Exp Rheumatol 2009;27(5):822–5.
68. Chung CP, Oeser A, Solus JF, et al. Prevalence of the metabolic syndrome is increased in rheumatoid arthritis and is associated with coronary atherosclerosis. Atherosclerosis 2008;196(2):756–63.
69. Pamuk ON, Unlu E, Cakir N. Role of insulin resistance in increased frequency of atherosclerosis detected by carotid ultrasonography in rheumatoid arthritis. J Rheumatol 2006;33(12):2447–52.
70. La Montagna G, Cacciapuoti F, Buono R, et al. Insulin resistance is an independent risk factor for atherosclerosis in rheumatoid arthritis. Diab Vasc Dis Res 2007;4(2):130–5.
71. Kiortsis DN, Mavridis AK, Vasakos S, et al. Effects of infliximab treatment on insulin resistance in patients with rheumatoid arthritis and ankylosing spondylitis. Ann Rheum Dis 2005;64(5):765–6.
72. Toms TE, Panoulas VF, John H, et al. Methotrexate therapy associates with reduced prevalence of the metabolic syndrome in rheumatoid arthritis patients over the age of 60- more than just an anti-inflammatory effect? A cross sectional study. Arthritis Res Ther 2009;11(4):R110.
73. Inaba M, Tanaka K, Goto H, et al. Independent association of increased trunk fat with increased arterial stiffening in postmenopausal patients with rheumatoid arthritis. J Rheumatol 2007;34(2):290–5.
74. Dessein PH, Norton GR, Woodiwiss AJ, et al. Influence of nonclassical cardiovascular risk factors on the accuracy of predicting subclinical atherosclerosis in rheumatoid arthritis. J Rheumatol 2007;34(5):943–51.
75. Bjornadal L, Brandt L, Klareskog L, et al. Impact of parental history on patients' cardiovascular mortality in rheumatoid arthritis. Ann Rheum Dis 2006;65(6):741–5.
76. Swanberg M, Lidman O, Padyukov L, et al. MHC2TA is associated with differential MHC molecule expression and susceptibility to rheumatoid arthritis, multiple sclerosis and myocardial infarction. Nat Genet 2005;37(5):486–94.

77. Farragher TM, Goodson NJ, Naseem H, et al. Association of the HLA-DRB1 gene with premature death, particularly from cardiovascular disease, in patients with rheumatoid arthritis and inflammatory polyarthritis. Arthritis Rheum 2008; 58(2):359–69.

78. Mattey DL, Thomson W, Ollier WE, et al. Association of DRB1 shared epitope genotypes with early mortality in rheumatoid arthritis: results of eighteen years of follow-up from the early rheumatoid arthritis study. Arthritis Rheum 2007; 56(5):1408–16.

79. Gonzalez-Gay MA, Gonzalez-Juanatey C, Lopez-Diaz MJ, et al. HLA-DRB1 and persistent chronic inflammation contribute to cardiovascular events and cardio-vascular mortality in patients with rheumatoid arthritis. Arthritis Rheum 2007; 57(1):125–32.

80. Panoulas VF, Stavropoulos-Kalinoglou A, Metsios GS, et al. Association of inter-leukin-6 (IL-6)-174 G/C gene polymorphism with cardiovascular disease in patients with rheumatoid arthritis: the role of obesity and smoking. Atheroscle-rosis 2009;204(1):178–83.

81. Vallve JC, Paredes S, Girona J, et al. Tumor necrosis factor-alpha -1031 T/C polymorphism is associated with smaller and more proatherogenic low density lipoprotein particles in patients with rheumatoid arthritis. J Rheumatol 2008; 35(9):1697–703.

82. Arlestig L, Wallberg Jonsson S, Stegmayr B, et al. Polymorphism of genes related to cardiovascular disease in patients with rheumatoid arthritis. Clin Exp Rheumatol 2007;25(6):866–71.

83. Dahlqvist SR, Arlestig L, Sikstrom C, et al. Tumor necrosis factor receptor type II (exon 6) and interleukin-6 (-174) gene polymorphisms are not associated with family history but tumor necrosis factor receptor type II is associated with hyper-tension in patients with rheumatoid arthritis from northern Sweden. Arthritis Rheum 2002;46(11):3096–8.

84. Holmqvist ME, Wedren S, Jacobsson LT, et al. No increased occurrence of ischemic heart disease prior to the onset of rheumatoid arthritis: results from two Swedish population-based rheumatoid arthritis cohorts. Arthritis Rheum 2009;60(10):2861–9.

85. Schillinger M, Exner M, Mlekusch W, et al. Inflammation and carotid artery–risk for atherosclerosis study (ICARAS). Circulation 2005;111(17):2203–9.

86. Solomon DH, Curhan GC, Rimm EB, et al. Cardiovascular risk factors in women with and without rheumatoid arthritis. Arthritis Rheum 2004;50(11): 3444–9.

87. Svenson KL, Pollare T, Lithell H, et al. Impaired glucose handling in active rheu-matoid arthritis: relationship to peripheral insulin resistance. Metabolism 1988; 37(2):125–30.

88. Sattar N, McCarey DW, Capell H, et al. Explaining how "high-grade" systemic inflammation accelerates vascular risk in rheumatoid arthritis. Circulation 2003;108(24):2957–63.

89. Hurlimann D, Forster A, Noll G, et al. Anti-tumor necrosis factor-alpha treatment improves endothelial function in patients with rheumatoid arthritis. Circulation 2002;106(17):2184–7.

90. Goodson NJ, Symmons DP, Scott DG, et al. Baseline levels of C-reactive protein and prediction of death from cardiovascular disease in patients with inflamma-tory polyarthritis: a ten-year followup study of a primary care-based inception cohort. Arthritis Rheum 2005;52(8):2293–9.

91. Gonzalez-Gay MA, Gonzalez-Juanatey C, Pineiro A, et al. High-grade C-reactive protein elevation correlates with accelerated atherogenesis in patients with rheumatoid arthritis. J Rheumatol 2005;32(7):1219–23.

92. Dessein PH, Joffe BI, Singh S. Biomarkers of endothelial dysfunction, cardiovascular risk factors and atherosclerosis in rheumatoid arthritis. Arthritis Res Ther 2005;7(3):R634–43.

93. Rho YH, Chung CP, Oeser A, et al. Inflammatory mediators and premature coronary atherosclerosis in rheumatoid arthritis. Arthritis Rheum 2009;61(11):1580–5.

94. Maradit-Kremers H, Nicola PJ, Crowson CS, et al. Raised erythrocyte sedimentation rate signals heart failure in patients with rheumatoid arthritis. Ann Rheum Dis 2007;66(1):76–80.

95. Xie JJ, Wang J, Tang TT, et al. The Th17/Treg functional imbalance during atherogenesis in ApoE(-/-) mice. Cytokine 2010;49(2):185–93.

96. van Es T, van Puijvelde GH, Ramos OH, et al. Attenuated atherosclerosis upon IL-17R signaling disruption in LDLr deficient mice. Biochem Biophys Res Commun 2009;388(2):261–5.

97. Liang J, Zheng Z, Wang M, et al. Myeloperoxidase (MPO) and interleukin-17 (IL-17) plasma levels are increased in patients with acute coronary syndromes. J Int Med Res 2009;37(3):862–6.

98. Eid RE, Rao DA, Zhou J, et al. Interleukin-17 and interferon-gamma are produced concomitantly by human coronary artery-infiltrating T cells and act synergistically on vascular smooth muscle cells. Circulation 2009;119(10):1424–32.

99. Feng W, Li W, Liu W, et al. IL-17 induces myocardial fibrosis and enhances RANKL/OPG and MMP/TIMP signaling in isoproterenol-induced heart failure. Exp Mol Pathol 2009;87(3):212–8.

100. Taleb S, Romain M, Ramkhelawon B, et al. Loss of SOCS3 expression in T cells reveals a regulatory role for interleukin-17 in atherosclerosis. J Exp Med 2009; 206(10):2067–77.

101. Martens PB, Goronzy JJ, Schaid D, et al. Expansion of unusual CD4 + T cells in severe rheumatoid arthritis. Arthritis Rheum 1997;40(6):1106–14.

102. Liuzzo G, Goronzy JJ, Yang H, et al. Monoclonal T-cell proliferation and plaque instability in acute coronary syndromes. Circulation 2000;101(25):2883–8.

103. Gerli R, Schillaci G, Giordano A, et al. CD4+CD28-T lymphocytes contribute to early atherosclerotic damage in rheumatoid arthritis patients. Circulation 2004; 109(22):2744–8.

104. Bryl E, Vallejo AN, Matteson EL, et al. Modulation of CD28 expression with anti-tumor necrosis factor alpha therapy in rheumatoid arthritis. Arthritis Rheum 2005;52(10):2996–3003.

105. Rizzello V, Liuzzo G, Brugaletta S, et al. Modulation of CD4(+)CD28null T lymphocytes by tumor necrosis factor-alpha blockade in patients with unstable angina. Circulation 2006;113(19):2272–7.

106. Loomans CJ, de Koning EJ, Staal FJ, et al. Endothelial progenitor cell dysfunction: a novel concept in the pathogenesis of vascular complications of type 1 diabetes. Diabetes 2004;53(1):195–9.

107. Schmidt-Lucke C, Rossig L, Fichtlscherer S, et al. Reduced number of circulating endothelial progenitor cells predicts future cardiovascular events: proof of concept for the clinical importance of endogenous vascular repair. Circulation 2005;111(22):2981–7.

108. Grisar J, Aletaha D, Steiner CW, et al. Depletion of endothelial progenitor cells in the peripheral blood of patients with rheumatoid arthritis. Circulation 2005; 111(2):204–11.

109. Herbrig K, Haensel S, Oelschlaegel U, et al. Endothelial dysfunction in patients with rheumatoid arthritis is associated with a reduced number and impaired function of endothelial progenitor cells. Ann Rheum Dis 2006;65(2): 157–63.

110. Ablin JN, Boguslavski V, Aloush V, et al. Effect of anti-TNFalpha treatment on circulating endothelial progenitor cells (EPCs) in rheumatoid arthritis. Life Sci 2006;79(25):2364–9.

111. Turiel M, Atzeni F, Tomasoni L, et al. Non-invasive assessment of coronary flow reserve and ADMA levels: a case-control study of early rheumatoid arthritis patients. Rheumatology (Oxford) 2009;48(7):834–9.

112. Surdacki A, Martens-Lobenhoffer J, Wloch A, et al. Elevated plasma asymmetric dimethyl-L-arginine levels are linked to endothelial progenitor cell depletion and carotid atherosclerosis in rheumatoid arthritis. Arthritis Rheum 2007;56(3):809–19.

113. Ruger B, Giurea A, Wanivenhaus AH, et al. Endothelial precursor cells in the synovial tissue of patients with rheumatoid arthritis and osteoarthritis. Arthritis Rheum 2004;50(7):2157–66.

114. Kumeda Y, Inaba M, Goto H, et al. Increased thickness of the arterial intima-media detected by ultrasonography in patients with rheumatoid arthritis. Arthritis Rheum 2002;46(6):1489–97.

115. Dierkes J, Westphal S. Effect of drugs on homocysteine concentrations. Semin Vasc Med 2005;5(2):124–39.

116. Merkle CJ, Moore IM, Penton BS, et al. Methotrexate causes apoptosis in post-mitotic endothelial cells. Biol Res Nurs 2000;2(1):5–14.

117. Choi HK, Hernan MA, Seeger JD, et al. Methotrexate and mortality in patients with rheumatoid arthritis: a prospective study. Lancet 2002;359(9313):1173–7.

118. Bernatsky S, Hudson M, Suissa S. Anti-rheumatic drug use and risk of hospitalization for congestive heart failure in rheumatoid arthritis. Rheumatology (Oxford) 2005;44(5):677–80.

119. Johnsen SP, Larsson H, Tarone RE, et al. Risk of hospitalization for myocardial infarction among users of rofecoxib, celecoxib, and other NSAIDs: a population-based case-control study. Arch Intern Med 2005;165(9):978–84.

120. Solomon DH, Glynn RJ, Rothman KJ, et al. Subgroup analyses to determine cardiovascular risk associated with nonsteroidal antiinflammatory drugs and coxibs in specific patient groups. Arthritis Rheum 2008;59(8):1097–104.

121. Fischer LM, Schlienger RG, Matter CM, et al. Discontinuation of nonsteroidal anti-inflammatory drug therapy and risk of acute myocardial infarction. Arch Intern Med 2004;164(22):2472–6.

122. Nashel DJ. Is atherosclerosis a complication of long-term corticosteroid treatment? Am J Med 1986;80(5):925–9.

123. del Rincon I, O'Leary DH, Haas RW, et al. Effect of glucocorticoids on the arteries in rheumatoid arthritis. Arthritis Rheum 2004;50(12):3813–22.

124. Hafstrom I, Rohani M, Deneberg S, et al. Effects of low-dose prednisolone on endothelial function, atherosclerosis, and traditional risk factors for atherosclerosis in patients with rheumatoid arthritis–a randomized study. J Rheumatol 2007;34(9):1810–6.

125. Davis JM 3rd, Maradit Kremers H, Crowson CS, et al. Glucocorticoids and cardiovascular events in rheumatoid arthritis: a population-based cohort study. Arthritis Rheum 2007;56(3):820–30.

126. Naranjo A, Sokka T, Descalzo MA, et al. Cardiovascular disease in patients with rheumatoid arthritis: results from the QUEST-RA study. Arthritis Res Ther 2008; 10(2):R30.

127. Prodanovich S, Ma F, Taylor JR, et al. Methotrexate reduces incidence of vascular diseases in veterans with psoriasis or rheumatoid arthritis. J Am Acad Dermatol 2005;52(2):262–7.

128. van Halm VP, Nurmohamed MT, Twisk JW, et al. Disease-modifying antirheumatic drugs are associated with a reduced risk for cardiovascular disease in patients with rheumatoid arthritis: a case control study. Arthritis Res Ther 2006;8(5):R151.

129. Suissa S, Bernatsky S, Hudson M. Antirheumatic drug use and the risk of acute myocardial infarction. Arthritis Rheum 2006;55(4):531–6.

130. Rho YH, Oeser A, Chung CP, et al. Drugs used in the treatment of rheumatoid arthritis: relationship between current use and cardiovascular risk factors. Arch Drug Inf 2009;2(2):34–40.

131. Reiss AB, Carsons SE, Anwar K, et al. Atheroprotective effects of methotrexate on reverse cholesterol transport proteins and foam cell transformation in human THP-1 monocyte/macrophages. Arthritis Rheum 2008;58(12):3675–83.

132. Popa C, Netea MG, Radstake T, et al. Influence of anti-tumour necrosis factor therapy on cardiovascular risk factors in patients with active rheumatoid arthritis. Ann Rheum Dis 2005;64(2):303–5.

133. Maki-Petaja KM, Hall FC, Booth AD, et al. Rheumatoid arthritis is associated with increased aortic pulse-wave velocity, which is reduced by anti-tumor necrosis factor-alpha therapy. Circulation 2006;114(11):1185–92.

134. Sidiropoulos PI, Siakka P, Pagonidis K, et al. Sustained improvement of vascular endothelial function during anti-TNFalpha treatment in rheumatoid arthritis patients. Scand J Rheumatol 2009;38(1):6–10.

135. Jacobsson LT, Turesson C, Gulfe A, et al. Treatment with tumor necrosis factor blockers is associated with a lower incidence of first cardiovascular events in patients with rheumatoid arthritis. J Rheumatol 2005;32(7):1213–8.

136. Macias I, Garcia-Perez S, Ruiz-Tudela M, et al. Modification of pro- and antiinflammatory cytokines and vascular-related molecules by tumor necrosis factor-a blockade in patients with rheumatoid arthritis. J Rheumatol 2005; 32(11):2102–8.

137. Dominguez H, Storgaard H, Rask-Madsen C, et al. Metabolic and vascular effects of tumor necrosis factor-alpha blockade with etanercept in obese patients with type 2 diabetes. J Vasc Res 2005;42(6):517–25.

138. Gonzalez-Juanatey C, Testa A, Garcia-Castelo A, et al. Active but transient improvement of endothelial function in rheumatoid arthritis patients undergoing long-term treatment with anti-tumor necrosis factor alpha antibody. Arthritis Rheum 2004;51(3):447–50.

139. Van Doornum S, McColl G, Wicks IP. Tumour necrosis factor antagonists improve disease activity but not arterial stiffness in rheumatoid arthritis. Rheumatology (Oxford) 2005;44(11):1428–32.

140. Irace C, Mancuso G, Fiaschi E, et al. Effect of anti TNFalpha therapy on arterial diameter and wall shear stress and HDL cholesterol. Atherosclerosis 2004;177(1):113–8.

141. Grundmann S, Hoefer I, Ulusans S, et al. Anti-tumor necrosis factor-{alpha} therapies attenuate adaptive arteriogenesis in the rabbit. Am J Physiol Heart Circ Physiol 2005;289(4):H1497–505.

142. Chung ES, Packer M, Lo KH, et al. Randomized, double-blind, placebo-controlled, pilot trial of infliximab, a chimeric monoclonal antibody to tumor necrosis factor-alpha, in patients with moderate-to-severe heart failure: results of the anti-TNF therapy against congestive heart failure (ATTACH) trial. Circulation 2003;107(25):3133–40.

143. Curtis JR, Kramer JM, Martin C, et al. Heart failure among younger rheumatoid arthritis and Crohn's patients exposed to TNF-alpha antagonists. Rheumatology (Oxford) 2007;46(11):1688–93.

144. Wolfe F, Michaud K. Heart failure in rheumatoid arthritis: rates, predictors, and the effect of anti-tumor necrosis factor therapy. Am J Med 2004;116(5):305–11.

145. Listing J, Strangfeld A, Kekow J, et al. Does tumor necrosis factor alpha inhibition promote or prevent heart failure in patients with rheumatoid arthritis? Arthritis Rheum 2008;58(3):667–77.

146. Peters MJ, Welsh P, McInnes IB, et al. TNF{alpha} blockade therapy reduces circulating NT-proBNP levels in RA patients with active disease: results from prospective cohort study. Ann Rheum Dis 2009. [Epub ahead of print].

147. Setoguchi S, Schneeweiss S, Avorn J, et al. Tumor necrosis factor-alpha antagonist use and heart failure in elderly patients with rheumatoid arthritis. Am Heart J 2008;156(2):336–41.

148. Solomon DH, Avorn J, Katz JN, et al. Immunosuppressive medications and hospitalization for cardiovascular events in patients with rheumatoid arthritis. Arthritis Rheum 2006;54(12):3790–8.

149. Kerekes G, Soltesz P, Der H, et al. Effects of rituximab treatment on endothelial dysfunction, carotid atherosclerosis, and lipid profile in rheumatoid arthritis. Clin Rheumatol 2009;28(6):705–10.

150. Gonzalez-Juanatey C, Llorca J, Vazquez-Rodriguez TR, et al. Short-term improvement of endothelial function in rituximab-treated rheumatoid arthritis patients refractory to tumor necrosis factor alpha blocker therapy. Arthritis Rheum 2008;59(12):1821–4.

151. Ikonomidis I, Tzortzis S, Lekakis J, et al. Lowering interleukin-1 activity with anakinra improves myocardial deformation in rheumatoid arthritis. Heart 2009; 95(18):1502–7.

152. Toms TE, Panoulas VF, Douglas KM, et al. Statin use in rheumatoid arthritis in relation to actual cardiovascular risk: evidence for substantial under treatment of lipid associated cardiovascular risk? Ann Rheum Dis 2009. [Epub ahead of print].

153. Panoulas VF, Toms TE, Metsios GS, et al. Target organ damage in patients with rheumatoid arthritis: the role of blood pressure and heart rate. Atherosclerosis 2010;209(1):255–60.

154. Flammer AJ, Sudano I, Hermann F, et al. Angiotensin-converting enzyme inhibition improves vascular function in rheumatoid arthritis. Circulation 2008;117(17): 2262–9.

155. McCarey DW, McInnes IB, Madhok R, et al. Trial of atorvastatin in rheumatoid arthritis (TARA): double-blind, randomised placebo-controlled trial. Lancet 2004;363(9426):2015–21.

156. Van Doornum S, McColl G, Wicks IP. Atorvastatin reduces arterial stiffness in patients with rheumatoid arthritis. Ann Rheum Dis 2004;63(12):1571–5.

157. Hermann F, Forster A, Chenevard R, et al. Simvastatin improves endothelial function in patients with rheumatoid arthritis. J Am Coll Cardiol 2005;45(3):461–4.

158. Tikiz C, Utuk O, Pirildar T, et al. Effects of Angiotensin-converting enzyme inhibition and statin treatment on inflammatory markers and endothelial functions in patients with longterm rheumatoid arthritis. J Rheumatol 2005;32(11): 2095–101.

159. Maki-Petaja KM, Booth AD, Hall FC, et al. Ezetimibe and simvastatin reduce inflammation, disease activity, and aortic stiffness and improve endothelial function in rheumatoid arthritis. J Am Coll Cardiol 2007;50(9):852–8.

160. Jick SS, Choi H, Li L, et al. Hyperlipidaemia, statin use and the risk of developing rheumatoid arthritis. Ann Rheum Dis 2009;68(4):546–51.

161. Wasko MC, Hubert HB, Lingala VB, et al. Hydroxychloroquine and risk of diabetes in patients with rheumatoid arthritis. JAMA 2007;298(2):187–93.

162. Munro R, Morrison E, McDonald AG, et al. Effect of disease modifying agents on the lipid profiles of patients with rheumatoid arthritis. Ann Rheum Dis 1997;56(6): 374–7.

163. Panoulas VF, Douglas KM, Stavropoulos-Kalinoglou A, et al. Long-term exposure to medium-dose glucocorticoid therapy associates with hypertension in patients with rheumatoid arthritis. Rheumatology (Oxford) 2008;47(1):72–5.

Index

Note: Page numbers of article titles are in **boldface** type.

A

B

Rheum Dis Clin N Am 36 (2010) 427–437
doi:10.1016/S0889-857X(10)00033-5
0889-857X/10/$ – see front matter © 2010 Elsevier Inc. All rights reserved.

rheumatic.theclinics.com

Moving?

Make sure your subscription moves with you!

To notify us of your new address, find your **Clinics Account Number** (located on your mailing label above your name), and contact customer service at:

Email: journalscustomerservice-usa@elsevier.com

800-654-2452 (subscribers in the U.S. & Canada)
314-447-8871 (subscribers outside of the U.S. & Canada)

Fax number: 314-447-8029

Elsevier Health Sciences Division
Subscription Customer Service
3251 Riverport Lane
Maryland Heights, MO 63043

*To ensure uninterrupted delivery of your subscription, please notify us at least 4 weeks in advance of move.

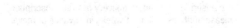

Printed in the United States
By Bookmasters